Childhood Cancer Survivors

A Practical Guide to Your Future

4th Edition

Editors:

Lisa Bashore, PhD, APRN, CPNP-PC, CPON
Oncology Nurse Practitioner
Cook Children's Health Care System
Adjunct Professor, Texas Christian University
Fort Worth, Texas

Joanne Quillen, MSN, APRN, PNP-BC
Pediatric Oncology / Neuro-oncology Nurse Practitioner
Oncology Survivorship Clinic
Nemours Children's Hospital
Wilmington, Delaware

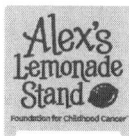

AlexsLemonade.org

Alex's Lemonade Stand Foundation for Childhood Cancer
Wynnewood, PA 19096 USA

Childhood Cancer Survivors: A Practical Guide to your Future, Fourth edition
Edited by Lisa Bashore and Joanne Quillen

© 2026 *Alex's Lemonade Stand Foundation*
333 E. Lancaster Ave. #414, Wynnewood, PA 19096

For information about special discounts for bulk purchases, please contact: familyservices@alexslemonade.org

ALEX'S LEMONADE® and ALEX'S LEMONADE STAND® are federally registered trademarks of Alex's Lemonade Stand Foundation.

DISCLAIMER:

This book is meant to educate and provide general information. It is not intended as, and should not be used as medical advice for individual patients or as an alternative for professional medical or psychiatric care. *Alex's Lemonade Stand Foundation* encourages those with questions concerning their or others' health or ongoing treatment to seek assistance from qualified medical practitioners. In researching for this book, the authors/editors have gathered information from sources they consider to be reliable and current and refer readers to relevant online resources for further study and information and guidelines. However, neither the authors, editors, nor *Alex's Lemonade Stand Foundation* guarantee or warrant the accuracy, completeness, or currency of the information provided in this book. In no event will the authors, editors, or *Alex's Lemonade Stand Foundation* be liable for any direct, indirect, consequential, or other damages resulting from reliance on or use of the information provided in this book.

Certain pharmaceuticals, devices, treatments, other products and services and companies have been referred to in this book by the trademarks, service marks, or trade names of their providers. Such references are made for the sole purpose of identifying the item or company in question and are not intended to indicate any affiliation with, sponsorship, or endorsement by the owners of the trademarks, service marks, or trade names referenced, and do not indicate any affiliation with, sponsorship or endorsement by the authors, editors or *Alex's Lemonade Stand Foundation* of any specific product, treatment, or resource, or indicate the legal or regulatory status of any product, treatment, or service.

Library of Congress Control number: 2024950984
Bashore, Lisa & Quillen, Joanne
Childhood cancer survivors: a practical guide to your future. 4th ed.
ISBN 978-1-7361662-1-5 (paperback)
ISBN 978-1-7361662-2-2 (digital)

1. Cancer in children/adolescents-popular works. 2. Cancer in children/adolescents complications/late effects of treatment 3. Cancer in children/adolescents – social aspects. 4. Cancer in children/adolescents – psychological aspects
Summary: A resource for survivors of childhood cancer and their families that includes information about medical late effects of treatment, necessary follow-up care, emotional aspects of survivorship, navigating the healthcare system, ways to maximize survivors' health, and resources of helpful organizations. Provided by publisher.

Dedications

To all the patients (survivors), parents, colleagues and friends that have given me the encouragement and motivation to be where I am today in my career. Also to Wendy Hobbie and other nurse pioneers who contributed to the growth and development of childhood cancer survivorship programs that now exist.

Lisa Bashore

To my husband, Dave, for his encouragement and support throughout my career and especially throughout the editing of this book. To my sisters, Diane and Colleen, who taught me what it really means to be a childhood cancer survivor. To Wendy Hobbie who influenced me to make a difference for the childhood cancer survivors that I encounter each and every day in my practice. Also a thank-you to Lisa for inviting me to join her as co-editor and her great insight throughout. She was a joy to work alongside.

Joanne Quillen

Acknowledgements

Childhood Cancer Survivors has been a valuable resource for survivors and families for the past 25 years since the first edition. We want to thank *Alex's Lemonade Stand Foundation* for giving us the opportunity to participate in editing and updating this fourth edition in collaboration with several new authors. The legacy of what Alex and her family started in 2005 lives on through the millions of dollars raised and given in support of survivors and families, and toward invaluable research. We thank ALSF for their vision and dedication to continue to update and revise this book which has been read and used as an invaluable resource for thousands of survivors and families. Alex's legacy lives on through this book and all the personal survivor stories that appear in this fourth edition.

We sincerely thank the previous edition authors, including Kathy Ruccione, for their incredible work and research. Our hope and intent was to build upon their excellent foundation and the information so clearly presented and to revise and introduce new information affecting survivors and their families. Both of us want to give a special thank-you to Wendy Hobbie who not only was one of the original coauthors but for her life and work in childhood cancer which inspired and motivated us to pursue careers in support of childhood cancer survivors and families.

Many people were involved in the production of this fourth edition. We especially thank our new authors for their excellent new contributions: Matthew C. Hocking, PhD (*Ch 3 Relationships*), Victoria E. Cosgrove, PhD (*Ch 2 Emotions*) Liron D. Grossmann, MD and John M. Maris, MD (*Ch 6 Genetic Testing in Childhood Cancer*), and Kasey Massa, LCSW (*Ch 4 Navigating the System*).

We especially want to thank the survivors and families who contributed personal stories about their own survivorship journeys: Lindsey, Margaret, Nick, Maggie, Gigi, Jennifer, Julia, Breeonne, Jason, Jeanette, Grace, Taylor, Ashley, Brittney, Shameeza, King, Trish, Lily, Yusef, and Daniel.

Each story is unique and very personal, sometimes gut-wrenching and painful and other times, uplifting and hopeful. These personal accounts are an integral part of the book and will greatly impact other survivors and families bringing hope and guidance as they navigate through their journeys emotionally and physically. We are deeply grateful for your candor and the legacy of truth and hope which will be such an inspiration to others, those just beginning their journey and for those yet to come.

We would also like to thank Katie Newell, Caroline O'Rorke, and the team at *ALSF* for their hard work and many hours spent interviewing survivors and families and collecting their stories.

And lastly, we thank our amazing project editors, Marty and Carole Wonsiewicz, who helped in the editing process, kept us on schedule, and kept the work flowing with ease.

Lisa Bashore & Joanne Quillen, co-editors

Contents

Contributors

Matthew C. Hocking, PhD
Division of Oncology
Children's Hospital of Philadelphia
Assistant Professor of Clinical
  Psychology
Perelman School of Medicine
University of Pennsylvania
Philadelphia, Pennsylvania
(Ch 3 Relationships)

Victoria E. Cosgrove, PhD
Assistant Professor
Director, StREaM Lab
Co-Director, Pediatric Mood
  Disorders Clinic
Division of Child and Adolescent
  Psychiatry
Stanford University School of
  Medicine
Stanford, California
(Chapter 2, Emotions)

Kasey Massa, LCSW, OSW-C, CCLS
Clinical Social Worker
Psychosocial Care Coordinator
Nemours Children's Hospital
Wilmington, Delaware
(Ch 4 Navigating the System - coauthor)

Lauren Gillespie, LCSW
Transition Social Work Coordinator
Nemours Children's
Wilmington, Delaware
(Ch 4 Navigating the System)

Liron D. Grossmann, MD
Physician-Scientist
Edmond and Lily Safra Children's
  Hospital
Sheba Medical Center, Israel
Scientist, Children's Hospital of
  Philadelphia
Philadelphia, Pennsylvania
*(Ch 6 Genetic Testing and
  Childhood Cancer)*

John M. Maris, MD
Giulio D'Angio Professor of Pediatric
  Oncology
Children's Hospital of Philadelphia
Perelman School of Medicine
University of Pennsylvania
Philadelphia, Pennsylvania
*(Ch 6 Genetic Testing and
  Childhood Cancer)*

Krista Krol-Buch, LGC
Genetics Counselor
Cancer Genetics Program
Nemours Children's
Wlmington, Delaware
(Ch 3 Relationships)

Foreword

Through our roles at Alex's Lemonade Stand Foundation, we've had the privilege of meeting childhood cancer survivors of all ages. We've encountered children years out from treatment who were still in elementary school, teens who were treated as toddlers, and young adults just beginning life after childhood cancer. We know their stories and we know their families, who always inspire us with their strength, honesty, humor, and hope. Their stories have shown us that childhood cancer doesn't end when treatment ends and taught us the motto that pediatric oncologists repeat in research labs and clinics, "a cure is not enough," should be a rallying cry for all of us.

In certain areas of the world, survivorship is growing, thanks to research and access to cutting-edge treatments. Over the past two decades, mortality rates continue to decrease and 80% of children diagnosed with cancer in the U.S. and Europe will survive. We believe research and efforts to improve access to treatment in underserved areas all over the world will increase that number to 100%. While scientists tirelessly work for cures, other researchers will continue to study the impact cancer and its treatment have on children.

The moment childhood cancer enters the family's picture, entire lives change. Life-saving treatments bring opportunities for cures but carry terrifying risks and possible late effects. Family dynamics change. Dreams for the future shift. Cancer leaves a mark on everything it touches: growing bodies, relationships, and futures. To those outside of childhood cancer, a cure might seem like the finish line. But to those on the inside, the children and the families, the cure is the start of the survivorship journey.

Childhood cancer survivors talk about the uncertainty and loneliness that comes in survivorship. Each diagnosis, even within the same cancer type, is as unique as the child impacted. For these children who have endured so much, the future should be healthy, productive, and happy.

The 4th edition of *Childhood Cancer Survivors* reflects years of progress, not just in scientific research, but in building a supportive community for families impacted by childhood cancer. Leading clinicians and researchers share their practical and science-based insights; while childhood cancer survivors and their families share their personal experiences navigating life after treatment ends.

This guide isn't just for survivors, but also for caregivers, community healthcare providers, and oncologists. Inside these pages, we hope that childhood cancer survivors and their families find community and camaraderie. We hope that pediatricians and other community healthcare providers use this resource as a guide to support their young patients as they transition from oncology patient to oncology survivor. We hope this guide continues to be the book families and survivors turn to as they navigate uncertain waters.

Finally, our hope is that someday, this book can be handed to every single child who battles cancer, along with the promise of a healthy future each one deserves.

Until there are cures for all children,

Liz and Jay Scott, Co-executive Directors,
Alex's Lemonade Stand Foundation

Preface

In 2022, there were an estimated 18.1 million cancer survivors in the United States. As of 2020 nearly 496,000 cancer survivors were first diagnosed when they were under age 20 (Armstrong G). The increasing large numbers of young adult childhood cancer survivors are a legacy to the hard work of physicians, advance practice nurses, nurses, other members of the healthcare team, and the scientific community of researchers who continue to develop new methods of cancer treatment and medications to minimize the late effects of treatment. Because of these advances in childhood cancer treatment over the past several decades, current statistics show that 85% of children treated will survive more than 5 years, and many are surviving well into adulthood. Survival rates among children with cancer vary widely depending on the type of cancer and other factors. (www.cancer.org). To best advocate for themselves, survivors must have specific knowledge of their cancer history and treatments to be informed and prepared for any possible late effects.

This new 4th edition does not minimize the potential reality of late effects and presents updated information/findings from the past 12 years, both what is currently known and that which remains unknown; for example, thousands of young women treated with chest radiation may *not* realize they are at increased risk for breast cancer over the course of their lifetime. Childhood cancer survivors who received certain chemotherapy drugs (anthracyclines) are at higher risk for heart problems over the course of their lifetime.

This edition presents the most recent medical and psychosocial information from updated literature/studies, most importantly, the updated *Children's Oncology Group (COG) October 2023, Version 6.0*

Long Term Follow-up Guidelines. This important resource is referenced throughout providing Healthlinks to important topics.

The ultimate goal of the book is to clearly present the latest medical information about late effects and to empower survivors to advocate for themselves in their healthcare. Being informed about potential late effects and problems, survivors and families are better able to cope with and treat them early if they do develop. We hope survivors with potential late effects will share this book with their healthcare provider to address all their concerns and make a plan for their future care.

- **Survivors' personal stories**: Survivorship is defined as "*the point in life when cancer treatment ends and the journey into the future begins.*" Every survivor's journey is unique but much can be learned from the shared experiences of other survivors. Survivor stories in this fourth edition are new and reflect the younger generation of survivors' perspectives amid the changing landscape of the past decade. Survivors and families share their personal emotions, fears, thoughts, and victories. Sharing these real experiences and concerns puts a human face to the scientific information and validates this information. These very personal stories provide reassurance, information and a sense of community for all survivors and helps survivors feel less isolated. You may identify with some of these stories, others you may not, but it should be comforting to know that you share many of the same concerns and struggles as others in the community of survivors.

- **New authors/chapter**: Several chapters have been updated by new authors who are experts in their fields: *Chapter 2,* by Dr. Matthew Hocking; *Chapter 3, Relationships* by Dr. Virginia Cosgrove. *Chapter 4, Navigating the System* includes a new co-author, Kacey Massa, LCSW who provided updated information relating to laws, regulations, and government policies protecting the rights of survivors in healthcare and the work place. *Chapter 6, Genetic Testing and Childhood Cancer* is a totally new chapter written by Dr. Liron D. Grossmann and Dr. John M. Maris, who explain genetic testing and biomarkers, what to expect in the process of genetic testing, and why it is so important for some survivors to undergo testing.

- **New glossary:** A new glossary of terms appears at the end of each chapter to help readers understand medical/scientific terms. Terms throughout the text are highlighted in *italics*. New Genetic Testing (Chapter 6) includes many terms that may be unfamiliar to survivors including *genetic testing, biomarkers* and the use of *precision medicine* which are changing the methods and protocols for treating some cancers. The term *subsequent malignancy* has replaced *second cancer* as the title of Chapter 20, although these terms are used interchangeably. *Hematopoietic stem cell transplant* or *stem cell transplant* replaces *bone marrow transplant* to include all types of transplants (e.g., bone marrow, cord blood, or peripheral blood).

- **Survivorship programs/clinics:** *Childhood survivorship program/clinic* is defined as "a program designed to provide long-term, multidisciplinary follow-up of successfully treated patients by a team of healthcare professionals (a nurse coordinator, pediatric oncologist, pediatric nurse practitioner, and sometimes a social worker, and psychologist) who are familiar with the potential late effects of treatment for childhood cancer and can help survivors monitor potential late effects and refer to specialists whenever needed (cardiologists, endocrinologists, orthopedic surgeons, and others). More childhood survivorship clinics are opening in regions of the United States at cancer treatment centers, but many survivors living in some areas may not live close to a childhood survivorship program and need to travel to them. *Chapter 4 Navigating the System* details how to locate a childhood survivorship program clinic near you.

As long-time oncology nurses dedicated to the care of childhood cancer survivors, we are honored for this opportunity to update the book. We are grateful to *Alex's Lemonade Stand Foundation* for producing another edition as this book continues to alter lives and give hope to childhood cancer survivors and their families and the healthcare professionals who care for them.

Lisa Bashore and Joanne Quillen

How the book is organized

This book organization follows the survivorship journey from immediately after treatment ends.

- *Chapter 1, Survivorship* describes the many emotions survivors and families feel and how they choose to celebrate being cured and the end of treatment and the transition from their cancer care team to a childhood survivorship clinic/program or post-treatment survivorship healthcare.

- *Chapters 2 Emotions and Ch 3 Relationships* address the varied emotions of survivors as they transition through childhood, adolescence and adulthood after treatment and how this greatly effects survivors' relationships with parents, siblings, friends, and spouses.

- *Chapter 4, Navigating the System* presents extremely helpful information about how late effects and a cancer history impact returning to school, going to college, finding a job, employment and workplace issues, and obtaining insurance. Resource lists are updated with current websites to access government policies, laws and agencies that protect cancer survivors (especially those with disabilities).

- *Chapter 5 Staying Healthy* gives the information regarding risk factors some survivors may have for developing other conditions or diseases as a result of their cancer treatment and steps survivors can take to develop the best possible future health.

- *Chapter 6, Genetic Testing* is a new chapter and explains the importance of *genetic testing, cancer biomarkers*, and *precision medicine* which are shaping cancer treatment and helping to develop new chemotherapy and radiation techniques and protocols. The chapter also outlines why childhood cancer survivors might want or need genetic testing, how to locate a genetic counselor, and what to expect in this process.

- *Chapter 7 Diseases* is an overview of types of childhood cancer and their respective treatment options and potential late effects and screenings for each.

- *Chapter 8, Fatigue*, provides an update on this nagging and challenging aspect of childhood cancer treatment and potential treatment options.

- *Chapters 9 to 19* address the various body organ systems and the late effects which can develop in each as a result of cancer treatment. Each chapter is organized under subheadings of organ damage, signs and symptoms, screening recommendations, and medical management.
- *Chapter 20, Subsequent malignancies* (*second cancers*) presents important information regarding risk factors for survivors for developing a subsequent malignancy (second cancer) and lifestyle and health habits that can minimize your risk.

Best ways to use this book

Survivors' information needs vary according to coping styles and where they are on their survivorship journey. Survivors who just ended treatment might want to read about others who coped with returning to school after cancer treatment rather than reading about potential late effects. A college student survivor who no longer routinely makes visits to their doctor might want to read *Chapter 5* about healthy lifestyle habits and how to find good survivor follow-up care. Another might want to locate a childhood survivorship program/clinic or other healthcare provider who will work collaborative with them to provide the best comprehensive healthcare (*Chapter 4*). Long-term survivors who are 30 years post end-of-therapy and confronting increasing physical ailments may be interested in learning the late effects of their cancer treatment received as a child.

Suggestions for positive ways to read/ use this book:

- **Consider reading only sections that apply to your present or immediate future**. Certain chapters/sections will not apply to you, for example, for a young adult who is dating, reading about when/how to disclose their cancer history makes sense, but not relevant for the parent of a preschooler who just finished cancer treatment.
- **Recognize that your need for information may change**. Every survivor has a different need for information, depending on their stage of life -- whether in school, going off to college, entering

the workforce, or getting married and starting a family. Survivors range from infants to baby boomers. Late effects of treatment may occur at any stage, never occur, or may become debilitating. Survivors need to be educated about late effects and how to get the healthcare they need if late effects develop.

- **Devise a strategy to screen for potential late effects and develop a plan to stay healthy and fit.** Realize that only a fraction of the late effects described in the book apply to you. This book contains information that pertains to a large group of people, but every survivor is different: some have no late effects, some have only a few, and some have life-changing problems. Take the information in this book to your healthcare provider along with a copy of your medical history and **Cancer Treatment Summary** (see Comprehensive Cancer Treatment form used by Children's Oncology Group (http://www.survivorshipguidelines. org/). Discuss this document with your healthcare provider to figure out your unique situation. Learn what late effects you are at risk for and those you shouldn't worry about. **Devise a strategy to screen for potential late effects and develop a plan to stay healthy and fit.**

- **Recognize that knowledge/information of late effects from cancer treatment, both psychological and medical, is growing daily.** The impact of today's treatments will unfold over the next 10 to 20 years. You should form a trusting relationship with a knowledgeable healthcare provider who is familiar with late effects of cancer treatment and thoroughly discuss your medial history and comprehensive cancer treatment summary.

- **Make yearly visits** to a comprehensive childhood survivorship program or healthcare provider who will work collaborative with the survivorship program to update new information as it becomes available and help you undergo appropriate monitoring/testing as prescribed by the Childhood Oncology Guidelines.

- **Consider which body system chapters (Chapters 9 to 19) to read based on your specific risks**. Dig into only chapters that relate to your particular situation on a need-to-know basis. Don't try to read straight through all 11 body system chapters or you may feel overwhelmed by information that may not pertain to your individual risks for late effects.

- **Share the book with family and friends as the need arises.** Often, they want to understand and help but just don't know how. This book can help educate them on best ways to be supportive.

1
Survivorship

LISA BASHORE, PhD, APRN, CPNP-PC, CPON
JOANNE QUILLEN, MSN, APRN, PNP-BC

From the time of discovery and for the balance of life,
an individual diagnosed with cancer is a survivor.
— National Coalition for Cancer Survivorship

OVER 80 PERCENT of the children and adolescents (under age 20) diagnosed each year with childhood cancer can now be cured. Survivors of childhood cancer often find that the illness and its treatment changed their lives in many powerful, and often positive, ways. There is much to celebrate.

However, long-term survivors of childhood cancer face an uncertain future. The surgery, radiation, chemotherapy, and stem cell transplants used to cure children sometimes affect growing bodies and developing minds. Complications from these treatments may occur later in life and are known as *late effects*. In addition, some survivors encounter job discrimination, difficulties obtaining insurance, and emotional or social difficulties.

During your (or your child's) journey through the many phases of survivorship, you may find yourself educating your family, friends, and healthcare providers about your physical and psychological responses to treatment and its after effects. Knowing about your disease, its treatment, and potential late effects will help you advocate for the care you need to maximize your health and well-being.

This chapter discusses some of the many stages of survivorship covering the transition from active treatment to going off treatment and the shift from childhood/adolescence to the independence of adulthood.

To take charge of your health, you need to collect information about your treatment and then assemble a team to help chart your medical course and help you monitor your healthcare. This chapter discusses ways to find the best healthcare providers for your unique needs.

Some survivors are fortunate to live near a major cancer center with a comprehensive survivorship clinic for their transitional and long-term health care after treatment ends. For others who don't, see specific guidelines on how to assemble your own health care team who is knowledgeable about the possible late effects and proper guidelines for follow-up, screening and testing (See section later in this chapter, Leaving your treatment facility and Creating your own health care team).

SURVIVORSHIP

The word *survivor* can have many different meanings depending on one's particular situation in time. There are many types of survivors but *survivor* refers to someone who survives an experience that has completely disrupted their life at a certain point in time, such as a personal tragedy or traumatic experience, a natural disaster (earthquake, tornado or flood), or those like you who have undergone treatment for an injury/cancer and been cured. In this book, we are going to refer to *survivorship* as the point in life when your cancer treatment ends and the journey into the future begins.

You are part of a growing community of children, teenagers, and adult survivors of childhood cancer who are pioneers in the post-treatment journey into adulthood. In the months and years after treatment ends, you may encounter physical late effects, emotional upheaval, and unexpected benefits.

Your journey may be easy or hard. It may take surprising turns and dips and reach dizzying heights. Although thousands of others make similar journeys, your path will be unique to you.

Life for all people is sometimes rocky and sometimes smooth. Being a survivor may throw a few unexpected stones in your path or may pave the way to new opportunities. Many survivors talk about how cancer opened their eyes and left them with an appreciation for life. They are able to shake off the small stuff and focus on the important things in their lives. They feel as if the cancer gave them perspective, and that this is a great gift. Others feel that the cancer was one small part of their lives and they prefer not to think about it. As time goes by, your feelings about the experience may change.

Being a childhood cancer survivor has shaped every aspect of my life, both the great parts and the hardships and is core to my identity. Enduring my diagnosis, treatment, and resulting complications, both physical and mental, has been and will continue to be the greatest challenge.

Despite these extreme difficulties, cancer either directly or indirectly has also brought me my greatest joys. My partner, my career, and the people and causes I choose to associate with have all come into my life as a direct result of my survivorship. These are people, activities, and causes I cherish and have given great meaning and purpose to my journey. Navigating these hardships is not as painful with the help of my support system. My advice is to embrace the survivorship club with open arms because it will lead you to great things and beautiful people.

My whole perspective on life has changed. I realize how precious life is and how much beauty can come from pain. It's a lesson I wish I could have learned in a different way, but it is also something I am thankful to have learned. I see so much more value in my life and what I can do to help others. I live every moment of my life to the best of my ability. Life is so short, and it can change in the matter of an instant.

I have learned that it's OK to have bad days, it's OK to be upset or angry, it's OK to let people help you. As a survivor, I am so much more than what I've lost – I am so much more than cancer.

Being a cancer parent is such a roller coaster of emotions. We struggle with sadness and anger about what cancer has done to our child and family and yet, at the same time, we are full of gratitude for how far she and we have come since the day of diagnosis.

Being a childhood cancer survivor is a unique experience. Some days I don't think about it much at all, while other days it's hard not to feel the effects of it. I have personally found the psychological side effects, like anxiety, depression, and guilt, to be harder to manage than my physical health. My advice to other survivors: try and seek mental health support, even if you don't think you need it. It is helpful to have someone to talk to and talk over your complicated feelings.

Being a childhood cancer survivor comes with a lot of responsibility. Like it or not, we are the ones looked up to by the children currently going through treatment. This can absolutely be daunting, stressful, and quite overwhelming. However, it can be an exceptional blessing. I was constantly inspired by the survivors I met and they allowed me to visualize myself as a survivor too someday.

Since being pronounced cancer-free, I have had wonderful opportunities to give back to organizations that helped me throughout my treatment. This has truly been life-changing for me and allowed me to fully embrace the responsibility of helping other children the way I was helped.

Part of surviving childhood cancer is dealing with and educating medical personnel, family, friends, and loved ones about the medical and emotional aspects of survivorship. You may find that family members want to pretend it never happened. You may be told to put it all behind you and not think about it. Or you may find people treating you as if you are a fragile piece of glass. Deciding what parts of your cancer history to explain and what parts to ignore may take some reflection, and will certainly involve planning how to communicate your thoughts and needs to loved ones. This topic is discussed more in *Chapter 2, Emotions, and Chapter 3, Relationships.*

Transition into survivorship

According to Webster's *New Collegiate Dictionary*, transition is a "passage from one state, stage, place, or subject to another." This definition expresses very well the road that survivors of childhood cancer travel, from active treatment, to off-treatment, and then from off-treatment to long-term survival. The definition also fits because the "place" of healthcare changes as the adolescent moves from pe-

After treatment I have been involved with two key organizations that were and are an important part of my support network, *The Hole in the Wall Gang Camp* and *Alex's Lemonade Stand*. These organizations brought the major members of my support network into my life. Those weeks at camp were always my happiest of the year. I spent time with and shared with other people my age going through similar experiences. Through those years, I met people that continue to be my best friends and my partner of 8 years. These people lift me up and support me every day. I owe a great deal to these communities for helping me through incredibly difficult transition periods. I encourage all survivors and their families to find similar support systems.

I found a lot of support through other childhood cancer families at *Alex's Lemonade Stand Foundation*. This was especially true when I was younger and continues to be. I also have support groups through my para-rowing sports and *Camp Hole in the Wall Gang*. Most kids there are cancer survivors which gives me joy because I don't need to explain myself or my life. There's no pressure because we're all there for the same reason.

diatric healthcare overseen by parents to self-designed and self-monitored adult healthcare. These periods of change can evoke anxiety and require a period of adjustment. For survivors, transitions involve medical, psychological, social, and educational changes.

People cope better with transitions if a period of planning occurs before the change happens. The transition from cancer patient to survivor should be acknowledged by all healthcare providers, and the psychosocial and educational aspects of survival should be addressed. For instance, if a teen's medical care shifts from a pediatric clinic to an adult clinic without discussions about his understanding of his disease, he may still have only the information that was given to him when first diagnosed as a young child. This is hardly the amount or depth of information needed by a survivor entering adulthood who will have to advocate for his own healthcare and make wise lifestyle choices.

The following sections discuss going off-treatment and moving from teen to adult healthcare.

End of treatment

The last day of treatment is a time for both celebration and fear. The protocol schedules and frequent appointments provided reassurance and structure. While most families are thrilled that the days of pills and procedures have ended, some fear a future without powerful medicines to keep the disease away. Concerns about relapse are an almost universal response, and family members often feel vulnerable after active treatment ends.

Many parents and survivors describe ending treatment as almost as wrenching an experience as the diagnosis. Families begin to experience the gamut of emotions—from elation to terror—months before the final day.

Survivors and their parents should anticipate that after months or years spent going through the rigors of treatment, they will have lost the feeling of a *normal* life. They may experience relapse scares and need to call the doctor to describe the symptoms and be reassured.

With diagnosis came the awareness that life can be cruel and unpredictable. Because many parents and children feel that treatment is keeping the cancer away, the end of treatment sometimes leaves families feeling exposed and vulnerable, and thoughts of "what's coming next?" When treatment ends, survivors and their parents must find ways to live with uncertainty, to find a balance between hope and reasonable worry.

I was diagnosed with acute lymphoblastic leukemia at age 4 and my treatment ended when I was 6. I went through some strange emotions then. I was happy because I felt better, could move better, and could do so much more than during my treatment. A lot of my first memories were of treatment years in the hospital, so when everything supposedly went back to "*normal*", it was a lot to adjust to.

My transition from being on a full-time treatment schedule to not having any at all has been overwhelmingly hard. I struggle a lot with anxiety, and knowing that I was not going to be getting life-saving treatment anymore made me very fearful that my cancer would come back. Of course, I was so happy to finally be done with the harsh treatments, but it also felt as though my safety net was gone. Our minds are powerful things, and anxiety creeps in whenever it wants to, so therapy was/still is an awesome outlet for me to express my worries and feelings.

Ending treatment was and still is a combination of relief and anxiety. Relief that treatment is complete, grief and sadness over all the internal damage and the loss of many loved ones to cancer including my grandmother. *"Normal"* does not exist for me, but I embrace being different and being me.

We have been so fortunate to have both healthy girls since finishing their treatment. They were both babies during treatment and have no recollection of the hell they went through. They are too young to know or worry about relapse. We are still uneasy at these follow-up visits but our confidence that there is no re-occurrence overshadows our fear of relapse.

It was a little strange to transition from being in-treatment to off-treatment. I was ecstatic to make the transition, but there were kids at school who still felt like they needed to walk on eggshells around me, even though I was in remission and could fully participate in whatever activities were taking place. After a few weeks, however, everyone began to adjust, and it was a much more inclusive and positive experience.

Transitioning off treatment was exciting, but also resulted in a bit of a culture shock. After spending a year almost entirely in the hospital surrounded by the same few people every day, transitioning back to a *"normal"* routine especially going to school regularly was a bit overwhelming. I was stuck in the middle of wanting to be treated as *normal* by my peers, while at the same time expecting to receive the same one-on-one attention from adults I was used to in the hospital. This dichotomy made me feel like I was being pulled in several directions emotionally and was tricky to navigate as a young girl.

End-of-treatment meeting with healthcare team

Doctors and nurses can help with the transition to survivorship by having a meeting with the family before the initial appointment with the *Survivorship Clinic*. The appointment should be long enough to allow a lengthy conversation.

Topics discussed during your first transition meeting to survivorship might include:

- The disease, the treatment, and possible late effects
- When and who to call with specific questions and concerns, including a written list of symptoms that should prompt a call
- Detailed discussion of the next steps: which healthcare providers will see your child, the appointment schedule, the follow-up schedule, and what (if any) immunizations to get.
- A detailed *cancer treatment summary* document (**Download a copy of Comprehensive Cancer Treatment form** used by the Children's Oncology Group (http://www.survivorshipguidelines .org/) that includes the name of the disease, date of diagnosis, place of treatment, total dosages of drugs, amounts of radiation, and necessary follow-up. This document will help survivors provide all future healthcare providers with comprehensive information about their unique medical histories.
- Access **Passport for Care**. Survivor Care Plans by Children's Oncology Group (V6, Nov 2023). Survivors and family can find online updated tailored long-term care plans which should be reviewed with their oncologist or health care provider. https://cancersurvivor.passportforcare.org
- Explanation of how to notify the treatment center of any change in address and/or how to share results of tests performed outside of the treatment center
- Realistic, but hopeful, portrayal of the future
- Praise for the child/teen for handling a very difficult time with grace (or courage, or whatever word is appropriate)
- Recognition of all of your family's hard work
- Thank-you and feedback to the healthcare team
- Acknowledgment that you may be relieved but also fearful of the future
- Discussion of any concerns parents or child might have

If any of these items are not mentioned in the last meeting, ask to have another meeting or phone call to address these or any other questions or concerns you may have.

Celebrations—or not

Some families enjoy having ceremonies to mark the end of cancer treatment. For younger children in particular, who have spent much of their lives taking pills and having procedures, ceremonies can help them grasp that the most active phase of treatment is truly over and the important transition to life as a survivor is about to begin. Following are ideas from many families about how to commemorate this important occasion.

- Take pictures of the hospital and staff.
- Give trophies to your child and any siblings.
- Throw a party for friends and family.
- Have friends and family send cards or messages of congratulations.
- Go on a trip or vacation to celebrate.
- If consistent with your beliefs, have a religious ceremony of thanksgiving.
- Organize a party at your child's school.

As you will discover in this book, every child, parent, and relative reacts differently to the phases of treatment and survivorship. The differences do not matter. What is important is that you recognize that all feelings are normal. Whether you feel joyful, relieved, fearful, or terrified, the end of treatment evokes strong emotions in every member of the family.

My class had a party for me, with ice cream and games, after I returned from my last round of chemo. Most of my treatment lined up with the school year, from diagnosis to end of treatment, so in a way that helped me transition out of the hospital mind set and into the home/summer mindset.

We had an end-of-treatment celebration in Times Square, New York City with my New York Police Department family, as well as family and friends, it was covered by our local radio station. My family and I have learned that every second in life is a gift and should be celebrated. Life is short and even shorter for survivors like me, so we celebrate every milestone big and small.

We had a big party for each child at the end of their treatment. Even if we didn't know what the future held, we decided to

(Continued)

celebrate each milestone. No one knows when we will die but that doesn't stop us from having birthday celebrations! We also knew so many friends and family members were praying and rooting for us, and we wanted a tangible way to give back to others and gather together in the spirit of gratefulness.

My daughter was diagnosed on my dad's birthday. He died 13 years ago. May 16 is a strange day for us—it kicks off a season of remembering and an entire summer of fear, upheaval, and trauma. But it is also the start of the end of the school, summer vacations and sunny days, and family trips. This year, my daughter receives a scholarship award on May 16. I think I try to find signs in the dates. Whether this is sane or not, I don't know. But finding meaning has helped me get through.

Our daughter had cancer during one of the hardest times the entire world has gone through - COVID. She was diagnosed with AML in March of 2020. Due to this, many things that usually come with cancer were elevated, including isolation. After months in the hospital, people raised money for her to take a limo ride home from the hospital as a safe celebration. We waited a few months after this to celebrate with family and friends. I would recommend a small celebration or surprise right after treatment, and then a bigger celebration when your kiddo can truly celebrate and remember it as a victory.

Return to normal

After years of treatment, families grapple with the idea of returning to normal. Unfortunately, most families don't really know what "normal" is any longer. Parents and children realize that returning to the innocent pre-cancer days is unrealistic, that life has changed. The constant interaction with medical personnel is ending, and a new phase is beginning in which routines do not revolve around being sick, taking medicines, and going to the hospital. Although it is true that the blissful ignorance of the days prior to cancer are gone forever, a different life, a new normal one begins—often enriched by friends and experiences from the past cancer years.

Overall returning to 'normal' for us meant having our own schedule, eating food we made ourselves, and being together as a family. Returning to work and routine helped too, instead of always feeling like we were at loose ends and often being stressed about money. Our hopes were that we could focus on creating memories and togetherness as a family, and we did. Traveling to see family members and friends and our daughter's make-a-wish trip were also really special. Oddly, going through the first sickness after treatment ended was even a special milestone. It brought back some feelings of anxiety remembering times we had to rush to the hospital with a fever, but this time we were grateful we didn't need the hospital visit.

Our family has not returned to "normal"; we have a "new normal." My daughter had a brain tumor which has left her with many long-term side effects – she has been forever changed physically and mentally by cancer. When she was diagnosed, I was told that there could be long-term side effects, but I didn't anticipate how they would constantly continue to impact our lives. Learning to live with these challenges has been hard. We did *not* have an end-of-treatment celebration because even though she was done with chemo, she still had a lot of rehabilitation to do (physical therapy, occupational therapy, and speech therapy). We do celebrate her diagnosis day. It's always hard, but we try to bring joy and gratitude to it.

It wasn't that hard for us. Our goal was to always treat her like a normal child. When her numbers were good, we took her out and had friends over as long as they were not sick. We did punish or not punish her because she was sick. She was treated exactly the same. She still had consequences for stealing a cookie out of the cookie jar if she wasn't supposed to - even if she just had chemo that day.

Open communication between parents and survivors

Parents and survivors need to talk to one another, examine their emotions, decide what course they want to chart, and work together toward a healthy life after cancer, recognizing that the journey will have twists and turns and ups and downs.

As survivors grow and mature, their understanding of what happened to them when they had cancer unfolds and expands. They are also ready for, and often desire, more detailed and current medical information concerning their diagnoses and treatments. The past is viewed from the perspective of an older individual with a broader world view, more education, and firmer values. They ask more questions of parents and medical personnel to more fully understand the past and its implications for the future. They will struggle to cope with, or make their peace with, any late effects from treatment that arise. And they do this on top of all the usual developmental challenges of growing up.

From childhood/adolescence to adulthood

The passage from adolescence to adult life may be a stormy one. The maturing teen must gradually separate from the protection of parents and home and become self-reliant and independent. This process is difficult for many teens and their parents. For survivors of childhood cancer, this task can be complicated by uniquely strong ties forged with parents or complex family dynamics that grew out of the turmoil of cancer treatment. However, the progress through adolescence into young adulthood is fairly normal for most survivors. Parents show great variability in how they feel as their teens begin to think about leaving home. Teens and young adults also show a mixed response to leaving the security of home for the first time.

By taking responsibility for your adult life, you can integrate the physical, emotional, intellectual, spiritual, and social parts of your life. In decades past, you might have been referred to as a "cancer victim." Now you can view yourself as someone who was victorious over cancer.

> My cancer treatment resulted in my decision to get a below-the-knee amputation, so for the rest of my life I have a permanent physical reminder of what I went through as a kid. I never regretted this choice and have been confident it was the right decision for me. However, having gone through it at such a formative age (9-12), it certainly influenced my transition into a preteen, teen, and adulthood.

I was adjusting to life as an amputee and life after treatment on top of all the emotions that come along with puberty and growing up. I felt uncomfortable in my changing body and also uncomfortable with a body that looked different from everyone else's. This was socially isolating not only for me but I'm sure for my parents with other parents as well. Fortunately, during these difficult periods, I had support from two incredible communities: *The Hole and the Wall Gang Camp* and *Alex's Lemonade Stand*. Both helped to connect me and my parents with other children and their families navigating similar circumstances.

My daughter was in kindergarten when she was diagnosed, and she's now a middle schooler. I feel like she is socially immature but mature in other ways. Going through cancer treatment taught her to know what she needs and how to advocate for herself. She has a slower processing speed so it's difficult for her to keep up socially-- middle school girls talk fast!

I was diagnosed as a freshman in college. I was living my life to the fullest and having the time of my life. After I was diagnosed, my world was completely different. After finishing treatment, I ever so eagerly wanted to return to college, so that is what I did. When I started my sophomore year, I thought everything would go back to exactly how it was before. When it wasn't, it took a big toll on me mentally. I was angry I couldn't do what I had been doing before and angry I was so behind compared to my friends. That adjustment was hard. To this day, it is something I deal with.

The transition has been weird but refreshing. I love being a wife and a mom, which are things I dreamed about and prayed for and wasn't sure would come to fruition. I love being normal and having normal experiences, like taking my son to school, going to work, coming home, eating dinner with my little family, and worrying about what's for dinner or if my son will eat it. I know it sounds dumb, but I prayed for this.

Being diagnosed at age 19 was really difficult. I was in college and my friends and I were enjoying first year. I tried really hard to stay, but when I got bronchitis, the doctors told me I was too sick and sent me home. All my life I was holding onto this idea

(Continued)

(Continued)

that I was the oldest child and would be the first to go to college. Then I was diagnosed and it was taken away in the blink of an eye. Being college-age, undergoing treatment is hard and there is little support for this age group. There are places for young kids with cancer and places for full adults, but not college-age. This is when your life is supposed to take off and for me it did not. It's important to have people who understand, but I didn't.

WORKING WITH HEALTHCARE PROVIDERS

All survivors need a long-term relationship with a knowledgeable and attentive healthcare provider (physician or nurse practitioner) whom they trust. If you are a cancer survivor, the provider you choose should oversee all of your medical care and refer you to specialists as the need arises. The provider should either specialize in treating survivors of cancer or be willing to work with you to keep up with the latest research and recommendations for care. Follow-up care for survivors of childhood cancer is lifelong. It is an investment in your future health, and perhaps your life, to spend time finding a healthcare provider who is capable of taking care of your particular needs.

As a survivor mom, I must constantly navigate medical situations and be an advocate for my daughter. I've learned that outside of her medical team, there is a lot of misunderstanding about childhood cancer, late effects, and things like hearing loss that affected my daughter. She lost high frequency hearing as a result of chemo. I wish there had been more supports available to me, but for the most part people have been supportive and understanding. I wish I had immersed my daughter in the deaf/hard of hearing community when she was young. I believe it would have provided a better support system there where she would have felt more comfortable, learned sign language, and been more confident in her communications with others. One thing I would tell other parents, is to always trust that voice inside you and if you feel something is not right, then don't ignore your gut feeling.

The challenges are from outside of pediatric oncology—from the "experts" who should know better, but they don't. Much like my struggles with non-cancer mothers, non-cancer health care providers don't understand it either.

The dentist wants to do constant x-rays—and we say no, she's had enough radiation to her brain. An optometrist is confused by her eye alignment—we have to share her entire story, again. The school nurse is annoyed we refuse the scoliosis check. Another school nurse doesn't want to clear her for sports after COVID, thinking my daughter might have cardiac dysfunction because of chemo, but she didn't receive chemo and doesn't have cardiac dysfunction. Even her pediatrician needs extensive education on what survivorship looks like.

Your cancer treatment history and medical records

Keep a copy of your Comprehensive Cancer Treatment document at home in a safe place, take a photo and keep on your phone, and give a copy to each of your healthcare providers. Also important to keep copies at home of reports (and actual scans) of key x-rays, scans, and important surgeries.

The first thing you share with a healthcare provider is your medical history, which includes your cancer diagnosis and treatment. Many of the 388,501 survivors of childhood cancer in North America do not know the specifics of their treatments. Some do not even know they had cancer. If you don't have a detailed cancer treatment summary, you need to get one as soon as possible.

The more time passes, the harder it will be to track down the specifics of your treatment. The easiest way to get a record of your treatments is to download a blank copy of Comprehensive Cancer Treatment form used by the Children's Oncology Group at (http://www.survivorshipguidelines.org/). Take it to the healthcare providers who treated you when you had cancer and ask them to fill in the information. Some clinics also have their own Oncology Summary

Template and will complete this for you. This health history will become an indispensable part of your medical records for the rest of your life. **You should keep a copy at home in a safe place, take a photo and keep on your phone, and give a copy to each of your healthcare providers.** When you leave home to begin your adult life, this document should go with you.

Essential information you need about your cancer treatment. If you do not have a copy of your cancer treatment history, request a doctor or nurse at the institution where you received cancer treatment to write down the following critical information:

- Name of disease
- Date of diagnosis and relapse, if any
- Place of treatment
- Dates of treatment
- Clinical trial protocol number and name, if applicable
- Names of attending oncologist and nurse practitioner
- Names and total dosages of chemotherapy drugs used
- Name of radiation center
- Dates radiation was received
- Amount of radiation and to what body part (for example, whole body, cranial, pelvis)
- Date and type of any surgeries
- Date and type of stem cell transplant(s), if any
- Any major treatment complications
- Any persistent side effects of treatment
- Recommended medical follow-up
- Contact numbers for treating institutions

Obtain copies of key x-rays and scans. It is also important to get copies of the reports for x-rays, scans, and major surgeries that were part of your treatment. Key reports would include any radiology tests such as chest x-rays or scans (CT, MRI, PET-CT) that show where the tumor was located, including those at diagnosis, at least one or two during your treatment to assess response to therapy, and those at the end of treatment.

Hospitals and clinics may not retain copies of your x-rays or scans or difficult to obtain copies years later or if you move locations. You may be charged a fee for copies, but it is well worth the price for the peace of mind that comes from having your own set of records. If you develop late effects from treatment, these early records are crucial for your current healthcare providers to review.

One area that was difficult for us was coping with the long waits for appointments with specialists and frustration with specialists who dropped the ball. One of our two survivors needed a neuropsychological appointment and it took months to get it scheduled. Once the assessment was complete, the doctor's office repeatedly forgot to upload the report. We never received documentation of the recommendations and diagnoses.

We also have had issues with our medical insurance cooperating with outside specialists, such as audiology. It took over a year for one of our children to get hearing aids after identifying they were necessary.

Dental care follow-up has also been hard, especially since it is completely separate from medical care. Some dentists have made comments about the number of times the kids go in for routine MRIs (right now, three times a year). These comments are stressful because these MRIs are necessary for monitoring for recurrence and we have no control over that.

COMPREHENSIVE FOLLOW-UP CLINIC OR SURVIVORSHIP PROGRAMS

In the past, survivors of cancer were often on their own after treatment ended. With increasing numbers of long-term survivors, it became apparent that these young adults faced complex medical and psychosocial effects from their years of treatment. Fitzhugh Mullan, MD, co-founder of the National Coalition for Cancer Survivorship, said, "It is as if we have invented sophisticated techniques to save people from drowning, but once they have been pulled from the water, we leave them on the dock to cough and sputter on their own in the belief that we have done all we can" (Mullan, 1984).

Some institutions, realizing the need for long-term services for survivors, started comprehensive programs, now called *survivorship programs*. There are many health care facilities that have survivorship programs but may have a different title, such as long-term follow-up clinics or comprehensive follow-up clinics. Other institutions have difficulty obtaining support and the financial resources to start and maintain survivorship programs.

For about a year after completing my treatment. I had monthly checkups at the oncology clinic with my oncologist which included blood work and scans (MRI, bone scan, CT, x-rays). After the first year those visits changed to every three months, then every 6 months, until I was about 5 years out from treatment, then just an annual visit. I also had frequent follow-ups with my orthopedic surgeon since all of my surgeries and my surgeon were located at a different hospital from where I received my cancer treatment with my primary oncologist.

The clinic where I received my post-treatment care had a well-established pipeline for patients finishing therapy, so from my perspective the follow-up was fortunately pretty straightforward. An area that was difficult for me was fully understanding why I still had to keep going back to the clinic, albeit less frequently. There was so much build-up to the end of treatment, and being so young, it was hard to wrap my head around why I had to return for follow-ups and frequently after I was "done." This was especially true around scan days which were very anxiety-inducing.

I don't remember much about the transition because I was only in 1st grade, but we continued to see my doctors fairly regularly after finishing chemo (maybe once a month) for a year, then steadily decreased until it was only once a year as part of a Survivorship Clinic. It was a comprehensive team and it was set up by the hospital, so we did not have to find doctors or ask for referrals.

I am impacted both physically and emotionally by late medical effects. I also have a rare blood disease, so it is very difficult. After treatment was complete, I am required to go to survivorship clinic also known as "forever care." I also have a doctor for every organ in my body to follow up yearly or more often if needed as symptoms present, which unfortunately is more often than I like.

We are lucky to have the Survivorship Clinic at CHOP. We keep in touch with the oncologist via email—this relationship is wonderful and extremely helpful as she has gone through the process to be classified as a para-rower, applied for grants to cover her rowing fees, applied for childhood cancer scholarships and struggled with some long-term physical issues. I also send regular updates to her doctor—I am so grateful, and I know her job is impossible. She has had an amazing impact on my daughter's life.

History of survivorship care

In 1996, the International Society of Pediatric Oncologists developed guidelines for the care of childhood cancer survivors and stressed the importance of psychological support and the education of patients about a healthy lifestyle. They stated, "We advocate the establishment of a specialty clinic oriented to the preventive medical and psychosocial care of long-term survivors . . . The goal is to promote long-term physical, psychosocial, and socioeconomic health and productivity, not merely to maintain an absence of disease or dysfunction." (Masera, 1996) In 2003, the Institute of Medicine published a book called *Childhood Cancer Survivorship: Improving Care and Quality of Life*, which stressed the importance of follow-up programs.

The Children's Oncology Group (COG) first published follow-up guidelines in 2004 to help survivors and the healthcare providers who treat them. COG guidelines are periodically updated as research and treatment evolve. The most recent COG updates Version 6 were published in 2023. In addition, the American Academy of Pediatrics published guidelines in 2004 for pediatric cancer centers, which stressed the importance of long-term follow-up and described survivorship programs as "An established program designed to provide long-term, multidisciplinary follow-up of successfully treated patients at the original treatment center or by a team of healthcare professionals who are familiar with the potential adverse effects of treatment for childhood cancer" (Corrigan, 2004).

As a result of these recommendations and a growing awareness of the needs of survivors of childhood cancer, some institutions began survivorship clinics using a multidisciplinary team to monitor and support survivors. The nucleus of the team usually includes a nurse coordinator, pediatric oncologist (physician), pediatric nurse practitioner, and sometimes a social worker and/or psychologist. They have a close working relationship with cardiologists, endocrinologists, orthopedic surgeons, and other specialists whose services are needed by some survivors.

What survivorship programs provide

Survivorship programs usually provide a review of treatments received, counseling about potential health risks, and any necessary diagnostic tests such as cardiac evaluations, hormonal studies, psychological evaluations, or testing for learning disabilities. These survivorship clinics not only provide comprehensive care for long-term survivors, but also participate in research projects that track the effectiveness of and late-effects from various clinical trials. In addition, members of the survivorship clinic team act as advocates for survivors with schools, health insurance agencies, and employers. The focus of these programs should be to educate survivors about strategies to maximize their health and well-being.

Finding survivorship clinics or comprehensive follow-up care

Many cancer centers do see long-term survivors, but do not have a survivorship or comprehensive program. Others have excellent survivorship clinics. The first step in finding a survivorship clinic is to ask your pediatric oncology provider for guidance and recommendations for transitioning to an adult program. Then try to find a survivorship program near you (for help, **see Resources** at the end of the chapter).

To assess the programs nearest to you, you can ask the following questions:

- How do you provide follow-up for childhood cancer survivors?
- Who is in charge of the program (doctor, nurse practitioner)?
- What is your experience in treating the late effects of childhood cancer?
- Which other professionals are part of the team?
- What is a typical visit to the follow-up clinic like?
- What transition services from child to adult care do you provide?
- Are there support groups or mentoring programs available?

Richard Klausner, MD, former director of the National Cancer Institute, wrote, *"We must move away from the 'take no prisoners' theory of cancer care and begin considering the sequelae of the treatment we are giving patients. We have to overhaul our programs so that we can follow survivors, ask the questions, and get the answers we need to evaluate the effects of cancer treatment on long-term health."*

Comprehensive follow-up not only improves the health and quality of life for survivors, but also helps physicians evaluate the long-term effects of cancer therapies and develop safer therapies for newly diagnosed children. Advocating for comprehensive follow-up not only helps you as an individual, but helps children diagnosed in the future.

Transition from your treatment facility to survivor follow-up healthcare team

It is sometimes difficult to leave your treating physician and staff for new healthcare providers. Often, the deep trust and strong ties you feel for the staff are hard to give up. However, sometimes continuing to see your treating oncologist for follow-up can create barriers to communication. Many survivors don't want to disappoint their doctors. They feel that discussing their complex feelings after treatment is not *worthy* of the doctor's time. Survivors are frequently reminded how lucky they are to be alive. Often gratitude for their life is the only socially acceptable emotion for survivors. The lack of support from society and the medical community for the difficulties that survivors often face can increase their distress and frustration.

Some survivors feel that to express their resentment or anger for having cancer will make the doctor think they are ungrateful. If you go to the oncology clinic and wait for your appointment with patients who are on treatment, you may feel that your problems are too insignificant to mention. And healthcare providers who treated you are sometimes—perhaps unconsciously—unwilling or unable to elicit all of the late effects information necessary to give good follow-up care. If you go to a specialist knowledgeable in late-effects who was not involved in your treatment, you will not feel like you need to protect your former healthcare provider's feelings. Such problems do not arise at institutions where treatment teams work closely with late effects specialists, such as cardiologists, endocrinologists, orthopedic surgeons, and other specialists whose services are needed by some survivors. At these locations, survivors get the benefits of seeing both kinds of healthcare providers without having to choose between them.

Creating your own follow-up healthcare team

If you do not live near a comprehensive follow-up clinic, you will need to assemble a team of healthcare providers in your community. The first and most important member of the team is a *primary healthcare provider*. This could be an internist, pediatrician, nurse practitioner, or women's health specialist (*gynecologist*). You may need to interview several healthcare providers to find the best fit.

The most important qualities to look for in your primary healthcare provider are the abilities to care about you, listen to you, work with you to assemble a team, and read the literature about late-effects. The provider should refer you to specialists as needed, organize your healthcare, and function as your medical case manager.

Try to find someone who is willing to work with you to address any health problems that arise and perform thorough checkups to find any problems early. You need someone who listens, provides plenty of time, and is interested in working with you to make a long-term

Our care team made sure our transition was smooth. We did not have to build our own team. We would see the oncologist every week at first. Then we went to biweekly, and eventually monthly. Four years after treatment, we still see the oncologist every three months, but we also go to the survivor clinic. The survivor clinic checks bloodwork, mental health, and side effects from chemotherapy treatments.

Our oncologist and pediatrician really helped inform us about issues we might face and give referrals when we asked for them. They have been great cheerleaders, supportive and helped us advocate well. I definitely think there will always be some ongoing anxiety that we aren't doing something, or we will miss something that will be crucial later on.

Late medical effects are difficult because there is so much unknown. The fear around late effects is a regular issue, as there are so many possibilities to watch for. Maintaining a positive relationship with my current care team and having access to my cancer treatment medical records, as well as staying aware of new research, have been helpful in alleviating the burden.

Our daughter's transition after the end of treatment was more gradual because of her follow-up MRI's. The first year they were every 3 months, then every 6 months, and now every year. The gradual decrease in visits really helped us transition. I used to get so anxious whenever scan appointments came up, but this has gotten a little easier with time. She also had a lot of rehabilitation appointments after treatment ended. Having that 5-year treatment plan was extremely helpful to know what to expect and when. Our clinic has a great comprehensive follow-up clinic where she has an annual visit.

health plan. Healthcare professionals who do not regularly care for survivors of pediatric malignancies are encouraged to consult with a pediatric oncology long-term follow-up center if any questions or concerns arise when reviewing or using these guidelines. If your current healthcare provider doesn't give you the time you need or stands with one hand on the doorknob while you are asking questions, it may be time to look elsewhere.

> Be informed about your own medical history and potential risk factors and communicate with your healthcare team when you have concerns or symptoms.

The more informed you are about your own risk profile, the better you can advocate for appropriate care. After you have educated yourself about your history and risks, do not hesitate to be a friendly advocate. Explain (in person, on the phone, or by email) your position and concerns, and state what you would like to have happen.

For example, if you know you are at risk for thickening of the wall of the heart and you are having chest pains, you can ask your primary healthcare provider for a referral to a cardiologist. If you then tell the cardiologist your history, symptoms, and what you are at risk for, you are much more likely to be properly diagnosed. It is well worth it to invest the time to find a caring healthcare provider to whom you go for a visit and say, "I'm having these symptoms," and allow her/him to investigate and get early treatment. Together you can work toward a healthy life.

Ways to advocate for the best possible medical care:
- Use a Cancer Treatment Summary (see example of blank Comprehensive Summary of Cancer Treatment form used by the Children's Oncology Group at (http://www.survivorshipguidelines. org/. Take this form to your oncology team that treated you to fill in and then educate your primary healthcare provider and all specialists about your treatments.
- Refer to the Children's Oncology Group's recommendations for follow-up care and Healthlinks for Patient Education (see Resource list, COG Long-term follow-up guidelines for survivors (Version 6, revised Oct 2023).
- Keep files containing copies of key x-rays, diagnostic tests, and reports.
- Keep your healthcare provider updated about any health concerns or symptoms you have.
- Find a resource person at a survivorship clinic or comprehensive follow-up clinic whom your healthcare provider can call for specialized information or advice. Phone consultations are common.

- Based on an accurate understanding of your treatment, know what medical services you require and what type of monitoring you need, and ensure that these are provided by your healthcare team. See Healthlinks for Patient Education at (**www .survivorshipguidelines.org**). If you are not getting the follow-up you need, consider having a frank discussion about your concerns or locating a primary care provider with a better understanding of survivorship.
- Learn what you need to know, surround yourself with knowledgeable professionals, and live your life to the fullest.

A nurse practitioner who runs a large, well-established survivorship clinic described: We really need to educate the community of healthcare providers. We have problems with healthcare workers who are attributing medical problems to cancer treatment that have nothing to do with the survivor's cancer treatment. The opposite problem happens, too. Many physicians and nurses miss obvious and sometimes life-threatening late effects. For instance, women who had high-dose radiation to the chest may develop heart disease at a young age. They are too often diagnosed with asthma or anxiety, when they really have restrictive pericarditis.

Another nurse practitioner said: I've been taking care of survivors for 18 years. Many of them apologize for "bothering me" when they call with a question or concern. Almost always they are calling with good questions about appropriate issues. Even if you think it is insignificant, if it bothers you, discuss it with your healthcare provider by phone, email, or during an appointment.

My care team prepared me very well! A follow-up team had already been formed for me before I was cancer-free, which was incredibly helpful. Immediately after end-of-treatment, I had monthly check-ups. After a year, the check-ups became bi-monthly, then every 4 months, then every 6 months, and eventually yearly. The check-ups were done to ensure that the cancer did not come back, and included bloodwork, EKGs, x-rays, and ultrasounds.

(Continued)

(Continued)

> The most helpful thing in working with my follow-up teams has been the consistency of the care providers. Seeing the same social worker, nurses, and specialists allowed me to feel comfortable and create a rapport with them over many different years. My physician ended up leaving at the end of high school and was replaced with a new doctor. This new physician is wonderfully qualified and cares a lot for me. It has all worked out, but it was definitely a difficult adjustment.
>
> My treatment took place from age 4 to 6. I made frequent visits to the hospital most of grade school for checkups. Immediately following treatment, we continued routine bloodwork and follow-up visits which became increasingly less frequent. My care team continued to follow-up with me until I was 18, at which point I was finally phased out of hospital visits. A week after my 18th birthday, my mom and I took our last trip to the hospital and walked out knowing it was the last one. It felt like stepping over a threshold into a new era. Now, my current team of doctors still follow up with occasional bloodwork.

REFERENCES

Chow EJ, Ness KK, Armstrong GT, et al. (2020). Current and coming challenges in the management of the survivorship population. *Semin Oncol.* 2020 Feb;47(1):23-39. doi: 10.1053/j.seminoncol.2020.02.007. Epub 2020 Mar 4. PMID: 32197774; PMCID: PMC7227387.

Corrigan JJ, et al. (2004). American Academy of Pediatrics' guidelines for pediatric cancer centers. *Pediatrics*, 113(6): 1833–35.

Hord J, Feig S, Crouch G, et al. Standards for Pediatric Cancer Centers. Section on hematology/oncology; *Pediatrics* (2014) 134 (2): 410–414. https://doi.org/10.1542/peds.2014-1526

Klausner R (Apr 1998). NCI Spotlights Survivorship. *The Bone & Marrow Transplant Newsletter*, 9(1), issue 41.

Long-Term Follow-Up Guidelines for Survivors of Childhood, Adolescent, and Young Adult Cancers, Version 6.0 (October 2023) http://www.survivorshipguidelines.org

Masera G, Chesler M, Jankovic M, et al. (1996) SIOP Working Committee on Psychosocial issues in pediatric oncology: guidelines for care of long-term survivors. Med Pediatr Oncol. 1996 Jul;27(1):1-2. doi: 10.1002/(SICI)1096-911X(199607)27:1<1::AID-MPO1>3.0.CO;2-K. PMID: 8614384.

Mullan F (1985). Seasons of survival: Reflections of a physician with cancer. *N Engl J Med*, 313: 270–273.

Phillips SM, Padgett LS, Leisenring WM, et al. (2015) Survivors of childhood cancer in the United States: prevalence and burden of morbidity. *Cancer Epidemiol Biomarkers Prev.* 2015 Apr;24(4):653-63. doi: 10.1158/1055-9965.EPI-14-1418. PMID: 25834148; PMCID: PMC4418452.

Song A, Fish JD. Caring for survivors of childhood cancer: it takes a village. (2018) *Curr Opin Pediatr.* 2018 Dec;30(6):864-873. doi: 10.1097/MOP.0000000000000681. PMID: 30124580.

RESOURCES

Website: ccgresources.org

All resources and references mentioned in this book are available on the website and will be routinely reviewed and updated.

Find a survivorship clinic near you:
Website: www.oncolink.org
Search bar: *Find a survivorship clinic, clinic search*

Alex's Lemonade Stand Foundation
Website: www.alexslemonade.org
Search, *childhood cancer families*
Alex's Lemonade Stand Foundation (ALSF) is changing the lives of children with cancer by funding impactful research, raising awareness, supporting families, and empowering everyone to help cure childhood cancer. ALSF offers many programs and tools to help families navigate the challenges of childhood cancer.

American Academy of Pediatrics (AAP)
Website: www.healthychildren.org
Search, *cancer survivors*
Resource for parents

American Cancer Society (ACS)
Website: www.cancer.org

Centers for Disease Control and Prevention (CDC)
U.S. Department of Health
Website: www.cdc.gov

Children's Oncology Group. (V6, 2023). *Long-Term Follow-Up Guidelines for Survivors of Childhood, Adolescent, and Young Adult Cancers*
Website: www.survivorshipguidelines.org

How to use this resource

This is a resource for healthcare professionals who provide ongoing care to survivors of pediatric malignancies. Healthcare professionals who do not regularly care for survivors of pediatric malignancies are encouraged to consult with a pediatric oncology long-term follow-up center if questions or concerns arise when reviewing or using these guidelines. Survivors who choose to review these guidelines should do this with the assistance of a healthcare professional knowledgeable about long-term follow-up care for survivors of childhood, adolescent, and young adult cancers. The screening recommendations in these guidelines are appropriate for *asymptomatic* survivors of childhood, adolescent, or young adult cancer presenting for routine exposure-based medical follow-up. For survivors presenting with signs and symptoms suggesting illness or organ dysfunction, more extensive evaluations are needed, as clinically indicated.

For survivors:

Download a copy of *Summary of Cancer Treatment (Abbreviated or Comprehensive)* and check *Health Links (Appendix II)* To access patient education materials on a variety of subjects listed alphabetically (ie. *bleomycin alert, breast cancer, chronic pain, dental health, eye health, mental health, precocious puberty*)

Passport for Care, Survivor Care Plans by Children's Oncology Group (V6, Nov 2023)

Website: https://cancersurvivor.passportforcare.org
Survivors and family can find online updated tailored long-term care plans which should be reviewed with their oncologist or health care provider.

Summary of Cancer Treatment form. Children's Oncology Group (V6, Oct 2023) *Long-Term Follow-Up* Guidelines for Survivors of Childhood, Adolescent, and *Young Adult Cancers.*

Website: www.survivorshipguidelines.org
Click on: *Summary of Cancer Treatment (Comprehensive or Summary)*

GLOSSARY

Comprehensive Summary of Cancer Treatment document, complete detailed medical history including type of cancer and all treatments with dates and specific treatments received (radiation, chemotherapy, and surgeries) www.survivorshipguidelines.org/ Click on : *Summary of Cancer Treatment (Comprehensive or Summary).*

gynecologist, a medical doctor who treats issues with female reproductive organs. They deal with all aspects of sexual health like preventive care, cancer screenings and physical exams. Some of the services and tests provided are: pelvic exams and external genital exams., Pap tests and cancer screenings, and testing for sexually transmitted infections.

healthcare social worker (or licensed clinical social worker), a professional provider with special education and training to help you understand your diagnosis and what it means for your future. They may help you adjust your lifestyle, housing or medical needs to live more comfortably and independently. For example, they may help you find home healthcare aids or support groups.

internist, doctor of internal medicine who only treats adults (over age 18) and specializes in the diagnosis and treatment of internal organs and systems of the body (not limited to those areas); they *do not* perform surgery.

late effects, physical, psychological or social problems/issues that arise after treatment and cure of cancer as a result of the treatment received; these effects can be immediate or develop/occur years after treatment completed.

nurse coordinator, a professional RN who oversees the work of a team of healthcare professionals in their department or unit. Clinical nurse coordinators provide both clinical and administrative leadership.

pediatric oncologist, a medical doctor who diagnoses and treats cancer in children and teens; many also specialize in *hematology* (treatment of blood disorders) and are referred to as pediatric oncologist/hematologist.

pediatric nurse practitioner (PNP), a specialized advanced practice nurse who cares for newborns, infants, toddlers, adolescents, and young adults. PNPs provide comprehensive care, including well-child and physical exams; diagnose illnesses and form treatment plans; and offer health education for patients and their families. They work closely with physicians and medical teams in hospitals, clinics, and schools. In some cases, a PNP may be the primary source of care for an individual or family.

nurse practitioner (NP), a registered nurse with advanced education/training to evaluate, diagnose, and treat various acute and chronic health conditions as part of a patient's healthcare team; they can interact with patients without supervision of a medical doctor for certain health conditions and manage patient caseloads and focus on communication and educating patients to become willing participants in their own healthcare.

primary care provider (PCP), a physician (MD or DO), nurse practitioner, clinical nurse specialist (nurse practitioner) or physician assistant (PA), as allowed under state law, who provides, co-ordinates or helps a patient access a range of healthcare services (healthcare.gov); also known as your *primary* doctor/nurse practitioner/PA.

psychologist, a professional trained and educated to help people with problems with their feelings and emotions including cognitive, emotional and social relationships

survivorship, the point in life when your cancer treatment ends and the journey into your future begins

survivorship program or clinic, a program designed to provide long-term, multidisciplinary follow-up of successfully treated patients at the original treatment center or by a team of healthcare professionals who are familiar with the potential adverse effects of treatment for childhood cancer. Teams include nurse coordinator, pediatric oncologist, nurse practitioner, and sometimes a social worker and psychologist. The team has a close working relationship with specialists such as cardiologists, endocrinologists, orthopedic surgeons, and other specialists whose services are needed by some survivors.

Adult survivorship program or clinic (for those over age 18) will include same team members as the pediatric except they will be adult oncologist and adult/family practice nurse practitioner

2
Emotions

VICTORIA E. COSGROVE, PhD

Emotions are like waves; they come and go.
Ride them out with courage and compassion.
– Tara Brach

IMPROVEMENTS IN TREATMENT for childhood cancer are a huge success story in modern medicine. However, survivors and their families often face many physical and psychological challenges after the end of treatment for their cancer. Late effects from treatment are common as is struggling to find a new *normal* in life. Survivors sometimes experience a range of strong emotions as they adjust to after-cancer life (i.e., fear of recurrence, anxiety, guilt, grief, gratitude, and joy). Some survivors experience these reactions even if they remember very little—or even nothing—about their cancer experience. Knowing that other survivors and members of their families share these emotions alleviates loneliness.

FEARS OF RECURRENCE

Survivors and their parents experience a whole spectrum of feelings about possible relapse. Some may never think about it, acknowledging its possibility in the future but deferring any worry. Cancer no longer is an active part of their daily, weekly, or monthly reality. Many feel anxious in anticipation of an anniversary date or medical checkup. And some, even many years after treatment, still have nightmares or anxiety attacks that may interfere with daily life.

Some survivors may be surprised to find that feelings about recurrence vacillate over time. They may experience periods of fearfulness, followed by longer times when they do not think about cancer at all. One mother said, "Funny how you think you've got the fear under control, then something happens and you again feel your head swimming, stomach churning, and your legs becoming spaghetti." It's normal to be at different places on this spectrum at different times.

Survivors may not normally be bothered by fears of relapse––until annual follow-up appointments arrive. Sometimes, visiting the hospital for blood work, x-rays, and an examination may cause dormant feelings to surface. This is a very common phenomenon, and each survivor has individual ways of dealing with these normal feelings.

Some survivors and some parents of survivors find that they continue to have deep fears of recurrence for a long time. For others, fear and distress are less about recurrence and more about the emergence of late effects. Psychosocial support from a professional therapist or psychologist familiar with the strain of cancer diagnoses and treatments often helps survivors and parents navigate complicated emotions.

Additionally, individual or family counseling and support groups may help to reduce isolation, allowing for sharing of suggestions for dealing with survivorship issues and channeling strong feelings in constructive ways. Mental health professionals can help you prevent problems from arising or deal with them if they do appear.

Fear of relapse has been one of the hardest things to deal with coming off of treatment. Relapsing crosses my mind almost every day. The thought of having to go through cancer treatment a second time is terrifying. There have been times when my fear has become debilitating. I do think my fear has lessened over time, but it has never really gone away. I think I have just learned to cope with it better.

I think of relapse often as I have memories of seeing my grandmother suffer from cancer for years and experience several relapses before she transitioned. She was my number one supporter throughout my cancer journey, so I was, and still am, heartbroken that she is no longer physically here with us. I feel survivor's guilt losing many friends and my grandmother to cancer, but every day I do something to give back and help others in her honor.

I didn't really think about the possibility of relapse until I was a teenager. At the 10-year anniversary, when I was 14, was the first time I thought about relapses. They were holding a blood drive at my school, and I realized I couldn't donate due to having had leukemia. The longer remission goes, the less likely relapse is, but there's always that thought in my head of "what if?"

I don't have panic attacks on a normal basis, but every time our daughter had a scan after treatment for the first cancer, I had anxiety that more cancer would be found. When the scans would come back clear, I'd feel relief until the next scan came up and the cycle started all over again. The moment our daughter was diagnosed with her second cancer, I thought, "This is it. This is the fear." After the surgeon removed the cancer, I hugged them and said, "I have to thank you. You removed her cancer, but also made my anxiety go away." I've never had anxiety since.

ANNIVERSARY REACTIONS

Anniversaries can be times of pain or joy and sometimes an inexplicable mix of both. There are different anniversaries for everyone: for some it is the date of diagnosis, while for others it is the last day of treatment. Some survivors celebrate the 5-year remission date. Whether or not any of these anniversary dates are *marked*, they are likely to touch off some kind of emotional reaction—and this is normal. One mother of a teen with cancer said, "I think that whenever we touch the same place in the circle of the year, we stop and look around us to see the different shapes and colors of reality. And it often takes our breath away."

For families of survivors with few or no long-term effects from their treatment for cancer, anniversaries are sometimes forgotten or sometimes celebrated. Some families file the memories away and skip rituals that tie them to the memories of hard times. Others remember and give thanks for their life and good health.

Families of survivors with numerous or serious late effects from treatment may have more evident daily reminders of their anniversaries. They often struggle with the urge to be grateful for life while simultaneously grieving the many losses. Sometimes it is not a specific date, but an entire month or season that is fraught with significance.

Cancer affects everyone in the family—often in different ways. It helps if family members share their feelings so they can create their own rituals to cope with or celebrate anniversaries. And each family should decide for itself when it is time to continue the tradition or let it fade into the past.

Typically, I use anniversaries as a time for reflection. My date of diagnosis is a time when I think of my struggles, but also remember the people whom I have met and would not have gotten to know without cancer – doctors, nurses, social workers, friends, and so many others who have been integral to my journey. On my cancer-free anniversary, I often think remember the friends I made in treatment who have passed away. This fills me with an overwhelming sense of sadness, but also gratitude that I had the opportunity to know them. I will carry their memories with me throughout the rest of my life.

Anniversaries are a hard thing for me, especially my diagnosis date. Each one is a reminder of how thankful I am to still be alive, but it is also a reminder of how much pain I've gone through. Around these times, I tend to remember all the sadness, anxiety, and fear I originally experienced. I often feel like I almost relive certain memories as time goes on when anniversaries come around. While I feel blessed to be where I am today, sometimes it feels like a curse, as well.

The diagnosis anniversary is very difficult, even 6 years later. I don't get more anxious but I just want to crawl in bed and lie

there for days that time of year. We have started trying to re-
frame the day. Instead of thinking of it as the worst day of our
lives, we are trying to think of it as the day that our daughter's
life was saved. We try to focus on the gratitude and usually get
a cake to "celebrate."

GRIEF AND LOSS

Although survivors were able to grab the ultimate *gold ring*—life—
they often suffer losses in the process. Losses come in all shapes and
forms and may emerge or continue to exist for many years or even
a lifetime. A universal loss is the sense that the world is a safe place.
Childhood cancer robs the entire family of that blissful belief in the
natural order of things—that children will have happy and carefree
childhoods and that children never die before their parents.

Treatment for childhood cancer also can result in the loss of abilities,
life prospects, skills, or body parts. A star baseball player can be rele-
gated to the bench. A skier might lose his leg. An "A" student might
discover when she returns to school that she is no longer gifted in
mathematics. And grief over the loss of normal developmental opportunities, such as missing the time when teens start to date or play
competitive sports on organized teams, are common. These losses put
survivors out of step with their peer groups, which in turn limits opportunities to develop friendships. Thus, survivors must cope not only
with physical changes but also with the alteration of their self-image.

The feelings most often associated with the normal grieving process are
denial, anxiety, fear, guilt, depression, and anger. These completely normal feelings are sometimes viewed by others as a problem when they are
actually a natural response to a life-changing event. It is important and
necessary to acknowledge these feelings in order to deal with what cannot be changed and to make the most of your life, even if it has changed.

Part of coping with grief involves sharing it with loved ones. In our
society, expressing these feelings is often socially unacceptable. Sur-

The biggest loss I think I experienced is what could have been. I'll never know what my life would have been like if I'd never been sick - maybe I'd be athletic, or taller, or more popular, or maybe my friends and interests would have been completely different. Because I got sick so young, I'll never know how much of my sense of self was formed by this experience. I feel like there is a whole different me that the world will never know, and it feels weird to grieve for a fake me when I have real friends who died, but I think about that a lot.

After my arm surgery, I remember thinking about how I would've continued on with the swim team if I hadn't had these problems. I tried joining after everything, and it just didn't work. Maybe I gave up too soon, but it just didn't feel right anymore. That was hard. I definitely lost a sense of who I was in that way because I had so many dreams to pursue. I tried going back to baton, as well and that didn't work. I felt a sense of uselessness because I wanted badly to fit in and be a part of a team. In the long run, I'm thankful for it because it clearly wasn't the path God had for me. And at my age now, it doesn't matter if I was on a sports team or that I didn't thrive in school. I wasn't included unless it was out of pity because I was sick. I just never felt like I belonged. I stuck to myself and a couple of my friends at the time and went on with life. I don't know what I would've done without those friends. It really makes you think about what is important, like having good friends and my family. There is grief over the life I could've had, but also gratitude for the life I have now.

We met many families whose children are no longer with us. It's terribly heartbreaking, and sometimes I do feel guilt, which contributes to my anxiety that something bad is still going to happen. Years ago, I read a poem called *On Children*, by Kahlil Gibran which describes that our children are really just on loan to us for a period of time. When I read that poem now, it always makes me feel better.

I definitely have felt grief in the sense that I miss so deeply who I was before cancer. I feel like who I am today and who I was before are two completely different people. I am missing my hair, missing my good health, missing how carefree I was, and missing my independence.

vivors and parents struggle to balance gratitude for life with sadness over the losses. However, parents and survivors may not view these issues in the same way, and conflicts may arise, creating an inability to rely on each other for support.

There is a need to educate relatives, friends, and professionals who work with families of people who have survived childhood cancer to enable recognition that grief over loss is very similar to the grief one feels when a loved one dies. Listening, understanding, and supporting the legitimacy of these feelings can be very powerful for the survivor and also help support the integrity of the relationship with the survivor. Suffering is diminished when it is shared. Siblings of survivors can experience negative long-term emotional effects and may need support and counseling (see details in *Relationship with Siblings* in *Chapter 3, Relationships*).

Parents of children who were treated at a very young age often have grief about things of which their children may not even be aware. In some cases, radiation at a young age can cause a change in personality and capabilities, so it may seem as if the child you knew and loved disappeared, and a new child replaced them.

You may find that at different ages, you view and feel your losses differently. A child of 10 may understand that his learning disabilities were the price he paid for cure from cancer, but a 20-year-old in college will probably have very different feelings as he is making career choices that may be affected by his disabilities. Similarly, a teenage girl may view potential infertility differently than an adult woman in love who is discussing marriage and contemplating having a family.

You can grieve fully, but later, still be stunned on occasion by a wave of grief. Everyone gets blindsided by a reminder of the loss. Stressors that can cause feelings to erupt include anniversaries, routine medical tests, or even a smell. Returning to the clinic for an appointment, developing an illness, or discovering a late effect can arouse strong feelings. The upsurge of physical or emotional responses doesn't mean you have to go through the whole process again, but it can feel overwhelming.

Survivors and their families describe a multitude of ways to work through the grief associated with childhood cancer. Some talk with family members and friends; others share their emotions by asking for hugs or a shoulder to cry on. Some join support groups (in person or online) to talk about their feelings with others in similar circumstances. Others prefer individual, private counseling to discuss their grief and feelings of loss. Some survivors describe taking better care of themselves or doing pleasurable activities whenever they felt sad about the changes in their lives. Others talk about the importance of their faith or religion in getting them through the tough spots. You can also ask loved ones for help during difficult times.

ANGER

In addition to the emotional reactions already discussed, many survivors and their families experience feelings of anger in the years after treatment ends. It is not unusual for survivors or family members to feel robbed of a "normal" life when they experience reminders of the costs of cancer and treatment.

Adolescents who are just beginning to understand the ramifications of physical differences, for example, might feel anger that waxes and wanes as they deal with questions like: "Why did this happen to me?" "When will I just be a normal kid?" "What do you mean this won't ever really be over with?" Parents, too, might feel bursts of anger as they watch their children continue to struggle with late effects of treatment. One father disclosed, for example, that even 20 years after his daughter's successful treatment for a brain tumor, he has weeks when he is incredibly angry that the possibility of independent living has been stolen from her, and that he must continue to worry about who will provide for his child when he is no longer able to do so.

It is important to keep in mind that feeling angry is a normal, healthy reaction to the losses caused by cancer. Survivors and their loved ones

I think I'm angry more often than I realize. I've lost friends, lost experiences, lost abilities, and lost time that I'll never get back. I didn't do anything to deserve my cancer, but I still have to deal with the consequences. I also don't like the idea that childhood cancer survivors should be grateful to be alive. I'm obviously grateful to the doctors and nurses and community members who supported me, but I'm not grateful to the universe for the fact that I survived. The universe dealt me a blow and I'm still standing, but I'm not going to thank it for that. All of that being said, I think it is useful to channel that anger into something more productive. I like to use the emotion I feel to support other causes, because the anger turns into drive and spurs me into action.

Anger has been a strange thing for me since being diagnosed. To this day, I am still angry that this happened to me, but I also feel guilty being angry because I often compare my journey to that of others who might have had it worse. It's an internal battle most days, going between feeling angry and feeling like I shouldn't feel that way because I am alive and doing fairly well since being diagnosed.

Survivors do experience anger and frustration but one must find ways to deal with it. I was constantly irritable because I had a newborn while navigating my 2-year-old through cancer treatment and surgery. I worked very hard not to take it out on hospital staff who were working their hardest to save my daughter's life. To this day, I still feel anger and frustration but as time passes, I am learning to let go and replace it with gratitude for her life and the people who made my days a little brighter during that very dark time period.

I didn't feel angry about cancer until I was older, reflecting on my childhood and realizing I had mostly memories of hospitals, tubes, and medicine. Knowing that it affected my siblings so much was hard too, realizing that none of us had normal childhoods.

As a parent, I really struggle with anger. I am angry at what cancer has done to my child. I even experience bitterness and feelings of resentment towards friends and family who have *"normal"* healthy children. My daughter was only 6 when she was diagnosed. She is now 12 and doesn't really remember much about what life was like for her before cancer. I wouldn't say she struggles with anger about having cancer per say, but one of the long-term effects of treatment is she has huge, angry outbursts over any variety of things. We never know what will set it off.

may feel bursts of anger at times when life changes or developmental demands remind them of the things lost to cancer. Anger may be present at one year or 20 years post-treatment. These feelings may occur alongside other feelings or in isolation. Survivors and their loved ones may even express anger, through behavior such as tantrums or angry, destructive actions.

When these angry periods come up, it may be useful for survivors and loved ones to recognize them for what they are—normal reactions to an unusual life situation——and to share the feelings of anger with supportive friends and family or psychosocial professionals (i.e., therapists, psychologists, etc.). If angry feelings or behaviors get in the way of everyday life or affect relationships, survivors and their loved ones could consider seeking additional support from a mental health professional, support group, nurse, nurse practitioner, or physician. Survivors and their family members have reported that once they feel supported in putting cancer and its inevitable effects in their place, they are able to more comfortably manage the anger without letting it derail them.

WORRY, SADNESS, AND DEPRESSION

Worry and sadness can be seen as two sides of the same coin. For many survivors, worry is fear related to losses that may occur in the future, while sadness is related to losses that occurred in the past. Both of these emotions are a normal part of anyone's life but both can become troublesome for survivors. In the case of worry, survivors can become focused on fear of a relapse or fear of late effects. If the worry grows too large, it may compromise a survivor's ability to seek appropriate healthcare. In essence, the survivor becomes afraid of knowing. Sometimes survivors become embarrassed or ashamed of their concerns about their health and body. After all, young adults aren't generally worried about things such as cancer relapse or heart problems. Routine health concerns for survivors make them out of step with their peers, potentially causing negative self-directed feelings.

Some survivors worry that they are hypochondriacs—that they are overly concerned about their health. They become fearful that their doctors will view them as complainers or find their health worries crazy. This may interfere with getting good, thorough follow-up care. Survivors who feel extreme worry may benefit from seeking help from a professional. There are many ways to reduce worry and not allow it to overwhelm your life.

Depression is distinguished from the normal sadness about the real losses that can occur from treatment. Sadness can arise from temporary losses (e.g., loss of hair) or permanent losses (e.g., loss of fertility or mobility). Depression takes over normal sadness when a survivor is only able to focus on losses and can no longer find any pleasure in life. It may become crippling and prevent the survivor from seeking and getting appropriate care and from enjoying the positive aspects of life. Survivors struggling with depression should consider seeking help with a mental health professional.

When people are profoundly depressed, they may feel life is not worth living, or that they are not worthy of care and help. They often lack the energy to participate in activities that used to interest them and they may withdraw from important relationships and social interactions. These feelings make it especially hard for them to get the help they need, both physically and emotionally. No one should have to suffer alone through depression; it can be successfully treated with counseling and/or medications.

I have been diagnosed with and treated for both anxiety and depression. My anxiety and depression have been daily issues for me. In many ways they are bigger problems than my physical side effects have been, as they impact my everyday life more evidently. For example, my cardiac health doesn't really affect how I interact with other people, but my anxiety can make it very hard for me to branch out and feel comfortable doing something different or making new friends. In that way, my anxiety and depression have been the hardest side effects for me to manage and control.

(Continued)

(*Continued*)

My family has been incredibly supportive and proactive about getting me help - I was seeing therapists within two years after ending treatment. I have gone to in-person therapists (including talk therapy, play therapy, and cognitive behavioral therapy) and I have seen psychologists and psychiatrists who have prescribed anti-anxiety and antidepressant medications. I've never done any support groups or online therapy.

During treatment, feelings of anxiety and depression were definitely present, but most of my focus and that of my family and care team was centered on getting better physically. It's worth noting that when I was undergoing treatment, the emotional toll of cancer on long-term mental health was poorly understood. After treatment, I think I expected those emotions to go away, and viewed the anxiety/worry as just a temporary result of what was happening at the time, but this was far from the truth.

My undiagnosed anxiety and depression persisted and intensified when I got to high school. That's when I made the decision to start seeking help regularly from a therapist. I was lucky to have friends that were very supportive, but in the beginning, it was very challenging to rationalize to my parents. Their generation feels a huge negative stigma around receiving therapy and medication for mental illness, and frankly the stigma was still quite strong at the time I sought help. They could not understand why an otherwise healthy and thriving teen girl would need to seek help in this way.

Now as a 26-year-old, I still regularly talk to my therapist and take prescribed medication for my anxiety and depression. Although a constant work-in-progress, I have made great improvements to my mental health and well-being. I now have the professional and personal support I need to continue this progress and to lean on if/when things get more severe. My parents, too, have made great strides in their respect and understanding of mental illness and are great supporters of the work I continue to do on my mental health.

Throughout my whole life I have struggled with anxiety and depression, both of which I feel have gotten harder to deal with since having cancer. I have put in a lot of hard work with different kinds of therapists to try and seek better ways to cope with anxiety and depression. Still, sometimes it's hard to cope by yourself, and I often look to my friends as a support.

Both times transitioning out of treatment, I felt a huge sense of relief, especially with our second during COVID policies where my children couldn't see each other the majority of a year. Each transition took about a year to begin to feel human again, have a sense of routine, normalcy as much as possible, and less full-blown anxiety. The second time I actually utilized anti-anxiety medication which helped a lot. It's hard not to assume the worst in any scenario, but I really tried to focus on "normalcy" and not hover over the kids or keep them from risky play that is a normal part of childhood.

Now as a Mom, I have an intense amount of anxiety about my little boy. When he gets bruises and even when he had the little "toddler tummy" my mind went to directly to negative thinking. It's a lot to deal with but it is bearable. What helps is talking about it with others that understand. Giving myself grace and allowing myself to feel the things I feel. And knowing that others that haven't been there, won't understand and that's okay. It doesn't mean I'm alone.

SURVIVOR GUILT

Some survivors feel guilty that they survived when so many others did not. Survivors who experience many late effects or have other disabilities or limitations feel guilty about how this creates a burden for family/friends they love. Some feel life is going to be short, so they must push themselves very hard. Because they feel they don't have much time, they want to squeeze in as much as possible. Some families have genetic forms of cancer passed from parent to child through inherited genes. Some of these parents feel very guilty that their genes are the cause of their child developing cancer. All of these negative feelings are referred to as *survivor guilt*.

Another variation on *survivor guilt* is that some survivors are burdened by what feels like extra-high expectations about what they will do with their lives and what they will achieve. They have the sense that they are expected to do more than the average person because they survived cancer. And they may feel guilty about just wanting to be themselves without the added weight of super-size expectations.

I have definitely dealt with survivor's guilt. I remember sending a wedding invitation to the mom of a friend that had passed away, and she said it would be too hard for her. I sobbed. I felt so awful. It was horrible. I can only imagine the pain she was feeling watching me live out a life her daughter should have. I try to remind myself that they would want me to live my life in the best way I can. And I try to, for them.

I have had some survivor's guilt. For me, the most upsetting thing has been feeling like I have to earn the fact that I survived. I sometimes feel like because I survived when others didn't, I have to do something worthwhile and big with my life, and that's a lot of pressure for a child/young adult to have while growing up.

I do have survivor's guilt. I saw children who were not even six years old die from the same cancer I had, yet I survived. It doesn't feel right. Because of that, I try to squeeze everything I can out of life so I can live with no regrets. Surviving resonates with me – I believe I'm here for a reason, and I will not throw away my shot.

Survivor's guilt is something I am incredibly familiar with. I have been dealing with it since I lost my best friend in treatment in third grade. First, I was overcome with sadness because I was unable to play with my friend anymore. But this sadness quickly turned to guilt, thinking, "What gives me the right to still be here while he couldn't be?" This feeling only intensified as I lost more and more friends throughout my life.

My biggest challenge dealing with survivor's guilt is the burden of high expectations. In my eyes, I consistently compare myself with what my friends would be doing if they were here. I feel responsible for carrying out their dreams, simply because I am here, and they are not. For example, my one friend was very into sports and wanted to play in college, so I joined my university's basketball team as a student manager. I joined a fraternity because my other friend always talked about doing that. Additionally, my school had an organization dedicated to childhood cancer research. Although I was personally helped by this organization, it was my friend's absolute dream to volunteer and be a leader, so that is exactly what I did. All of these experiences were integral to my college experience, but I joined them to have the experience that my friends couldn't. It allowed me to stay connected to them. With that being said, it can be incredibly taxing and unfair to compare yourself and your life to others, especially when doing things you may feel obligated to do. I finally realized my friends would not want me struggling like I have.

In order to combat this guilt, I spend the first and last five minutes of everyday reflecting on my friendships with those who have been lost. That way, I'm able to keep them front of mind, but I am not overwhelmed with grief throughout the course of the day. Since I have started doing these reflections, my mental health has greatly improved and the constant guilt I felt has mostly subsided. It is still there, but much more manageable.

This cancer journey is life-changing. I don't take one day for granted and thank God every time we wake up as a complete family. We went through it twice with two of our children. There is some survivors guilt that I carry. It is hard knowing so many families who lost children while both of ours survived. Each has different ongoing and unique struggles; one with intellectual struggles and the other wears hearing aids and has other physical setbacks. My advice is to take each challenge as it comes, try to acknowledge "survivor problems" for what they are, but always remember how far you've come."

COMPLICATED EMOTIONS AFTER TREATMENT ENDS

During treatment, patients are engaged in an arduous battle against their cancer. They direct all of their time, energy, and strength toward dealing with immediate survival. But when the treatments stop, the drugs aren't necessary, and the scars heal, many survivors come to realize there is also an emotional price to pay and that being free of cancer does not mean their emotions are cancer-free.

Some survivors and their parents are able to set their feelings aside during treatment, but are left to come to grips with the experience and what it means in life when treatment ends. That process can be very difficult. Family, friends, and doctors may brush off concerns, saying it's time to "get on with your life." Ignoring the feelings is unlikely to cause them to disappear. Unresolved emotions usually don't just vanish—they may even grow stronger and surface unexpectedly.

After people experience a traumatic event, they may have symptoms of anxiety that persist over time. Just like soldiers returning from combat, survivors of childhood cancer and family members may experience symptoms of *post-traumatic stress*.

Post traumatic stress syndrome (PTS)

Some of the most common symptoms are:

- Avoiding people, places, and thoughts that remind you of treatment
- Being hypervigilant (feeling constantly "on alert")
- Difficulty falling or staying asleep

Other symptoms include irritability or angry outbursts, difficulty concentrating, or having an exaggerated startle response. Some people tend to have intrusive recollections or dreams of the event, or feelings that the trauma is recurring (flashbacks). Survivors and their family members may have only some of these symptoms or they may have enough symptoms to meet criteria for a diagnosis of *post-traumatic stress disorder (PTSD)*. Rates of PTSD among survivors and their parents are generally low, but many survivors and their parents have some symptoms of post-traumatic stress (Cook JL, 2021 and Tremolada M, 2016). The good news is that treatments are available to help people recover from PTSD or manage post-traumatic stress symptoms.

I was diagnosed with PTSD several years ago. I have a terrible startle response and lots of recurring memories. I always hated when my kids would ride in cars with other people, and I have lots of anxiety now that they drive. However, I made a decision that I would not keep them from doing these things because of my fears. That would be so unfair. I think it may always be with me, but it does not keep me from living my life, nor would I consider it debilitating. You have to keep putting one foot in front of the other for your children. As a parent, you don't have the luxury of indulging your pain all the time, nor would it be good for you.

I have far more anxiety than I think I ever would have had. Mainly I worry about the death of one of my children. I have never been able to find any therapist that has a background to deal with this, although I know they exist. Family and friends are supportive, but this experience is so unique that it is often hard to share. I have not engaged in support groups, etc., because it is also hard to relive that trauma and it is just not something I would be comfortable doing in a group setting.

It has impacted where I choose to work, what I watch for in my own child, and how I react to certain situations. It's definitely life-changing. PTSD is real and extremely hard. I have the weirdest triggers. Getting in the car before 8 am, feeling sick if I eat when I first wake up (I was NPO [nothing-by-mouth] a lot so I think it stems from this), the smell of the hospital and the sound of IV pumps and hand sanitizer are all things that trigger me. The smell of the soap my mom used to use in the hospital makes me physically want to be sick. Just the thought of having to be admitted in the hospital sends me into a panic. I don't like the thought of being trapped there. I sobbed the last day we were in the hospital with my son after we had him. I wanted out and I wanted out right then. The poor nurse came to do an echocardiogram on me, and I think I scared her. I was so over that place.

PTSD has played a big role in my life since diagnosis. Cancer is a scary thing. During treatment, there are very many unknowns and a lot of things that can go wrong. Unfortunately, I experienced many times when I thought it would be the end for me.

(Continued)

(*Continued*)

After I finished treatment, I noticed myself having extreme flashbacks to those times, along with other symptoms. PTSD has impacted many parts of my life and is something I actively try to work on and cope with.

I have not officially been diagnosed with PTSD, but I do have many of the symptoms. I have long-term anxiety (often in the form of repetitive, intrusive thoughts), anger/a quick temper, ADHD/concentration issues, etc. These symptoms are treated alongside my anxiety and depression, though my doctors are aware of my history and could be taking the possibility of PTSD into account when treating me.

NETWORKING FOR SUPPORT

Peer support networks can help survivors regain control of some aspects of their lives, learn how others have coped with similar problems, and share feelings. Exchanging information, experiences, and thoughts with others who have similar life experiences may help forge close ties. Even survivors with close families and friendships often seek out peer support.

The sense of community can help dispel the isolation felt by too many survivors. Support can profoundly affect the way you view yourself and how you manage your life after cancer.

Networking for support can occur in many ways: talking with fellow survivors, attending survivor conferences and camps, joining a survivor support group, organizing or attending educational workshops, or participating in online discussion or support groups. Some survivors and family members have reported feeling so strongly about the lack of support in their lives that they volunteer with an existing group or organize their own group to address the needs of those treated for childhood cancer.

The need many survivors have for support from fellow survivors' changes over time. Some may embrace emotions head on, consider giving back to the community, and perhaps sense the need to move on.

As a child, I attended Camp Can Do (a camp for kids with cancer) for nine years, and have been a staff member for five years. I met a lot of campers who were actively going through treatment, and not all of these campers made it. When I was younger, these campers were my friends. Nowadays, these are the campers that I am responsible for. It is always difficult to lose a friend or a camper you have gotten to know. I have found it to be very important to lean on your support system when this happens. There are plenty of people, including campers, staff members, friends, and family, who are dealing with these same losses. Talking with others and keeping their memory alive is the most important thing. It has allowed me to work through my grief.

I learned just how deeply people can care for one another. We had and still have so much support from the people around us: family, friends, neighbors, the towns where she grew up, our church, and more. The way that people showed up for us shaped me for the better. It also taught me how to be there and support others who are going through a hard time.

We met so many great families at Ronald McDonald House and at the hospitals who were going through the exact same thing we were. We would talk, ask questions, compare experiences, and look forward to seeing each other at our next visits. We still keep in touch with some of these connections!

My family is my biggest support network. I didn't have many survivor friends growing up, but made a friend when I got to college who was also an ALL survivor. It was one of the first times in my life I met someone like me, and we spent a lot of time discussing our cancer journeys. She had gone to a survivorship camp and had a lot more friends to talk about everything with. Now that I am working at a childhood cancer foundation, I've met a lot more people with similar experiences. It is so important to connect with other survivors.

I did try therapy with a few people! The therapist I really liked was only offered through the college I attended, so after graduation I could no longer use that resource. I tried a few others, but they just did not fit. I felt like they were trying to fix me, but

(Continued)

my experience is not just something you can fix. My friends and family are extremely supportive and try so hard to understand, but they can't. Knowing they still try is comforting, though. I have a friend I met at the children's hospital through treatment that I talk to almost every week. That friendship has been a huge blessing for us both.

Online support groups

Online support groups often offer a unique type of support for survivors, their parents, and family members. Any time of the day, support is just a keystroke away on a multitude of social media sites. There are multiple moderated groups and spaces available where survivors and parents can connect with others who may be enduring similar challenges. Thousands of survivors and their family members use these mechanisms to connect with others around the world traveling a similar emotional path. Discussing concerns, fears, and triumphs may help make sense of what has happened to them, heal, and move on with their lives. Support groups for parents are widely used.

A word of caution: if medical information is shared in support groups—in person or online—survivors and their caregivers should question the accuracy. Before acting on medical information obtained from a layperson, individuals should check with their healthcare provider.

I have felt it is pretty easy to network with other childhood cancer survivors. There are Facebook groups and online forums that are easily accessible. Additionally, the network I have from knowing people through treatment has been extraordinarily steady, and the people I have forged a bond with are some of my best friends today.

Staying involved in things like camps for kids with cancer or other events where I can help as a survivor has led me to some incredible people who have made an impact on my life. From my experience, this brotherhood/sisterhood of survivors is a strong one, and the support system is truly second to none.

EMOTIONAL EXPRESSION AND HEALTH

Emotions—of all kinds—are inevitably part of experiencing cancer, its treatment, and survivorship. Being able to recognize feelings and find healthy ways of expressing, channeling, and learning from them are keys to creating a balanced life. Not having tools for managing emotions can make life more difficult.

Research has shown that survivors with high levels of psychological distress are more likely to engage in risky health behaviors such as substance use and abuse (Ji X, 2021 and De R, 2020). Unhealthy habits may complicate and worsen late effects from cancer treatment. So, in addition to the value of seeking support from healthcare professionals and networks of people with similar experiences, some other available tools for dealing with strong emotions include blogging or journaling, physical activity, meditation, and yoga, among others. Chapter 5, *Staying Healthy*, includes more information about this topic.

All of our family receives professional help to deal with our daughter's cancer journey. There is no shame in discussing our experiences with an outside party. Our daughter has many mental health issues due to her cancer diagnosis and treatment. Some of these include anxiety, fears, big emotions, and reverting back to immature behaviors similar to those of a toddler.

I think about my daughter's time in treatment all the time. Things that happen change you as a person and you live with that. Seeing your child suffer continuously, come close to the brink of death, and then survive has a profound impact on your emotions. At least for me, the hurt and pain of that time does not leave you, although things do get better. When you run on adrenaline, lack of sleep, poor eating habits, and caring for another child, you do experience PTSD. Even once treatment is complete, the fear and anxiety each time your child has tests or scans can be debilitating. The silver lining of that time in my life is that you get to see the good in people, in medical professionals, and in your community.

FUTURE PLANNING

Cancer treatment forces many youths and their families to drop future plans to focus on surviving the present. When treatment ends, an adjustment in mindset occurs. Some survivors resume working toward pre-cancer goals—athletics, studies, relationships. Others find that they avoid thinking about the future because expectations of a long, healthy life have been changed by cancer. Commitment to a relationship or a long-term goal may be difficult. Thinking about having children may be complicated. Previously-mentioned resources such as support groups or counseling with mental health professionals may support future-planning efforts. Sometimes survivors alter their life plans because cognitive or physical disabilities limit future possibilities. It may be difficult for survivors, their families, and friends to accept that the price they paid for life has irrevocably changed the future.

In contrast, sometimes the cancer experience opens up new visions of the future. For example, cancer often gives children or teens their first glimpse of the medical world. Exposure to the helping professions and the medical world sometimes sparks an interest that blossoms into a career.

My treatment ended right before I applied to colleges. After I was diagnosed and met the other patients at the hospital, I was inspired to go into immunology and choose a major that would put me on a life path that would enable me to give back to the cancer community. Instead of learning about astrophysics in my free time, I started watching videos on microbiology. The doctors recommended taking a gap year and stopping soccer for a year, but I was really stubborn back then, and continued everything. Surviving cancer has given me a sense of purpose, a goal of giving back to the community that supported me, and helped me appreciate the special people in my life.

Being a childhood cancer survivor comes with a lot of responsibility. Like it or not, we are the ones looked up to by the children currently going through treatment. This can absolutely be daunting, stressful, and quite overwhelming. It is a duty that you may not have signed up for. However, it can be an exceptional blessing. Looking back to my own treatment, I was constantly being inspired by the survivors I met. It allowed me to visualize myself as a survivor someday too and gave me encouragement that helped me push through to the finish line. These were people who could relate to what I was going through.

Since being pronounced cancer-free, I have had wonderful opportunities to give back to organizations that helped me throughout my treatment. This has truly been life-changing for me. Getting to meet current childhood cancer patients has allowed me to fully embrace that responsibility of helping children the way I was helped as a child. If I could give one piece of advice, it would be to look into ways to give back. It can make such an incredible impact on not only your life, but the lives of so many children as well.

BREAKS IN THE CLOUD: POSITIVE IMPACTS

Many studies of the effects of the cancer experience on survivors have focused on negative effects. However, the positive impacts are also routinely recognized by survivors and their caregivers. Many survivors and their families eventually find great meaning from their suffering. Often, survivors and families discuss in reassuring and hopeful terms a renewed appreciation for life and an awareness of the value of each day.

While mom says initially there is no silver lining, one positive that came out of our experience is all the amazing people, organizations and charities whom are all truly selfless and go to great lengths to help and care for people they've never even met! We are a family with ties stronger than steel. Our experiences have been exponentially trying and have only made our ties stronger.

Making friends that understand the unique experience of childhood cancer has been the highlight. During our daughter's

(Continued)

treatment before COVID, we connected with a lot more people, but even after COVID-policy restrictions, passing in the halls, we would swap numbers with families and made sure to give words of hope and encouragement to each other where possible.

I think the journey was what taught me about faith and trust in God. The journey still affects me daily, mentally, physically, and emotionally. I have anxiety, depression and PTSD. I have long term effects from chemotherapy and surgeries. But it was all worth it to be where I am now. I am so thankful to have the opportunity to live a life, so many didn't.

It's so hard to know what to tell other survivors, because each one is so unique. But I guess my broad statement would just be that giving up and quitting is not an option. Staying positive is so important. Don't compare yourself to others and remember that you are worth every second of the fight.

I grew up knowing how hard things could be and how bad I could feel. It made me very grateful for life and helped me understand my own place in the world at a young age. It gave me great empathy for others and helped me to keep moving forward, because that's the only option you have.

I believe navigating my daughter through her cancer and treatment made me a better person --- a more compassionate, loving person, yet also a "harder core" person, if that makes sense. Not much makes me cry and small things no longer bother me. I feel incredibly lucky and blessed to be a mother. I possess strength and resilience that I never had before. I never knew I had the strength in me to do this. I was seven months pregnant with my son when my daughter got sick. Shortly before her diagnosis, I had a dream that I was crawling on my stomach in some type of hardcore military drill. Anyway, it felt impossible to me, and I recall deciding that I wanted to quit I remember thinking "there is always an out to this type of activity," and knowing that I would end it. When I attempted to get out, however, I learned that there WAS no way out. I think that dream was preparing me for what was to come, and sending me a message that I would be able to survive it. I remember feeling that this was one of the few times in my life where I had literally had NO choice.

REFERENCES

Cook JL, Russell K, Long A, Phipps S. (2021) Centrality of the childhood cancer experience and its relation to post-traumatic stress and growth. Psycho-oncology. 2021 Apr;30(4):564-570. doi: 10.1002/pon.5603. Epub 2020 Dec 15. PMID: 33232545; PMCID: PMC9125987.

De R, Zabih V, Kurdyak P, et al. (2020) Psychiatric Disorders in Adolescent and Young Adult-Onset Cancer Survivors: A Systematic Review and Meta-Analysis. *J Adolesc Young Adult Oncol.* 2020;9(1):12–22. DOI: 10.1089/jayao.2019.0097.correx. PM-CID: **PMC7313201**. PMID: 32379518

Ji X, Cummings JR, Mertens AC, et al. (2021) Substance use, substance use disorders, and treatment in adolescent and young adult cancer survivors-Results from a national survey. Cancer. 2021 Sep 1;127(17):3223-3231. doi: 10.1002/cncr.33634. Epub 2021 May 11. PMID: 33974717.

Tremolada M, Bonichini S, Basso G et al. (2016) Post-traumatic stress symptoms and post-traumatic growth in 223 childhood cancer survivors: Predictive risk factors. *Frontiers in psychology 7*. Feb 2016, DOI:10.3389/fpsyg.2016.00287

RESOURCES

Website: ccgresources.org

All resources and references mentioned in this book are available on the website and will be routinely reviewed and updated.

Children's Oncology Group (V6, Oct 2023). *Long-Term Follow-Up Guidelines for Survivors of Childhood, Adolescent, and Young Adult Cancers.*
Website: www.survivorshipguidelines.org
Healthlink: *Mental health*

American Childhood Cancer Organization (ACCO)
Website: www.acco.org
ACCO provides support, education, and advocacy for children and adolescents with cancer, survivors of childhood/adolescent cancer, their families and the professionals who care for them.
P.O. Box 498, Kensington MD 20895

Cancer Care
Website: www.cancercare.org
A nonprofit organization that provides a variety of services, including counseling, education, referrals, publications, and financial assistance.
275 Seventh Ave, New York, NY 10001
(800) 813-HOPE or (800) 813-4673

Chai Lifeline

Website: www.chailifeline.org

A non-profit organization with the mission of providing critical support to children and families around the world who are impacted by serious illness, crises, and loss.

151 W. 30th St., New York, NY 10001

Phone: (212)465-1300

Camp Simcha

Website: www.campsimcha.org

Special summer camps for children with cancer, other blood disorders, and chronic illness.

Family Voices

Website: www.familyvoices.org

National organization and grassroots network of families and friends of children and youth with special health care needs and disabilities that promote partnership with families, including those of cultural, linguistic and geographic diversity in order to improve healthcare services and policies for children.

561 Virginia Road, Bldg 4, Suite 300. Concord, MA 01742

Phone: (888) 835-5569

Momcology®

Website: https://momcology.org/

National community-based patient advocacy and support organization founded in 2011 by mothers of children with cancer.

Passport for Care, Survivor Care Plans by Children's Oncology Group (V6, Nov 2023)

Website: https://cancersurvivor.passportforcare.org

Survivors and family can find online updated tailored long-term care plans which should be reviewed with their oncologist or health care provider.

Ulman Cancer Foundation

Website: https://ulmanfoundation.org

UCF supports, educates, connects, and empowers young adult cancer survivors. It raises awareness of young adult cancer issues and helps ensure all young survivors and their families have a voice and the resources necessary to thrive.

Ulman House, 2118 E. Madison Street, Baltimore MD

Phone: (410) 914-0202

GLOSSARY

anxiety, a normal human reaction to stressful situations when one feels nervous, has worried thoughts and/or feelings of dread, and some physical changes like heart pounding or sweating. Anxiety usually is temporary and ends when the stressful situation is over. But for some, anxiety can persist and can even get worse over time. If anxiety persists and begins to interfere with school, work, and social situations, one should seek help from a healthcare professional or psychologist. There are effective treatments for persistent anxiety.

depression, a profound and prolonged feeling of sadness and lack of energy that prevents one from seeking appropriate care and engaging in activities of daily life and enjoyment from once pleasurable experiences

post-traumatic stress disorder (PTSD), a disorder that develops in some people who have experienced a shocking, scary, or dangerous event that disrupts their life and emotions (fear, anxiety, depression); people may experience a range of reactions after trauma, and most people recover from initial symptoms over time. Those who continue to experience problems may be diagnosed with PTSD.

psychologist, a trained mental health professional who helps people learn healthy ways to handle mental health challenges. They can help people living with specific conditions, like depression or anxiety, or those who are going through a tough time in life, like grieving the loss of a loved one

survivor guilt, feeling guilty or shame over surviving cancer while others have lost their lives; and having the feeling of pressure to accomplish or excel in life since they have been given the gift of life; feeling guilty because they just want to live an ordinary normal life

3
Relationships

MATTHEW C. HOCKING, PhD

Love looks not with the eyes, but with the mind.
– *Shakespeare, A Midsummer Night's Dream*

A DIAGNOSIS OF CHILDHOOD cancer can involve tumultuous changes in relationships. Every survivor has stories to tell of lost or strained friendships and altered relationships with family members. Yet we are social creatures, reliant on a web of love and support from family, friends, and neighbors.

Cancer is a life-changing experience, and family dynamics inevitably shift during and after treatment. This chapter begins with a discussion about survivors' relationships with their loved ones. It then covers lost friendships, how survivors make and keep new friends, and romantic relationships. Dating opens up new worlds and sometimes old wounds. Rejection due to health history or altered appearance can occur, but deeply satisfying romantic relationships can develop. This chapter also contains many stories of how and when survivors disclosed their medical history to friends and partners. Finally, the chapter looks at marriage, fertility, health of offspring, and adoption.

RELATIONSHIPS WITH PARENTS

Childhood cancer affects the entire family. At diagnosis, the family system undergoes intense stress and reorganization. Roles and responsibilities are adjusted as parents try to balance taking care of their ill child with the needs of the rest of the family. Major financial decisions often need to be made; one parent sometimes must take leave from or quit a job to help the child through treatment. Parents strain to find ways to support one another emotionally and manage their own strong feelings of fear and uncertainty.

Shifting roles

Interactions between parents and a child with cancer also dramatically shift. Family rules may change to adapt to behaviors caused by disease, medication, or emotional reactions. Parents need to become the medical overseers for their child—monitoring temperatures, side effects, and reactions to medication. Children often shift to spending more time with family members than with peers. When treatment ends, interaction patterns and roles among family members may have permanently shifted. While survivors and parents often report increased closeness as a result of the survivor's cancer and treatment, these changes may impact important developmental processes of the survivor.

> We ended up being really permissive parents during treatment. That was hard to shift from afterwards. I feel we have a closer bond with our children than some parents because of our cancer journey, since our care and time together was so much more intimate in many ways. Watching our children being so brave during treatments and dealing with adult situations, like intense medical treatments and the death of some friends, gave them a maturity that a lot of kids don't have. I respect them a lot as people and survivors, not just little kids.

> It was a little difficult to return to normal, but my family made it much easier. They threw a surprise end-of-treatment celebration with all my friends and extended family, and it was a truly touching and special event. I really felt loved. Moving past it, there were times when my family was a little overbearing because they were nervous about me. For example, I was not allowed to play football until a year or two after treatment, despite there not being a real reason to keep me from playing. Over time we were able to find a happy medium. My grandmother, the constant worrier and whom, I'd like to mention, I love very much, would fuss over me whenever I saw her, always worrying that

a speck of dust would bring the cancer back. It took a while for everyone to adjust, but after some time, things returned to "normal."

My parents were an incredible support system throughout my time with cancer. They juggled job responsibilities and caring for my brother, yet still managed to always have one or both of them in the hospital with me at all times. After treatment, their parental roles stayed relatively the same.

Cancer in adolescents may disrupt their normal developmental process of emerging autonomy. At a time when they are gradually withdrawing from the family and beginning to function independently, they suddenly become dependent upon medical personnel to save their lives and on their parents to provide emotional and physical care. This can add considerable stress to the already turbulent teen years. After treatment ends, some parents continue to feel protective and have difficulty when their children begin or resume their journey toward independence. Conversely, some teens may have difficulty initiating this process towards independence and may feel more inclined to stay near family.

Parents and their survivor children often have different views about how prominent a role the cancer experience should play in life after cancer treatment ends. Some surviving teens and young adults want to leave the cancer behind and get on with their lives. If their parents share this view, a smooth transition to adulthood can occur. If the parent has established deep ties in the cancer community, he or she may have difficulty accepting the child's decision to relegate the disease to the past. On the other hand, some parents want the child to pretend the cancer never happened or accept that it is over now and time to move on. Parents' long-term responses to their children's survival vary widely and can fluctuate over time.

In some cases, cancer results in disabilities that affect the survivor's ability to live independently. Some survivors are never able to live on their own, while others return intermittently to live with their parents for financial or health reasons. These situations create a tremendous challenge for the family. Parents need to adapt to having an adult child as a temporary or permanent resident in their home, as well as make arrangements for care when they are no longer able to provide it.

I grew up feeling very close to my mom after spending countless hours with her in hospitals and cars going back and forth to appointments. My sister told me she grew up feeling a lot closer to our dad, since our mom was not at home as much.

My mom and I were always really close. The one it really affected the most was my dad. My relationship with him changed --my cancer brought us closer. He gave me so much empathy and support where previously we didn't have that kind of relationship. I saw how hard it was for him to see me sick. It made me feel like "oh, maybe he does love me because this is making him sad." My mom did everything in her power to make me comfortable. If I was able to eat that week, she was making whatever I wanted. She provided constant support and helped me through it all.

My relationship with my parents was impacted for the better as a result of my battle with cancer. Spending that much time one-on-one with your parents or caregivers for such long stretches of time built a level of trust, love and honesty between us that I think few people are lucky enough to have. Making hard decisions together when I was young has allowed me to always be very honest with my parents, allowing us to maintain a strong and special relationship into adulthood.

We both had a lot of animosity about her experience, but were not good at expressing it. We would get in arguments, but eventually we realized that, yes, we were handed really crappy cards, but we still won the deck. It wasn't until recently that we worked through a lot of our issues. I was projecting on her that we did not or could not have certain things because she was sick, but that is not her fault. She was mad at me for being sick in the first place, but that is not my fault. My relationship with my youngest daughter was easier because we have never had any animosity toward each other. Our relationship revolved around going places and having fun together, whereas my time with my oldest daughter centered around all her medical appointments. They would both get annoyed when I brought up issues with the other at their doctor appointments. But the doctors needed to know our family's medical cancer history.

My relationship with my parents is very complex. Even though they are loving, we also fought a lot. Although I am now an adult, I feel like they are still very involved in my life. They say that they would like me to be more independent and live on my own, but they continue to try and have a say. I understand that it is because they feel protective and concerned, and a large part of me does not mind, but another part of me would like to be truly independent for the first time.

I was close to my parents before, but I was also only 11 at the time I was diagnosed. I think we are so close now because of my experience with cancer. I think they also became spiritual people because of it. I think they show emotions more than they did prior because they know how important this life that we've been given is. I truly don't know what I'd do without them.

Both times that our oldest daughter was diagnosed with cancer, my husband and I were on the same page, always loving and understanding toward one another. The experience of our young daughter surviving two childhood cancers strengthened our marriage. My husband had to bear the financial burden, and I took on the emotional burden. We understood the challenges of each other's responsibilities and were never angry with one another about it.

My mom took off work throughout my entire treatment. As we went through the treatment together, it gave me a deeper level of love and appreciation for her. There were good and bad days of treatment. One weekend when I stayed home, I felt really sick. My mom let me play FIFA with my brothers for hours upon hours. Usually, my mom would have wanted us to spend our time in more beneficial ways, but I know she adjusted the rules a bit depending on how treatment was going. If it was a good day, she would encourage me to do my homework while I felt

(Continued)

(Continued)

good, which helped me stayed on top of everything. Without her guidance, I don't know that I would be at UCLA. She was very good at understanding what I needed in the moment. I finished treatment at the end of my junior year.

Adult survivors sometimes revisit their cancer experience by asking their parents questions and soliciting their memories. This can be especially helpful if they experienced cancer at a very young age...some might have no memory at all. Such parent-survivor conversations may help survivors gain an understanding of the trauma from their parents' perspective. One method is to sit down together and compare recollections. Individual views of the same experience can be incredibly different. Another method to explore one's cancer memories and feelings about them is to join an online discussion group, chat room, or survivor support group.

RELATIONSHIPS WITH SIBLINGS

Siblings can be significantly affected by a childhood cancer diagnosis. The diagnosis, treatment, and aftermath can all create an array of conflicting feelings in siblings. Intermixed with the feelings of concern for their brother or sister are feelings of resentment and anger about how their family has been affected. They feel jealous of the gifts and attention showered on the sick child, yet feel guilty for having these emotions. Some siblings feel that the child or teen with cancer continues to consume most of the parents' attention long after treatment ends. Additionally, siblings are impacted by the changes to family routines and roles. However, siblings still often report deep and close relationships with the child with cancer.

The most common reactions of siblings to their brother or sister's cancer are concern, fear, jealousy, anger, guilt, fear of abandonment, sadness, and worry about their parents. Younger children may also feel that something they did caused their brother or sister's cancer. These feelings can cause academic and social problems or feelings of anxiety and depression.

Brothers and sisters within the same family can have markedly different reactions to their sibling's cancer treatment and survival, depending on their age, temperament, and social support. Some siblings can demonstrate difficulties with emotions and behavior. Risk factors for poor adjustment can include poorer family functioning, lower social support and family income, and shorter time since their sibling's cancer diagnosis (Long KA, 2018).

Family therapy can be very effective in exploring the various reactions of members of the family and working out ways to communicate well and support one another.

Our children are five years apart in age. Our youngest is the cancer survivor and our oldest is the cancer sibling. During diagnosis and treatment, it was extremely hard for our oldest. She tried to keep all her feelings inside. She missed us being a family, as well as time with Mommy while Mommy had to be in the hospital with her younger sister for a month or so at a time. This was made worse as treatment was during COVID, no one but Mommy could be in the hospital room.

We set up a "wishlist" for our oldest so she would not feel left out. We also set up a friends-and-family activity sign-up so friends could take her on special adventures and spend time with her. Our youngest then had to have a bone marrow transplant since the chemo wasn't working. Her sister was a half match! We sat our oldest daughter down and asked her if she would donate her marrow. We made it her decision, as we knew how much of a burden and responsibility this would become. She chose to save her sister's life. My girls still do not realize the magnitude of one sibling saving another's life. I look forward to the day that they both are able to discuss this and bond as true sisters and friends.

My sister and I have a good relationship, but it has been rocky at times. I think she felt like she did not get the attention she needed or deserved at times because my parents devoted more attention to me, even after I was off treatment. Sometimes this affected our relationship because I think she felt that I wanted

(Continued)

or sought that attention, even when I didn't. I know she has also had caregiver/people pleaser anxiety. Overall, though, we have a good relationship, and it has gotten better as we have grown up and gotten further away from my cancer days.

My younger brother is my best friend. He always has been. However, when I was going through treatment at the ripe age of seven, my brother was five and having difficulty understanding what was happening. He saw everyone constantly fussing over me and caring for me. He felt very left out. He was always spending the night at other people's houses and jumping around between grandparents and various friends. This caused him to ask my mom once, "Why doesn't anybody love me?" Even recalling that story seventeen years later, my heart breaks. From then on out, my family made sure to include my brother in everything so he would feel loved and properly appreciated. It is imperative to include siblings whenever possible.

I was away from my brother for a long time, and I felt sad but at least I got to play a bunch of video games with dad and have fun and do special things. I was angry at him when he first got home. I still feel angry a little because we don't get to do as many special things as we did before he got cancer. I just feel kind of sad and anxious now. But my brother is fun and cute and snuggly, and I love playing with him, especially in the snow in winter and the flowers in spring. I do feel anxious about him going back to the hospital.

Her sister was born into a cancer family, so that's all she has ever known. She went to all of her sister's scans and appointments and was there throughout it all. We planned "treat" activities for the whole family. The idea wasn't that her older sister got a treat after treatment, but that the whole family enjoyed a treat because we were going through it together as a family. For the most part it has not affected our daughters' relationship with one another. They are normal sisters and act like it. They both have sympathy for each other when they get sick. Our youngest has a lot of compassion for her sister because she grew up going with us to all her appointments during and after treatment. She still worries about her when she gets sick.

My relationship with my sisters has been complicated since my diagnosis. I am the youngest of three girls, and when I was diagnosed, my eldest sister was 17 and my other sister was 13. My oldest sister, given her age, her personality and her role as the oldest, assumed a huge amount of responsibility and a caretaker role during my treatment. With my parents being away at the hospital so much with me, she spent a lot of time taking care of our other sister, and took care of me whenever my parents had other things that needed their attention, or simply just needed a break. I think this strengthened my relationship with her, because I knew I could count on her as a caregiver, and as a result I really looked up to her.

My cancer diagnosis affected my relationship with my other sister much differently because we are so close in age. The attention I received throughout my treatment made her feel pushed aside and forgotten. Although I know my parents tried the best they could to give her the attention she needed, I do not think it felt like enough to her, and she harbored a lot of resentment and jealousy toward me. In recent years, we have both been doing a lot of work on ourselves and our relationship, and have been able to address some of the feelings that we both had during and after this difficult time in our lives. Our relationship is something we're still constantly working on together, but things have gotten much better in the last couple of years now that we are mature enough to seek help for ourselves and talk through things together.

Siblings also learn important lessons about compassion, sharing, and coping skills. Most realize that should they ever become as sick, the same attention would be paid to them and that all possible efforts would be made to help them survive. That can be a comfort when jealousy or feelings of neglect arise. Their empathy and compassion may grow through the crisis. Brothers and sisters of children with cancer sometimes feel they have benefited from the experience in many ways, including:

- Increased knowledge about health and disease
- Empathy for the sick or disabled
- Sense of responsibility

- Self-esteem
- Maturity and coping ability
- Family closeness

Many of these siblings mature into adults interested in the helping professions such as medicine, social work, or teaching. Survivors themselves often have strong feelings about the effect their cancer had on family functioning and the long-range effects on siblings.

RELATIONSHIPS WITH FRIENDS

Cancer can affect friendships and new relationships in a variety of ways. While some friendships can be strengthened, cancer can disrupt relationships with friends and interfere with developing new friendships.

I was fortunate enough that the friendships I had going into treatment remained intact after treatment. I was relatively young, so the majority of my friends were family friends, but even the ones I met at school were very loyal to me. I was constantly visited by friends in the hospital, and they made my life much more manageable. If anything, I gained friends through the community of childhood cancer patients, and they have stayed my friends to this day. If someone left my side while I was going through treatment, I probably would not have wanted to be their friend anyways.

I have two friends from high school that I am still friends with. They were both there for a lot of my cancer journey, but one was there for me the most. She and I are best friends now. We live down the street from each other and have babies the same age. It's such a special thing and I don't know what I'd do without her.

I had plenty of friends before cancer treatment, but once I started my treatments and everyone saw me less, I felt invisible, almost like a ghost. Toward the end of treatment, I started making new friends online. These friends accepted me for me, not as some kid with cancer.

> Since I was diagnosed so young, I didn't have many friends before treatment. It was hard to make friends during and after treatment because I had limitations, but I am very grateful to my elementary school friend, Julia, for always being a friend and letting me be a normal kid.

Losing friends

Unfortunately, childhood cancer occurs at a time when friendships normally change rapidly. When the diagnosis occurs in elementary school, friendships often depend on what classroom you are assigned to or who shares your lunch table. If you are gone for an extended period of time, the group may welcome you when you return, or the groups may have shifted so that you are now on the outside. When cancer strikes middle-school-aged children, friendships often dissolve. Social groups are forming, peer pressure is at an all-time high, and compassion is often a temporary casualty of puberty. In many cases, high-school-aged adolescents are more mature and understanding, and friendships remain strong throughout treatment.

Friends disappear for many reasons—they can't think of what to say or are afraid they will cry or say the wrong thing. Or they simply grow unfamiliar with the child who in the midst of a rapidly changing social scene misses huge chunks of time with friends. The friends may even think they can catch cancer. Many survivors have painful stories to tell of lost friendships.

Survivors also lose friends to cancer, and this is very difficult for children and their parents. During treatment, children and teens become extremely close to others going through treatment for cancer. And some of these children and teens die.

> Losing some of my friends was very sad and disturbing. I still pray that they will have a good time in Heaven and I'm hopeful to see them there. I'm so glad to be home from all that cancer and I'm so glad I survived. It was a miracle for me from God and angels. Making some new friends is probably the best part.

(Continued)

> I have had both good and bad experiences with friendships since having cancer. I have lost friends, which has been really hard. I think it's hard for some people to understand what to do for or say to someone who is living with cancer, so they just leave. It's hard not to take it as a punch to the face, but I have come to terms with it and now feel like maybe it was for the best.

Making new friends

Friendships in childhood are fluid; they depend on what class, school, neighborhood, church, or sports team you are involved with. Some survivors renegotiate or rekindle friendships and others make new friends during and after treatment.

Children being treated for cancer also miss key times for socialization and the development of social skills. Further, motivation to initiate new relationships or interact with others may be impacted due to physical issues such as fatigue or cognitive issues. Children whose parents take an active role in encouraging social interactions tend to do better socially. They can ask their child whom they like the most in their class at school and invite that child over to play or watch a movie. They can befriend parents of children with similar interests and invite the whole family over for dinner. Encouraging participation in school, music, church, or athletic activities exposes the child or teen survivor to new groups of peers.

Some survivors worry about making new friends because they don't want to cause their friends pain in the event the cancer returns. Some survivors blend back into their peer group after treatment while others, even many years later, still feel different. Some survivors feel that they are rejected socially due to their cancer history, while others feel mature beyond their years because of what they have experienced. This can create differences in interests and value systems between survivors and their peers.

In hindsight, I realize there were some people who did not support me the way I expected. My oldest friend was at a different place in her life and was distant. She came into my life after treatment. Another good friend came to visit all-day, every-day and would just sit with me. He has since passed away, but it was very special knowing how much time he spent with me in the prime of his life. Those friends kept me going. They didn't try to coddle but just stayed with me so I wasn't alone. I didn't really connect with other survivors. I just focused on getting through it.

Making friends that understand the unique experience of childhood cancer has been the highlight. During our daughter's treatment before COVID, we connected with a lot more people, but even after COVID-policy restrictions, passing in the halls, we would swap numbers with families and made sure to give words of hope and encouragement to each other where possible.

When she was 5, we sent her to a childhood cancer camp. Although she did not have any recollection of the diagnosis and treatment of her neuroblastoma as a baby, she met and was able to talk with other kids who had extensive follow-up care and secondary side effects. We stay in contact with a lot of them through Facebook.

Late effects from cancer treatments can create additional barriers. Issues such as skin problems, thin or absent hair, very short height, or amputation may affect survivor's engagement in social interactions. Additionally, sensory issues like hearing or vision loss, or disrupted social skills from neurological side effects, can impact the ability to interact with peers and make friends.

Cranial radiation at a young age or high-dose radiation to the brain at any age can affect a survivor's social skills, including ability to attend to socially relevant information in conversations and interpret nonverbal behavior. Parents can help their children by getting them involved in social activities, role-playing social skills, enrolling them in social skills classes, and encouraging friendships with schoolmates.

Peer support groups for teen and young adult survivors can provide a safe place to make friends, talk about feelings, and have fun.

Having other survivors as friends

You may find that you don't get the support and understanding you need from your friends who do not have cancer. Perhaps you need people who are willing to listen without judgment when you talk about your cancer, or you may not like to talk about it at all. You may feel strongly that you need to live a healthy lifestyle to lessen the chances of late effects, and your friends may not respect your decision not to smoke or drink. For a variety of reasons, you may seek out or continue friendships made during treatment with other people who had childhood cancer. This shared experience can create deep and long-lasting bonds.

Dating

Close and intimate relationships are difficult at times for everyone, whether or not they had cancer. Some survivors have a more difficult time starting relationships than others. Whether you are merely looking for some fun or searching for a partner for life, you may find that your cancer history is an impediment. If you missed months or years of middle school or high school, re-entering the dating world can be especially complicated if your appearance is altered by baldness, weight gain, or scars. People you are attracted to may avoid you due to phobias about cancer or because of peer pressure. You may not feel ready to date after enduring the physical pain and social isolation that usually accompany cancer treatment. Or you may just pick up where you left off pre-cancer.

> During my treatment, I met this guy that transported me to an MRI, and he asked me for my number so I gave it to him. We dated, but I constantly got in my own way in relationships. Being bald really messed up my head. I would ask him, "why do you want a sick person? I'm bald, and there are all these other women who don't have this life." I projected so many things onto him that weren't actually his feelings. I would break up with

him, then get back together, then break up again. Eventually he just said he couldn't do it anymore. I ruined a lot of relationships with just being wild. Mentally, I was shoving everything down. My ruthlessness was a cover for my feelings, and I never dealt with them. I just didn't care about my relationships, and when I did care it was too late. I didn't fully have a connection to anyone.

Dating as a survivor is strange. Something I have struggled with when meeting new people, especially when dating, is how much or how little I should share with someone about my experience. Cancer has been a big part of my life and it is something I will always struggle with. Leaving it out of conversations, especially with a potential love interest, is a tricky thing to navigate. Opening up about it to some people is hard.

I disclosed my cancer through social media and through my family and friends because I felt too sad to share it in person, face-to-face. I shared the news pretty quickly after being diagnosed, but I never shared intimate details unless I felt safe enough to do so. With my boyfriend at the time, it was uncomfortable to share certain aspects because I was scared to be looked at differently, but he was so comforting and supportive. Sharing with anyone can be scary, but feeling supported enough to share with someone is really beautiful.

When I met my partner, I told her right away that I was a cancer survivor. Her response was very positive: "We will navigate and figure it out together." Re-entering the dating scene has been complicated at times. I feel like I'm a burden due to my health issues, but then I remember that I have an amazing girlfriend who accepts me and will be by my side no matter what. Trying to keep that in mind is sometimes hard but I'm reminded every day that I'm loved.

BODY IMAGE, SEXUALITY, HORMONES

Cancer can change not only your physical appearance, but how you view yourself. You may have an obvious difference (amputation) or a more private one (loss of a testicle). You may have scars on your face that can be seen by anyone you meet or scars only seen by loved ones (such as, on your lower abdomen from a laparotomy). Even if you have no physical scars, you may have an altered sense of your own appearance. If you don't think you are attractive, it may be hard to convince yourself that someone you want to date will be attracted to you. On the other hand, many survivors and those who love them feel that the scars represent life and thus are beautiful.

Healthy adult sexual relationships have psychological, interpersonal, and physical aspects, one or more of which can be affected by treatment for cancer. Most studies of childhood cancer survivors show that overall emotional well-being is good (Kazak, 2010; Brinkman, 2013). However, some areas can become problematic, including sexuality. People with histories of cancer can view the body mostly as a source of health concerns rather than a source for sexual pleasure. Some young men and women have positive dating experiences during or after treatment that help them feel better about their appearance. Others may have other sexuality/sexual function concerns. One recent study showed that most childhood survivors are similar to their non-cancer peers in terms of sexual satisfaction and sexual function (Priobi, 2023). Another study from the Children's Oncology Group found different results that "survivors reported worse sexual function overall" (Cherven, 2021). More research is needed in this area. Clearly, some survivors face difficulties with sexuality/sexual function after cancer treatment which cause anxiety and stress and negative effect on overall emotional health. Survivors should feel comfortable discussing such sexuality concerns with a trusted member of their healthcare team and seek help.

Losing my hair was probably one of the most heartbreaking things I have ever experienced. I had beautiful dark brown long hair before I lost it to chemo. Going bald was deeply traumatic for me, and I rarely let anyone see me without a wig or beanie on. I felt embarrassed and ugly most times and worried about how sick and bad I looked. It definitely affected my self-confidence and self-esteem. To this day, it is something I struggle with, even now that my hair is growing back.

> I always hated the way I looked and the scars from all my surgeries. I came to realize the scars meant and showed I won the hard battle. I didn't truly love them until I met my husband. He pointed out all the things he loved about me and those scars were one of them.

Others especially those who have visible scars or disabilities may have to learn to adjust to some negative reactions from others. Although disability awareness is changing, there are still plenty of people who stare, make rude remarks, or just act uncomfortable around people with disabilities.

Some sexual problems can be caused by hormone imbalances (see *Chapter 10, Hormone-producing Glands* for details). These are normal late effects from treatment for which help is available. Survivors with hormonal problems should be evaluated by an endocrinologist or obstetrician/gynecologist with experience treating cancer survivors.

How to find help for your questions/concerns

The healthcare provider at your follow-up clinic should discuss any sexual concerns you have. They can also suggest therapists who help individuals or couples understand and deal with sexual problems. The American Association of Sexuality Educators, Counselors, and Therapists (AASECT) can suggest accredited therapists in your area. The website address is https://aasect.org and check resource list at the end of the chapter. Another resource that contains a wealth of information about sexuality after cancer is Leslie Schover's article, *Sexuality and Fertility After Cancer* (see reference).

The Livestrong Foundation has information about female and male sexual late effects Website: www.livestrong.org Click on Resource Center, then download the Livestrong Guidebook, Search for *late effects*.

Telling your cancer story

No one else can decide the right time for you to disclose your cancer history. You might want to find out right away if someone you are interested in is cancer-phobic. On the other hand, you may wish to establish a relationship first so the person already cares for you and will be less likely to respond negatively. Some survivors feel strongly that quick honesty is the best policy, while others feel equally strongly that it's better to wait awhile. Only you can decide when the time is appropriate to share such an important part of your life.

If you have obvious scarring or a disability resulting from cancer treatment, you might not have a choice of when to share the information. Some survivors enjoy educating the public about disabilities or differences. Others say there are days when they don't mind explaining and days when they just wish strangers would keep their stares and personal questions to themselves.

Disclosure may be especially problematic for survivors at risk for fertility problems. Having cancer as well as losing the ability to have children can be a crushing blow. It can also undermine relationships if having biological children (rather than adopting) is an important life goal of the partner. Some survivors choose not to get fertility tests to avoid the necessity of dealing with the issue before marriage. Others do not disclose the possibility of infertility due to fear of rejection.

When and how to disclose your cancer history to friends or partners is a purely personal choice. Most survivors opt for sizing up the person and deciding on a case-by-case basis. Often survivors adopt the concentric circle method of sharing information. Those in the innermost circle know the entire history, those farther out are given a little information or only what they need to know, and those on the outer perimeter know nothing. Some survivors find it helpful to practice what they will say when disclosing their cancer history.

Some survivors just pick up their lives where they left off. They find that their cancer history makes no difference in their social lives.

Disclosure of cancer history to potential employers or coworkers is a completely different matter covered in detail in *Chapter 4, Navigating the System*. Health care providers of adolescent and young adult survivors should initiate discussions regarding the possibilities of infertility, options for fertility preservation, and suggest fertility counseling when appropriate.

> I told my husband about my cancer around the 3rd or 4th date, but he already knew because everyone in my town knew. I cried when I told him, and he didn't understand why. It didn't change how he felt about me.
>
> ———
>
> I don't openly talk about my cancer story to everyone because I don't see the point in that. I have told some people in our lab when the topic of cancer comes up, but I don't bring it up out of the blue.
>
> ———
>
> I have no problem talking about my cancer. I talk about cancer so nonchalantly that it shocks people. Once someone asked me if cancer was contagious. My partner now is very supportive of me and everything I have told him about my cancer journey. I don't tell him everything though. I keep a lot of feelings inside. There are things I haven't told anyone.

Communication

Communication about cancer history is very important for those who live with the memories and late effects of their treatment. Sometimes survivors have one or two close friends from the hospital with whom they continue to share their thoughts and feelings about the past and their hopes and worries about the future. Joining a support group for survivors is a way to connect with others who have lived through similar experiences. These groups are a great resource for talking over practical matters with people who have traveled the same path. If there is no peer support at your hospital or follow-up clinic, ask a social worker or nurse to connect you with someone in similar circumstances. You could also train to become a counselor at the closest camp for children with cancer. Most of the young adults who are counselors at the camps share a history of cancer and many form lifelong friendships there.

The Internet is a way to contact those who have lived through cancer. There are numerous support groups and websites where survivors can connect, chat, and share stories and advice. The Internet is a great leveler—it doesn't matter what you look like or whether or not you have any disabilities— you are valued for the thoughts, words, and ideas you choose to share.

> Returning to work was extremely difficult for me. Coworkers can sympathize, but they will never truly understand what you went through. It helps to talk to other cancer moms and dads during and after your journey. Get back to your routine slowly and don't be afraid to reach out to people who understand your journey. Also, don't be afraid to let people know when you want to talk, don't want to talk, or want to take a "breather."

MARRIAGE/LIFE PARTNERSHIPS

Marriage (or a lifetime commitment) is one of life's major events. But for survivors of childhood cancer, making a life-long commitment may take on even greater meaning. A lingering fear of recurrence makes some survivors hesitant to link their future to another. Coming to terms with uncertainty, however, allows you to acknowledge you have a future that includes love and companionship.

Some young adults rush into relationships while they are feeling vulnerable and uncertain of who they are or what they want. Others feel that having cancer gave them a maturity that helped them find a partner who shares their values.

Fertility

A big concern of some childhood cancer survivors is whether they will be able to have healthy children. Evidence indicates that cancer survivors are not at greater risk of having children with disabilities or cancer when compared with those who never had cancer (see the "Health of offspring" section later in this chapter). The vast majority of survivors remain fertile, and many have one or more healthy children. In some cases, however, the treatment used to save lives takes away the ability to create new life. This is an especially poignant and difficult loss. Health care providers of adolescent and young adult survivors should initiate discussions regarding the possibilities of infertility, options for fertility preservation, and suggest fertility counseling when appropriate.

> The conversations that my husband and I had while dating were some of the most difficult ever. Fertility was probably one of the biggest conversations we had. It was terrifying, but he said it didn't change how he felt about me. He never cared. It didn't make a difference for him. He loved me for me, and that's all I wanted. There were many ways to grow a family. We did try IVF and it failed, but we then got pregnant naturally.

Those most likely to be infertile or have impaired fertility are:

- Survivors who had high doses of alkylators—cyclophosphamide, carmustine (BCNU), lomustine (CCNU), busulfan, melphalan, ifosfamide—and/or total body radiation
- Male children and teens who had direct radiation to their testes
- Female children and teens who had direct radiation to their ovaries

Children treated before puberty tend to have fewer fertility problems than those treated after puberty, and girls usually are less affected by treatment than boys. For more information about the effects of radiation and chemotherapy on fertility, see *Chapter 10, Hormone-Producing Glands.*

In addition to the treatments listed above, many other factors affect the nature and degree of fertility. These include the type of cancer, its location, the treatment, gender of the survivor, and age at diagnosis. Physical and psychological late effects also impact the desire and ability to have children.

Fertility is affected if female survivors have an early menopause. Normally, fertility tends to decrease when women are in their mid-30s. In some women treated for cancer, this decrease in fertility can occur much earlier.

Those most at risk for early menopause are:

- Adolescent girls treated after puberty.
- Female children or teens treated with both cyclophosphamide or other ovarian toxic drugs (ifosfamide, BCNU, or the combinations of medicines called MOPP and COPP) and radiation below the diaphragm.
- Girls who had an early puberty due to cranial radiation.

If you are at risk for early menopause, talk with your healthcare provider about family planning. You may be fertile for fewer years because of your treatments. If your periods become irregular or stop completely, see your gynecologist. Fertility can decline even with regular periods, so survivors at risk of early menopause should not rely on their periods as evidence of fertility—they need to have hormone levels monitored by their healthcare provider. Survivors who experience early menopause should get routine medical care to check for osteoporosis (thinning bones) and heart disease. These medical issues are covered in *Chapter 10, Hormone-Producing Glands,* and psychological issues are discussed in *Chapter 2, Emotions.*

There may be factors other than physical problems that affect childbearing. Some women worry that pregnancy may be risky because of their treatment for cancer—a true medical concern for those who had certain treatments, such as pelvic radiation. Others fear they may pass on cancer to their children, a fear that is, in most cases, unfounded. Yet other survivors are concerned about relapse or secondary cancers and may hesitate to bring a child into the world whom they might not be able to parent into adulthood.

Some survivors who are told they are infertile from their treatments are surprised to find out that they or their partners are unexpectedly pregnant. Even if it is likely that you are infertile from treatment, it is best to use birth control if you do not desire children.

Discussions regarding infertility should be initiated at the time of diagnosis and be ongoing throughout the course of treatment and survivorship. Some adult survivors were never told or do not recall hearing that infertility was a potential consequence of treatment for their cancer. Prior to the early 1970s, many parents were advised not to discuss the cancer with their children. Young children knew they were sick, and when treatment was complete, the family acted as if the cancer had never invaded their lives. Many young adults do not learn that their ability to have children may have been compromised or destroyed until they have spent several emotional and expensive years trying. Learning the truth can unleash overwhelming feelings of anger and devastation. Survivors who were told of their probable infertility have varying feelings, and these may shift over time. Counseling from an expert in grief and loss can be of immense help to those struggling with these strong feelings.

Support and empathy from family and friends may not occur if you are infertile. Leslie Schover, in her article, *Sexuality and Fertility After Cancer*, writes:

The most profound loss is giving up the dream of having one's own, genetic child. Cancer survivors are often told by physicians, family, and well-meaning friends that they should be glad to be alive. Their pain at being infertile is dismissed as ingratitude. But many people see having a child as a very concrete way of defeating death and leaving a part of oneself for the future. Many men and women grow up assuming they will be parents one day. For a couple, that longed-for child was to be the blending of their individual strengths and the product of their love. Mental health professionals who treat infertile couples often point out that it is difficult for them to grieve adequately or to get true understanding and support from family and friends because what has been lost is potential, rather than an actual child. The loss is no less real, however. (Schover LR, 2005)

In order to make informed decisions about childbearing, you need to ask questions and get thorough, understandable answers. Start off by asking yourself the following questions, and then consult a medical professional at a comprehensive follow-up clinic to get an honest evaluation of your individual situation.

Questions to ask yourself before considering having children:

- Am I in a stable relationship and do we both want children? Not having children is a choice made by many couples, with or without a cancer history.

- Am I experiencing any anxiety about the health of my future children? The next section discusses health of offspring, and for the vast majority of survivors, the news is very encouraging.

- Am I worried about my ability to physically carry a child? Pregnancy places additional stresses on the heart and lungs. If you received anthracycline drugs (doxorubicin, daunorubicin, idarubicin, or mitoxantrone) or lung, heart, or uterine radiation, you may have a higher risk for pregnancy complications. Prior to pregnancy, obtain expert advice about your actual risks so you can make an informed decision. If you do have any increased risk, get obstetrical care from a specialist in high-risk pregnancies during your pregnancy.

- If I wait to try to get pregnant, will I have problems conceiving? Much is known about risks to fertility from various treatments. Opinions from your caregivers will be about risks to groups of survivors, not you as an individual. Fertility is a complicated matter, and your healthcare provider will consider your type of cancer, age at diagnosis, your gender, and your treatment. Keep in mind that you are getting an educated opinion (or two), but not having your future told. The honest answer is that knowledgeable healthcare providers can give you their best guess, but no one can accurately predict your future.

- If I am infertile, what technologies are available to help me become pregnant? Donor sperm, donor eggs, in vitro fertilization, and surrogate mothers are methods of reproduction for infertile survivors. To find out about the most up-to-date techniques available, contact Livestrong Fertility https://www.livestrong.org or RESOLVE at www.resolve.org.

- What are the costs of the various options—adoption, infertility treatments— and how will they be financed?

- Would we rather adopt a baby, go through infertility treatments, or choose not to have children? Spend time talking over your priorities before making these important decisions. Consulting a mental health professional with experience helping couples cope with infertility may help you clarify your feelings and sort out your options. Infertility clinics in your area or your oncologist can provide the names of skilled therapists.

Explore whether there are local support groups for infertile couples in your area. Sharing experiences and talking over your situation with others can yield understanding and empathy you may not get from family or friends.

Health of Offspring and Genetics Counseling/Testing

Cancer survivors often worry about the health of their future children. They are afraid that a child conceived after surgery, radiation, or chemotherapy might be born with serious or life-threatening health problems. They also sometimes wonder if they could pass on their cancer genetically to their children.

The results of studies looking at the rate of birth defects in children born to childhood cancer survivors are very encouraging. In general, children born to survivors are just as healthy as those born to people who never had cancer. Health care providers should initiate discussions with young adult survivors contemplating having children regarding any concerns over health of their offspring and possible infertility options and refer to fertility counseling or genetic counseling/testing when appropriate.

Certain risk groups do require close monitoring during pregnancy such as those who received pelvic radiation or received drugs that can damage the heart.

A study of 4,699 children of 1,128 male and 1,627 female childhood cancer survivors provided strong evidence that the children of cancer survivors are *not at significantly increased risk* for congenital abnormalities resulting from their parents' cancer treatments (Signorello LB, 2011). This was encouraging news for the survivors treated in the 1970s and 1980s. Results about the effects of newer treatment protocols will unfold over the next 2 decades as survivors reach adulthood, marry or enter committed relationships, and have children.

Physical changes in the bodies of some female Wilms tumor survivors can cause health problems in offspring. Women who had abdominal or pelvic radiation may have a uterus that does not expand well during pregnancy. This can cause spontaneous abortion (miscarriage), low-birthweight infants, and a higher rate of babies who die in the uterus or soon after birth. Any pregnant survivor with a history of radiation that included the uterus should be followed by an expert in high-risk pregnancies.

Pregnancy is a stress on the heart, so if you were treated with drugs that can weaken the heart (see *Chapter 13, Heart and Blood Vessels*), you should have your heart evaluated prior to pregnancy and be cared for by a specialist who can monitor your heart during pregnancy and labor.

Genetics counseling and testing

Our knowledge about cancer predisposition syndromes continues to grow every year. We know that certain types of cancers are more often associated with a cancer predisposition, such as retinoblastoma, hereditary retinoblastoma, hepatoblastoma, familial adenomatous polyposis, and rare tumors like adrenal cortical carcinoma and Li-Fraumeni Syndrome (clusters of different types of cancers such as breast cancer, leukemia, brain tumors, and sarcomas in a family). Other cancers are not as likely to be caused by an inherited mutation unless you have a family history. For example, neuroblastoma and most types of leukemia are less likely to be caused by an inherited genetic mutation, unless you have a family member diagnosed with a similar cancer.

If you are one of the survivors whose family history puts you at higher risk for having a child with health problems, you might want to consider genetic counseling and possibly genetic testing. Prior to the testing, take steps to protect the confidentiality of the information. One way to do this is to learn about the Genetic Information Nondiscrimination Act (GINA), a federal law passed in 2008 to limit disclosure of genetic information without your permission. Consumer factsheets about GINA are available at *www.ginahelp.org*.

Genetic counseling is a multi-step process with several sessions during which a genetic counselor discusses your family history, your risks (if any), and helps guide you through the decision whether to pursue genetic testing or not. If you choose to pursue testing, a genetic counselor will also follow-up to thoroughly explain the report, what it means, any recommended medical management, and how these risks may affect future children. Your test results and counseling sessions should be confidential.

Genetic testing is a rapidly evolving field. To learn more about genetic testing for cancer, view the National Cancer Institute slide program, Gene Testing at https://www.cancer.gov/about-cancer, and Click on, Cancer Basics, then Screening. *See Chapter 6, Genetic Testing and Childhood Cancer* for more detail.

Finding a genetic counseling program

Make sure you go to a well-respected genetic counseling program. You can get a referral from your doctor, your nurse practitioner, or find one in your area at the website for National Society of Genetic Counselors (www.nsgc.org) Click on *Find a Genetic Counselor*. Various resources related to genetics are also available at www.geneticalliance.org.

Adoption

Whether to adopt children is an intensely personal decision. If you wish to adopt an infant, you may find it a difficult and time-consuming process. Choose your agency or attorney carefully to ensure that your emotional and medical situation is clearly understood. Try to put together a team that works well together to give you the best chance to adopt.

If you are open to adopting a toddler, older child, or a child of mixed-race background, the waiting time is almost always shorter. Many of these older children are healthy and well adjusted, although others have medical needs, disabilities, or emotional issues. When applying to adopt, you may face barriers from agencies based on your health history. Nevertheless, many adoptive parents describe the process as worth every second once they fold their new infant or child into their family.

Domestic or international adoptions can be arranged through public or private licensed adoption agencies. Title III of the Americans with Disabilities Act prohibits agencies from discriminating against cancer survivors based solely on their cancer history. They must consider applicants on an individual basis. You can also arrange adoptions privately through an attorney.

Home study and your medical history

During the adoption process, a home study is done by the agency involved. This study will require a medical exam by the prospective parents' physicians. Make sure your doctor explains your medical history in an honest yet positive way and stresses the length of time you have been off treatment and your current health status.

REFERENCES

Aloaoui-Lasmaili KE, Nguyen-Thi PL, Demogeot N, et al. Fertility discussions and concerns in childhood cancer survivors, a systematic review for updated practice. Cancer Med. 2022 Oct 12(5):6023-6039.

Bjornard KL, Howell CR, Klosky JL, et al. (2020) Psychosexual Functioning of Female Childhood Cancer Survivors: A Report from the St. Jude Lifetime Cohort Study. J Sex Med. 2020 Oct;17(10):1981-1994. doi: 10.1016/j.jsxm.2020.06.005. Epub 2020 Jul 25. PMID: 32723681; PMCID: PMC7552816

Cherven B, Sampson A, Bober SL, et al. (2021). Sexual health among adolescent and young adult cancer survivors: A scoping review from the children's oncology group adolescent and young adult oncology discipline committee. *CA: A Cancer Journal for Clinicians, 71(3), 250-263. https://doi.org/10.3322/caac.21655*

Kazak AE, Derosa BW, Schwartz LA, et al. (2010) Psychological outcomes and health beliefs in adolescent and young adult survivors of childhood cancer and controls. J Clin Oncol. 2010 Apr 20;28(12):2002-7. doi: 10.1200/JCO.2009.25.9564. Epub 2010 Mar 15. PMID: 20231679; PMCID: PMC2860405

Lehmann V, Gerhardt CA, Baust K, et al. (2022) Psychosexual Development and Sexual Functioning in Young Adult Survivors of Childhood Cancer. J Sex Med. 2022 Nov;19(11):1644-1654. doi: 10.1016/j.jsxm.2022.07.014. Epub 2022 Sep 8. PMID: 36088275.

Long KA, Lehmann V, Gerhardt CA, et al. (2018) Psychosocial functioning and risk factors among siblings of children with cancer: An updated systematic review. Psycho-oncology. 2018 Jun;27(6):1467-1479. doi: 10.1002/pon.4669. Epub 2018 Mar 15. PMID: 29441699.

Newton K, Fuchsia Howard A, Thorne S, et al. Facing the unknown: uncertain fertility in young adult survivors of childhood cancer. Journal of Cancer Survivorship (2021) 15:54-65. https://doi.org/10.1007/s11764-020-00910-x

Priboi C, van Gorp M, Maurice-Stam H, et al. Psychosexual development, sexual functioning and sexual satisfaction in long-term childhood cancer survivors: DCCSS-LATER 2 sexuality substudy. Psych oncology. 2023 Aug;32(8):1279-1288. doi: 10.1002/pon.6181. Epub 2023 Jun 26. PMID: 37365748.

Sankila R. Olsen JH, Anderson H, et al. (1998). Risk of cancer among offspring of childhood cancer survivors. N Engl J Med 1998; 338:1339-1344. DOI: 10.1056/NEJM199805073381902

Schover LR. (2005) Sexuality and fertility after cancer. Hematology Am Soc Hematol Educ Program. 2005:523-7. doi: 10.1182/asheducation-2005.1.523. PMID: 16304430.

Seppänen VI, Artama MS, Malila NK, et al. (2016) Risk for congenital anomalies in offspring of childhood, adolescent and young adult cancer survivors. Int J Cancer.

2016 Oct 15;139(8):1721-30. doi: 10.1002/ijc.30226. Epub 2016 Jun 30. PMID: 27280956.

Signorello LB, Mulvihill JJ, Green DM, et al. (2011) Congenital anomalies in the children of cancer survivors: a report from the childhood cancer survivor study. J Clin Oncol. 2012 Jan 20;30(3):239-45. doi: 10.1200/JCO.2011.37.2938. Epub 2011 Dec 12. PMID: 22162566; PMCID: PMC3269950.

RESOURCES

Website: ccgresources.org

All resources and references mentioned in this book are available on the website and will be routinely reviewed and updated.

Alex's Lemonade Stand Foundation

Website: www.alexslemonade.org

Search, *childhood cancer families*

Alex's Lemonade Stand Foundation (ALSF) is changing the lives of children with cancer by funding impactful research, raising awareness, supporting families, and empowering everyone to help cure childhood cancer. ALSF offers many programs and tools to help families navigate the challenges of childhood cancer.

American Association of Sex Educators, Counselors, and Therapists (AASECT)

Website: www.aasect.org

AASECT is devoted to the promotion of sexual health by the development and advancement of the fields of sexual therapy, counseling, and education. AASECT's mission is the advancement of the highest standards of professional practice for educators, counselors and therapists.

35 E Wacker Drive, Suite 850, Chicago, IL 60601

Ph: (202) 449-1099

Genetic Alliance

Website: https://geneticalliance.org/

Genetic Alliance a non-profit organization founded in 1986, is a leader in deploying high tech and high touch programs for individuals, families, and communities to transform health systems by being responsive to the real needs of people in their quest for health.

Genetic Information Nondiscrimination Act (GINA)

Website: www.ginahelp.org

The Genetic Information Nondiscrimination Act of 2008 (GINA) is a federal law that protects individuals from genetic discrimination in health insurance and employment. Genetic discrimination is the misuse of genetic information. This resource provides an introduction to GINA and its protections in health insurance and employment. It includes answers to common questions and examples to help you learn.

Livestrong Fertility

Website: www.livestrong.org

Click on Resource Center, then download the *Livestrong Guidebook*, Search, *late effects*

National Cancer Institute

Website: www.cancer.gov

Scroll down to topics: *Find Cancer type*;

Select, *childhood cancer* & other general topics

National Council of Genetic Counselors

Website: www.nsgc.org

Click, *Find a Genetic Counselor*

RESOLVE: The National Fertility Association

Website: www.resolve.org

Provides access to care, advocacy, support and community, education, and awareness.

4
Navigating the System

KASEY MASSA, LCSW, OSW-C, CCLS
JOANNE QUILLEN, MSN, APRN, PNP-BC
LISA BASHORE, PhD, APRN, CPNP-PC, CPON

The best prescription is knowledge. — *C. Everett Koop*

HAVING A CANCER HISTORY continues to create challenges for survivors even in the 21st century. Knowledge, networking, and advocacy are necessary to overcome barriers to obtaining an appropriate education, health insurance, and a job. Although some disabilities are physical and visible, others (such as educational and social competence) may not be as obvious. To help children and teens reach their true potential, changes in intellectual functioning and social skills must be diagnosed early and addressed. It helps to have a map for the cancer survivorship journey. This chapter offers basic information to help guide you on your journey and covers the following areas:

- education from elementary school through vocational training or college including your legal rights and specific suggestions about how to understand and use the system to get the most appropriate education for yourself (or your child);
- how to obtain comprehensive and affordable life and health insurance;
- how to obtain free or low-cost medications;
- how to handle job interviews and strategies for avoiding discrimination;
- ways to enter the armed services;
- individual and group advocacy

EDUCATION

Childhood cancer and its treatment can leave survivors with unique educational needs. Treatments that sometimes affect school performance are brain radiation, brain surgery, intrathecal methotrexate, and high-dose systemic methotrexate. *Chapter 9, Brain and Nerves*, covers these possible late effects in detail. In addition to these treatments, learning potential can be impacted by numerous or lengthy hospitalizations, persistent fatigue, hearing or vision loss, fine or gross motor impairments, and social difficulties.

Families and survivors who have access to a comprehensive survivorship follow-up program/clinic and *survivorship visits* will have skilled personnel to help them work with school systems to get the best possible education for their children. But many individuals and families do not have access to these resources and must navigate the special education system on their own. You have many legal rights, and knowing what they are can help you advocate for yourself or your child.

> Since I was so young, I thankfully bounced back pretty well after treatment ended. I had a great support system and terrific teachers in school who had taught my siblings and did a great job of accommodating me and helping my family through treatment.
>
> ---
>
> Our girls are still in daycare. There is potential for reduced vision so support services could come into play in the future, but given their prognosis, we are hopeful their educational careers will not be affected by their cancer or their treatments.
>
> ---
>
> In first grade, she was having reading issues. In second grade, she was diagnosed with a secondary cancer, so addressing the reading issues fell to the back burner. In third grade, she was tested and diagnosed with dyslexia. The doctors were unsure if the dyslexia was genetic or caused by the earlier chemotherapy. Her neurologist suggested she could benefit from working with a tutor, so we hired a tutor that worked with her during sixth and seventh grades. She read 10 different series of books, and before starting eighth grade, she was reading at a 10th grade level.

Legal rights regarding school

The *Individuals with Disabilities Education Act (IDEA)* requires every public school to provide a free and appropriate education in the least restrictive environment to all disabled individuals between the ages of 3 and 21. That means providing, without charge, special education programs, speech therapy, occupational therapy, physical therapy, psychiatric services, assistive communication techniques and technology, and other interventions as needed to help children learn. This law has been extended and modified by the *Individuals with Disabilities in Education Improvement Act of 2004 (IDEA 2004) and updated regulations published in 2006, 2008, and 2018 website: https://sites.ed.gov/idea/*

The major provisions of these laws are the following:

- All children, regardless of disability are entitled to a free and appropriate public education and necessary related services. Schools are required to provide an individually designed instructional program, called an Individual Educational Plan (IEP) for every eligible child, including early intervention programs for at-risk toddlers.
- Children will receive fair testing to determine if they need special education services. This testing can be done either by the school district or privately arranged by the family.
- Parents of a child with disabilities participate in the planning and decision-making for their child's special education.
- Children with disabilities will be educated in the least restrictive environment possible, usually with children who are not disabled.
- The decisions of the school system can be challenged by parents with disputes resolved by an impartial third party.
- Planning for transition to postsecondary schooling, work, or independent living must start by the time the student turns 16 or younger if appropriate.
- Parents have the right to withdraw consent for special education and related services, but they must do so in writing.

These laws cover survivors of cancer whose medical problems affect their educational performance, and eligibility is usually obtained using the categories known as "other health impaired," "traumatically brain injured," or "learning disabled." Special education services are also available if the child's medical condition limits energy, alertness, or strength. Many survivors do not need special help in school but those who do have a legal right to it.

Children on-and-off treatment may also be eligible for services and accommodations under *Section 504 of the Federal Rehabilitation Act (1973)*. This law applies when the child does not meet the eligibility requirements for specially designed instruction but still needs accommodations (provided through a *504 Plan*) to perform successfully in school. For example, special accommodations to address health needs can include a water bottle on the desk, reduced homework during periods of illness, waiving regular attendance/tardy policies and procedures, or allowing additional time to get to class. Another example is a child off therapy with cognitive impairments that do not meet the IDEA requirements might need to have accommodations that eliminate timed tests or provide more time to finish written assignments. Your healthcare team can provide a letter to outline recommendations for accommodations to support your child's specific needs.

Special education in Canada

A similar special education process is in place in Canada. Children between the ages of 6 and 22 may qualify for special education assistance under the Designated Disabled Program (DDP), the Special Needs Program (SNP), or the Targeted Behavior Program (TBP), depending on the evaluation.

Provincial guidelines are established by the national Ministry of Education and governed by the Education Act, but most decisions are made at the regional, district, or school level. Evaluations are performed by a team that may include a school district psychologist, a behavior specialist, a special education teacher, other school or district personnel, and in some cases a parent, although the latter is not required by law as required in the United States.

Referral for services

The steps necessary to obtain services in the United States are referral, evaluation, eligibility, development of an individualized education program (IEP), annual review, and triennial assessment.

Neuropsychological evaluation

Usually in survivorship clinic, a psychologist is available to meet with the survivor and parent. A baseline neuropsychological evaluation is performed which is a test to measure how well a person's brain is working. This evaluation includes reading, language usage, attention, learning, processing speed, reasoning, remembering, problem-solving, mood, and personality. The psychologist is an important member of the oncology survivorship team who can provide essential school guidance. Insurance plans often dictate what testing will be covered; thus, survivors may need to seek testing within the community or at school. Neuropsychological testing results can be provided to the school from the parent to support identification of learning needs.

Who makes the referral

Social workers/counselors also play a key role in referrals and support for survivors with educational needs. These individuals are vested in the care of cancer survivorship and their academic success, but close collaboration with school districts is important.

Parents or teachers can make a referral by writing the school principal to request special education testing. Some school districts automatically set up an IEP for any child who had cranial radiation during cancer therapy, while other school districts are extremely reluctant even to evaluate struggling children for possible learning disabilities.

Therefore, it is best for the parent or physician to send a *written request* to the principal or other school personnel stating that the child is "health impaired" due to treatment for cancer, listing the child's problems, and requesting assessments and an IEP meeting.

> Make sure that in all written correspondence with the school, you clearly express your desire to be present at all meetings and discussions concerning your child's special education needs.

Multidisciplinary team evaluation from school district

Once the referral is made, an evaluation is necessary to find out if the school district agrees that the child needs additional help, and what types of help would be most beneficial. Usually, a multidisciplinary team consisting of the teacher, district psychologist, speech and language therapist, and resource specialist will meet to administer and evaluate the testing. Your written consent is required prior to your child's evaluation, and you have the right to obtain an independent evaluation if you believe the school's testing is biased or flawed in any way. However, you may be responsible for this cost. The evaluation usually includes a review of educational, medical, social, and psychological status.

If you pay for the neuropsychological evaluation, you can choose how much of the information to share with the school. You can hide or cover over portions of the report you wish to remain confidential and make a copy to give to the team.

After the evaluation, a conference is held to discuss the results and reach conclusions about what actions will be necessary in the future. Parents should attend this meeting and can bring a doctor, therapist, educational liaison, professional advocate, or friend with them. *Make sure that in all written correspondence with the school, you clearly express your desire to be present at all meetings and discussions concerning your child's special education needs.* You know your child best and have the right to be there. The school can still have the meeting if you choose not to attend or if you do not show up.

Individualized education program (IEP)

The IEP describes the special education program and any other related services specifically designed to meet the individual needs of a child with learning differences. It is developed collaboratively between parents and educators to determine what the student will be taught and how and when the school will teach it. Students with disabilities need to learn the same things as other students: reading, writing, mathematics, science, history, and other preparation for college or vocational training. The difference with an IEP in place all specialized services are stipulated––such as small classes, home schooling, speech therapy, physical therapy, counseling, and instruction by special education teachers. These services are available to children with subtle learning difficulties, not just those with severe late effects. Parents must monitor the situation to make sure stipulated services are actually provided.

The IEP includes the following:
- Parental concerns, medical history, and information about the disability
- Statement of present levels of academic achievement, social, behavioral, and physical functioning, academic performance, and learning style
- Annual goals, objectives, benchmarks, and methods of evaluation
- Services that will be provided and any program modifications or supports for school personnel that will be provided
- Projected date when services/modifications will begin, and frequency, location, and duration
- Plans for standardized testing and graduation requirements
- Description of the least restrictive setting in which the above goals and objectives can be met
- Any individual accommodations needed for state and district-wide assessments
- A statement of parental rights and responsibilities

At least once a year, and more frequently if requested by a parent or teacher, a meeting is held (which your child can attend) to review the progress toward meeting the short- and long-term goals and objectives of the IEP. Some states have limits on the number of IEP meetings per year. Someone from the school system is appointed to carry out and monitor each part of the IEP. However, the parent needs to know what it contains and work with the school if included services are *not* being performed. A written copy of the plan is given to the family.

> **It is helpful to keep a binder or folder of assessments and communications to support the growth and needs of your child.**

Communication between parents and school system

It is best to create a positive relationship with the school so you are able to work together to promote your child's well-being. If communication deteriorates for whatever reason, and you feel your child's IEP is inadequate or not being followed, there are several facts you need to know and steps to resolve the situation:

- Changes to the IEP *cannot be made without parental consent.*
- If parents disagree with the school about the content of the IEP, they can either withdraw consent and request *(in writing)* a meeting to draft a new IEP or they can consent only to portions of the IEP with which they agree.
- Parents can request to have the disagreement settled by an *independent mediator* and *hearing officer.*
- Parents can hire a *special education advocate*—a person with special training and expertise whose profession is helping families get appropriate special education services for their child. The advocate will attend all meetings and give advice about legally mandated services and how to obtain them.

For more information about *IEPs,* visit Center for Parent Information & Resources (CPIR) at https://www.parentcenterhub.org/ or American Childhood Cancer Organization website: www.acco.org. Download free copy of the book, *Educating the Child with Cancer, A Guide for Parents and Teachers, 3rd ed.* edited by Ruth I. Hoffman, MPH. See Resources end of chapter.

Canadian laws related to IEPs

IEPs in Canada are almost identical to those used in the United States. In Canada, the IEP is updated yearly, or more frequently if needed. A formal review is required every 3 years. In Canada, if disputes arise between the school or district and the parents, the School Division Decision Review process is available to resolve them. The concept known as *due process* in the United States is usually referred to as *fundamental justice* in Canada, meaning that all citizens are entitled to the same treatment by law.

Individualized transition plan

Special education students also have a right to be prepared for graduation, higher education, and work in ways that fit their needs. For some survivors, extra support is needed to make the transition from high school to adulthood go smoothly. Under IDEA 2004, when a student with an IEP turns 16, the annual IEP meeting must include discussion about transition service needs, and the child must be invited to attend. IEPs must include a transition plan for students ages 14 years or older. The statement of transition goals and services must be written into the IEP.

Transition plans should include the following:

- Desired post-school outcomes
- Necessary documents and support services
- List of transition resource team members
- Career preparation activities
- Transition services for instruction, community experiences, employment, post-school living, and daily living skills
- Vocational evaluation
- Summary of agency responsibilities
- Summary of designated instruction and services for transition

A statement about the rights that will transfer to the child when s(he) reaches the *age of majority*, beginning at least 1 year before that date. Age of majority is determined by state statute.

In most states when children turn 18, they are considered an adult. As a legal adult, a child may assume some or all of the education rights previously held by the parent or guardian.

Obtaining a high school diploma usually requires passing a certain number of specified courses. Students sometimes need changes in the required courses for graduation, for example, a deaf student might ask that the foreign language requirement be waived or that fluency in sign language be allowed to substitute for foreign language proficiency. Some students need extra coursework to make it through high school, such as special instruction in computers or study skills. These abilities will also help with higher education or future employment.

Some students will not be able to earn a regular diploma. A special form of graduation called an *IEP diploma* is also available. If a student earns an IEP diploma, that means s(he) has completed all of the objectives set out in his IEP for graduation. Passing a series of four tests (language arts, math, social studies and science) called the *general educational development (GED)* may be an option for other students. Passing these four tests demonstrates the student has the same knowledge as a student attending 4 years of high school. The GED is a 7-hour test and generally takes a year or more for a student to prepare for the test. The GED test can be taken any time after age 16. Most colleges and employers view the GED and high school diploma the same.

In the United States, many states have implemented high school exit exams that must be passed to graduate. In some states, exemptions are available for students with an IEP or *504 Plan*.

Students planning to attend vocational/technical school, a 2-year community college program, or a 4-year (or longer) college program need information far in advance about which high school courses required for admission. This is especially important for those students with disabilities who carry a lighter course load, as they may need to make up credits/courses in summer school or via correspondence or online courses.

Transition programs should address the move from high school to vocational-technical school, community college, or a 4-year college program. Students are eligible for publicly funded education and/or services until age 22, if needed.

VOCATIONAL TRAINING

Preparing for the world of work means gaining appropriate skills, such as typing, filing, driving, filling out forms, and using tools. These skills may be gained in school-based vocational-technical classes, classes taken at a community college or vocational school while still in high school, union- or employer-sponsored apprenticeship program, an internship, or on the job. Vocational career planning is mandatory for special education students in the United States by age 16 as part of an Individualized Transition Plan, but should begin much earlier.

Transition-to-work services

Transition-to-work services may include moving into the public vocational rehabilitation system which trains and places adults with disabilities into jobs. However, in many states, the vocational rehabilitation system is severely overloaded with waiting times for placement ranging from 3 months to as much as 3 years. There are a range of different work environments. *Sheltered workshop* jobs are segregated facilities where disabled people go to work for very low sub-minimum wages (e.g., sorting recyclables, light assembly work) and are meant to be temporary workplaces that prepare them for finding and working regular jobs.

Another type of job placement is *supported placement* which provides people with severe disabilities the appropriate, ongoing support necessary for success in a competitive work environment. These are jobs within the community such as grocery clerks, office helpers, and factory workers. Often the survivor works with a *job coach* for a period of time. The job coach is a person who helps them learn work skills, workplace rules/regulations, and how to handle workplace stresses. In some cases, the job coach may accompany the survivor on the job for a period of time or only make periodic visits to see how the survivor is getting along and resolve any problems.

For more information about various work programs for disabled: https://www.dol.gov/agencies/odep
U.S. Department of Labor, Office of Disability Employment

School districts may sponsor their own supported work opportunities, such as learning to run an espresso coffee cart or student-run horticultural business. Many schools have vocational programs that connect students with a *mentor* in their chosen field which may include actual work experience with local employers.

Some public and private agencies may offer help with job training and placement, such as the state employment department, or the U.S. Department of Labor, (https://www.dol.gov/agencies/eta/). Goodwill Industries operates a job placement service in most larger cities.

Students with disabilities should receive appropriate vocational counseling, including aptitude testing, discussion of their interests and abilities, and information about work possibilities. Parents need to ensure that students with the potential for higher level skilled jobs are not shunted into jobs that leave them financially vulnerable and possibly unhappy as adults.

State vocational rehabilitation agencies

Every state has a vocational rehabilitation agency that provides services to individuals who live in that state. The federal Rehabilitation Act requires states to provide the following minimum services:

- Evaluation of potential for rehabilitation
- Counseling
- Placement services
- Physical accommodations (the state does not have to provide equipment but is required to help determine what equipment is needed)

Some states have *vocational rehabilitation scholarship money* that provides an amount comparable to tuition at a state university that can be used for vocational training. They also provide information about private vocational rehabilitation programs within the state. The Rehabilitation Act requires that state vocational rehabilitation agencies work with schools to provide transition from high school to the workplace for youth with disabilities. For information about accommodations on the job, see resources below.

Resources for vocational rehabilitation

- Job Accommodation Network Website: http://askjan.org. Phone: (800) 526-7234 (Prompt #2)
- To file a complaint if you feel *your home state* is denying or inadequate response for rehabilitative services/accommodations, Website: www.advocacyinstitute.org
- Rehabilitation Services Administration, U.S. Department of Education, Office of the Commissioner, 400 Maryland Avenue SW, Washington, DC 20202-7100 Website: https://rsa.ed.gov

SEVERELY DISABLED SURVIVORS

Some survivors, primarily those who had brain tumors, can suffer devastating late effects that leave them unable to work or live independently. Families dealing with this situation face a difficult future, one that is not often discussed. In some cases, nothing can be done to improve the survivors' functioning, and families may feel isolated and desperate. They must cope with complex medical, social, and psychological issues because so many body systems can be affected by tumor location, extent of surgery, and cancer treatment to the brain. They must seek out professionals to meet all of the survivors' needs and are often frustrated by the many gaps in services. This can be a relentless and exhausting job.

In some communities, parents can find resources that address their needs, while in other locations they are left on their own. One method of support is finding respite care, which allows parents or guardians to have a break from caring for their child. This can be arranged through local social services, regional programs for the developmentally disabled, or privately. Some families network and take turns taking small groups of survivors on outings.

One way for caregivers to get respite time is to try to link the disabled survivor with a part-time job or a volunteer position that matches an area of interest. Some examples are walking dogs in the neighborhood, working with animals at farms or shops, or helping at a daycare center. These jobs allow the survivor to earn money and improve self-esteem, as well as provide a connection to the community and opportunity for socialization for those who feel isolated.

Parents can contact local head-injury groups for possible organized outings/social events or other local resource organizations that might help. Some comprehensive follow-up clinics provide monthly activities for adult disabled survivors. In some areas, social groups have been established to provide a social community for disabled survivors.

Parents may also need help to ensure that a plan is in place to provide care for their adult child when they are no longer able to do so (such as a *limited conservatorship*). Making arrangements prior to illness or old age with the help of an attorney who specializes in estates and trusts can ease parents' minds about this most crucial transition.

> Most of the planning and communication at this level will require your child to self-advocate. Student Disability Services will want to work directly with your child to develop the appropriate accommodations to meet his/her needs.

COLLEGE FOR DISABLED SURVIVORS

Most survivors have no cognitive difficulties and continue their education through the level they would have reached if cancer had not been part of their lives. However, survivors with cognitive late-effects may need some help applying for and attending college. They need to carefully evaluate colleges and apply to those that will best address their special needs.

Chemo brain and chemo fog definitely got the best of me at times, especially because I jumped right back into college after treatment. I was lucky enough to have amazing social workers and a support team who helped me get testing to ensure I got the best results when trying to finish my college degree.

Since my daughter has a shunt which could randomly fail at anytime, she has selected her college options based on proximity to a major medical institution. When she goes to college, we'll have pre-meetings with the local neurosurgery team, a plan in place with her RA, and information where to take her in case of failure and all the appropriate legal forms to ensure we can support and guide her healthcare. I never would have thought about the latter—but it is important. An 18-year-old is hardly in a place to manage the crazy complications of cancer survival and healthcare. I am 46 but hardly in a place to do it.

When visiting colleges, you must talk with admissions personnel or staff in Disabled Student Services Office about your special needs and additional help you may require.

Resource: Learning Disabilities Association of America Website: https://ldaamerica.org

Steps when visiting colleges

Every college and university has a Disabled Student Services Office. When visiting colleges, you must talk with admissions personnel or staff in this special office about your special needs and additional help you may require. Survivors with disabilities that affect mobility may need to pre-plan class schedule before registration to allow for crossing campus to get to classes on time.

Some colleges offer learning-disabled students special study majors designed around the student's strengths, special help (e.g., untimed tests, tutoring, notetakers), lighter class load, or waivers from course requirements.

It is against the law to deny admission to students based on disabilities; of course, other admissions criteria generally must be met.

Public universities and community colleges may waive some admissions criteria for disabled students on a case-by-case basis if the student can show they are capable of college-level work. For example, if a student's poor hand/eye coordination is the reason for a low score on the SAT® or ACT® exam, but the student will have a classroom aide available at college to help with note-taking and test-taking, admission might be granted despite the low score on SAT® or ACT®. Standardized test requirements might also be set aside if high school grades or the student's work portfolio look good.

Schools that normally require all freshmen to live on campus may waive this requirement for a student with special needs. If living at home is not an option, a group home or supervised apartment near campus might be the next best choice. Before your child leaves for college in another city, make sure you have secured safe and appropriate housing, found competent local professionals to provide ongoing care, and rehearsed daily life activities such as grocery shopping and visiting the laundromat. You should also work out a crisis plan with your child in the event that a problem arises, and he/she knows exactly who to call and where to go, especially in an emergency situation.

Paying for college

Paying for college is difficult for many families. For most students, with or without disabilities, the best place to start is at the financial aid office at colleges being considered. A discussion with the high school guidance counselor may also yield information about scholarships. Check with your own survivorship program for more information on scholarships for survivors.

Many scholarships are given based on the student's unique endeavors or obstacles they have overcome. You may wish to share with the college of your choice the values and perspectives you gained from facing and overcoming cancer.

The following organizations provide information about ways to pay for college:

- Federal student aid programs provide various types of student loans Website: https://studentaid.gov

- FastWeb (www.fastweb.com) is an Internet site that matches individual students with eligibility requirements for more than 1.3 million scholarships. It also contains a college directory of more than 4,000 schools with information about admissions, financial aid, and other topics.
- The American Cancer Society can connect you with its state affiliates, some of which sponsor scholarships for survivors or you can check the website at www.cancer.org (search for *college scholarships*).

INSURANCE

Survivors of childhood cancer frequently encounter discrimination when trying to obtain adequate insurance. Some survivors are unable to get insurance and others pay increased premiums because of their cancer history. Securing insurance coverage requires research and persistence.

> Resource for help to obtain adequate insurance:
> Website: https://triagecancer.org/state-laws

Life insurance

Many companies have strict medical requirements that sometimes exclude survivors no matter how long they have been cured.

Before shopping for life insurance, consider first whether or not you need it. Three important reasons for having life insurance are:
- To replace wages if the family wage earner dies
- To support an aged parent if the family wage earner dies
- To provide burial expenses for a child

You probably ***do not*** need life insurance if:
- You have no dependents (e.g., spouse, children, elderly relatives who require financial support)
- You are married, have no children, and your spouse will not suffer financial hardship if you die

The easiest way to get life insurance if you have a cancer history is during open enrollment at your place of employment. Most companies have a period in which you can sign up without providing your medical history.

There are several ways to obtain life insurance:

- **Through place of employment.** If you or your spouse/partner work for a large corporation, organization, or government agency they provide a group plan. These plans do **not** make individual evaluations of employees or their dependents in order to grant coverage. They may provide good coverage at reasonable rates and often have no waiting period for pre-existing conditions.

- **You can hire an independent insurance agent** (one who does not work for a specific insurance company) to act as your broker and research estimates from several companies. Your state insurance department can provide you with a list of all the licensed insurance brokers in your area. The broker can check with many companies to find the best policy for your particular needs.

- **You can purchase a *graded policy*** that will refund the premium and a percentage of the face value of your plan if you die within a certain number of years (called a *waiting period*). After the waiting period has passed, you will have full benefits.

Filling out application for life insurance

When applying for life insurance, the company usually first asks you to fill out a health questionnaire. You should answer all questions truthfully, but be careful to only answer the questions asked. For instance, if asked "Do you have cancer?" you can truthfully answer "no" if you are now cured. However, if asked, "Have you *ever* had cancer?", you must answer "yes."

If an insurance company learns that you have lied about your health status in your application, you or family members could lose some or all of their benefits.

Legal advice directs survivors when filling out insurance applications to only answer the specific questions asked. Do not volunteer any additional information. The company will decide after reviewing your application whether you qualify for insurance benefits and how much coverage will be provided.

Health insurance

As survivors mature, seek employment, and move away from home, many have encountered barriers to obtaining health insurance, such as rejection of application based on cancer history, policy reductions, policy cancellation, pre-existing condition exclusions, increased premiums, or extended waiting periods. Recent U.S. healthcare reform legislation, the *Patient Protection and Affordable Care Act (ACA) of 2010* and its companion amendments, has the potential to relieve many of these problems for survivors.

The ACA offers the following provisions that are relevant to childhood cancer survivors:

- Young adults are allowed to stay on their parents' insurance plan until they turn 26 years old. One exception (in 2014) is that "grandfathered" group plans do not have to offer coverage for a young adult up to age 26 if the young adult is eligible for group coverage outside the parents' plan.
- Certain preventive services are covered, including services that are important aspects of survivorship care.
- If you are unemployed with limited income, you may be eligible for health coverage through Medicaid. Criteria for eligibility may vary state-to-state.
- If an employer doesn't offer health insurance, you will be able to buy it through a *Health Insurance Marketplace Exchange*, which will offer a choice of health plans.
- You may get tax credits to help pay for insurance if your income meets certain government defined income requirements.
- Health plans cannot limit or deny coverage for a child younger than age 19 simply because the child has a pre-existing condition. This protection will be extended to people of all ages.
- The Pre-existing Condition Insurance Plan (PCIP) makes health coverage available if you have been denied health insurance because of a preexisting condition, and you've been uninsured for at least 6 months.

Key provisions of the law have been phased in over several years, and were affected by court challenges and legislative actions. There may be further changes over time. Some companies consider a 5-year remission acceptable, while others exclude all cancer survivors from their life or health insurance policies. Most companies evaluate risk based on the type, grade, and stage of cancer, and how long you have been in remission. If you had a policy prior to diagnosis, it cannot be canceled because of your cancer as long as you pay your premiums.

The three main types of health insurance in the United States are *group policies*, *individual policies*, and *public health insurance programs*. Group and individual policies are either traditional indemnity policies or some variation of managed care. Publicly funded health insurance options include Medicaid, Medicare, state programs for low-income residents or residents with disabilities, county health programs, or state high-risk insurance pools.

Group policies

The easiest way to get insurance is if you or your spouse/partner work for a large corporation or government agency that provides a *group health insurance policy*. The larger the pool of employees, the less likely you are to be rejected for health coverage. In many cases, you will not be required to answer any questions about your health.

If you do not work for an employer with hundreds or thousands of employees, you may be eligible for group policies through other organizations such as labor unions, fraternal organizations, professional or business organizations, student associations, church groups, or other special interest groups. If their risk pool is large, the organization may be willing to provide you with adequate coverage if you are a member.

Individual policies

If you explore all of the groups with which you are affiliated and cannot obtain group coverage, check out individual policies. But be forewarned, individual health insurance policies can be exorbitantly expensive. An insurance broker may be able to help you find all options available to you. You might also consider the following options:

- Your parents can extend their policy to cover you if you are *disabled* or *handicapped*.
- Regardless of your abilities, your cancer history may qualify you as *disabled*.
- Your parents' policy will allow you to obtain a policy with the same company when you are no longer eligible for coverage on their policy.
- Your state might have a *catastrophic insurance pool*. Your state's Department of Insurance or Insurance Commissioner's office can tell you whether this is an option.
- You can get coverage through your spouse's/partner's employment.

If you cannot obtain group or individual insurance, it's time to evaluate government programs.

Insurance during and after has been an utter nightmare. We were supposed to be worrying about the health of our daughters, but we were often forced to spend long hours on the phone making sure services would be covered or straightening out billing errors. We explained the same thing over and over to different people in different departments. Not to mention the added stress and distraction at work trying to figure out how to cover costs of necessary treatment, figure out payment plans, or arguing benefit terms with the insurance company.

My wife had to quit her job due to all the medical appointments and treatments for both girls. I had extreme fears of seeking a new job because we had already met our insurance deductible for the year and didn't want to start a new insurance plan, especially having no idea whether a new insurance company would cover a pre-existing condition that required out of network treatments/specialists.

(Continued)

I own my own business now and was able to get health insurance through the state. There were a few times where I needed to pay out of pocket, but I never paid. I cannot get life insurance. I was on the cusp of getting it when I got my second cancer at 27, so my chances are even lower now.

I have not had barriers obtaining insurance. I have insurance through my employer, and since I work for a healthcare network the insurance is pretty good. This is my first insurance plan outside of my parents' insurance plan, and it was a bit stressful making the change, but I haven't experienced any issues so far.

I have health insurance through the market place because I work part time as a nurse, and you can't get insurance when you're part time. If I got it through my husband it would go up to $800 a month. I do not have life insurance because no one will accept me. I've tried a couple times.

She is not eligible for life insurance. When she turns 18, she could have gotten an off-name plan but she cannot get one now because she has had two cancers. We have not had any issues with medical insurance. Even when my husband's job was terminated during COVID and we lost his insurance, we paid for a plan that included her doctors in network.

Government healthcare plans in the United States

The United States government does supply low-cost health insurance to some citizens through the *Medicare* and *Medicaid* programs. It also has healthcare plans for those in current military service and, through the U.S. Department of Veterans Affairs, for former military personnel. In addition, some states have healthcare plans.

Medicaid. Medicaid is a federal program that provides free or low-cost health insurance coverage to certain individuals with limited income, but it is administered at the state level. The federal government requires all states to provide a minimum level of benefits, but states are allowed to apply for exceptions. Medicaid programs must follow federal rules, but the coverage, costs, and other details may differ in each state. Keep in mind that Medicaid programs have different names from state-to-state. For a full list of specific Medicaid state names and laws, visit the website below and learn particulars for your state, how to apply, and updated information online. Website: https://triagecancer.org/state-laws/medicaid

Supplemental Security Income (SSI). SSI or *disability insurance* is administered by the Social Security Administration (SSA). If a person is diagnosed with a chronic or serious illness and undergoing treatment or unable to work because of this illness/injury, SSI can provide some financial aid. To qualify for SSI, there are income limits if you do work part-time. In 2025, the limit is $2,000 in countable resources. Too much family income, may not always bar a disabled child from qualifying for SSI and Medicaid. In some cases, family income will reduce the amount of SSI received to as low as $1 per month, but the beneficiary will still get full medical coverage. Individual state rules also affect eligibility. See further guidance from a social worker or your state Medicaid office since guidelines change over time. To find out how to apply and check current amounts of assistance in your state contact your local SSA, check online: Website: https://triagehealth.org/quick-guides/ssi or call: Phone: 1-800-772-1213

Representative Payee. You can appoint someone as your Representative Payee if you need help managing your SSI benefits, often a parent or family member. Since 2014, several states offer a savings account for SSI recipients called ABLE (Achieving a Better Life Experience) accounts which allow SSI recipients to save above the $2,000 dollar earning limit and stay eligible for SSI and other benefits. Find out more at: Website: https://www.ablenrc.org

Disabled Adult Child (DAC). An adult survivor who has a qualifying disability that began before the age of 22 and meets the definition of disability for adults, may be eligible for benefits based on their parents' Social Security earnings record if the DAC is unmarried and age 18 or older. The parent must be deceased or receiving retirement or disability benefits themselves. Even if the DAC has never worked, benefits are paid based on the parents' earnings record. For more information: https://www.ssa.gov/benefits/disability/qualify.html

At the time of writing this you cannot apply for DAC benefits online. To file for DAC benefits, you must call SSA at 1-800-772-1213 (TTY 1-800-325-0778) and request an appointment or find your local office and call for an appointment. See Resources.

Qualifying for Aide at home. If a disabled adult cannot perform activities of daily living (ADLs) such as showering, grooming, eating, using the toilet, they can qualify for Home and Community Based Services. In some cases, a family member may be paid to provide care in lieu of an aide. These services are state-based and vary widely depending on state where you live. The family member/caregiver must qualify financially, and depends on Medicaid status. For more information, you can contact your State's Center for Independent Living (CIL) or your local Intellectual/Developmental Disability (IDD) agency. Website: https://acl.gov/ or locate your state agencies, Website: https://dial.acl.gov/home

Comprehensive health insurance plans

The majority of states offer high-risk individuals, such as survivors, access to *comprehensive health insurance plans (CHIPs)*, also called *high-risk pools*, are a means for individuals to obtain insurance regardless of their physical condition or medical history.

> For more information about CHIPs, call your state insurance commissioner or department and check the following: https://www.hhs.gov/answers/medicare-and-medicaid/index.html
>
> Legal aid assistance: ask for pro bono (free) legal help. https://triagecancer.org/

If you have specific problems getting appropriate medical benefits under Medicaid, state health plans, or other public healthcare plans, a social worker at your treating hospital or survivorship program may be able to help. If your problems are of a legal nature, such as outright refusal of services or discrimination, talk to a disability attorney or call your state bar association and ask for its *pro bono* (free) legal help referral service.

Legal protection in obtaining health insurance

Before the ACA, although neither states nor the federal government mandated a legal right to insurance, there were some legal remedies to insurance discrimination.

COBRA. The Comprehensive Omnibus Budget Reconciliation Act (COBRA) is a federal law that requires public and private companies employing more than 20 workers to provide continuation of group coverage for 18 months to employees if they quit, are fired, or work reduced hours. Coverage must extend to surviving, divorced, or separated spouses, and to dependent children. You must pay for your continued coverage, but it must not exceed by more than 2 percent the rate set for your former co-workers. By allowing you to purchase continued coverage, you have time to seek other long-term coverage.

Some states require COBRA benefits from employers with fewer than 20 employees. Check with your State Insurance Department to see if your state has a *mini-COBRA* law.

> Maintaining continuous health insurance coverage is critical to prevent being locked out of healthcare due to pre-existing conditions.

If you are leaving a job that provides you with health insurance for one that does not, pursue a COBRA plan. These plans allow you to continue your coverage after leaving employment. You will pay the full rate, including the contribution previously made by your employer, but it will still be less than what you'd pay as an individual customer.

ERISA. The Employee Retirement and Income Security Act (ERISA) is a federal law that prohibits employers from discriminating against an employee for the purpose of preventing the employee from collecting benefits under an employee benefit plan. For example, an employer may violate ERISA by firing a cancer survivor to exclude him from a group health plan. ERISA also prohibits employers from encouraging a person with a cancer history to retire as a *disabled* employee. ERISA does not apply to job discrimination (e.g., denial of new job due to cancer history), discrimination that does not affect benefits, and employees whose compensation does not include benefits.

Health Insurance Portability and Accountability Act of 1996 (HIPAA, also known as the "Kennedy-Kassebaum law"). This law allows individuals to change to a new job without losing coverage if they have been insured for at least 12 months. It also prevents group health plans from denying coverage based on medical history, genetic information, or claims history, although insurers can still exclude those with specific diseases or conditions. It also increases portability if you change from a group to an individual plan.

- **Pension and Welfare Benefits Administration of the U.S. Department of Labor** This agency enforces laws related to COBRA, ERISA, and parts of HIPAA and ensures that disabled are entitled to receive healthcare (866) 487-2365 or 866-4-USA-DOL

  Website: https://www.dol.gov/agencies Go to: *Employee Benefits Security Administration (EBSA)*

- **Consult the Cancer Legal Resource Center (CLRC).** The CLRC provides free information and resources about cancer-related legal issues to cancer survivors, caregivers, healthcare professionals, employers, and others coping with cancer. Contact the national office at (866) 843-2572 or Disability Rights Legal Center: Website: https://thedrlc.org Scroll to: *cancer justice*

Canadian health insurance

The *Canada Health Act* ensures coverage for all Canadian citizens and non-citizens who require medically necessary (as defined by provincial and territorial health insurance plans) hospital and doctors' services. Healthcare regulations are the same nationwide, although providers can be hard to find in less-populated provinces. A wide variety of specialists is available through the Canadian health system. Many of the best are affiliated with university hospitals. Some services not covered under the *Canada Health Act* (e.g., drugs prescribed outside hospitals, ambulance costs, and hearing, vision, dental care) may be funded by supplementary benefits from provinces and territories, by an employer-based group insurance, or by purchasing private insurance.

More information about Canadian healthcare coverage is available at: https://www.canada.ca/en/health-canada.html

FREE OR LOW-COST MEDICINE PROGRAMS IN THE UNITED STATES

Resource: https://www.needymeds.org/

Survivors often need expensive medications that they sometimes cannot afford. Most major drug companies have patient-assistance programs, and you can apply to obtain free or low-cost prescription drugs. Although each company has its own criteria for qualification, in general, you must meet the following criteria:

- Be a U.S. citizen or legal resident
- Have a prescription for the medication you are applying to get
- Have no prescription drug coverage for the medication or high premiums
- Meet income requirements or program eligibility

> Because the application process takes time and includes obtaining information from your physician, plan ahead so you do not run out of medication.

You may qualify even if you have health insurance, if it does not cover the medication prescribed to you. For expensive medications, the income cut-off is high, so it is worth investigating whether or not you qualify. Organizations that can help you find and apply to patient-assistance programs are listed in *Resources*.

JOBS AND WORKPLACE

The population of adults who have survived childhood cancer is growing at a rapid rate. There are an estimated 496,000 childhood cancer survivors in the United States (National Cancer Institute, 2020). Thousands of survivors are staying well, growing up, graduating from high school or college, and successfully entering the workforce. Survivors of childhood cancers are educators, sports figures, radio announcers, nurses, doctors, social workers, dancers, lawyers, receptionists, computer programmers, and workers of all types.

Work fulfills many needs for adults, including financial security, health insurance, and self-worth. Despite the high numbers of survivors, some still face job discrimination. Cancer survivors' right to work is better protected than ever before by federal and state laws that protect employment rights. However, a cancer history can still create barriers to finding, keeping, or changing jobs.

Interviews

Careful preparation for job applications and interviews can help you avoid job discrimination. Make an honest assessment of your skills and job history when deciding what job to apply for. A job counselor can help you prepare your résumé and practice interviewing skills. Apply only for jobs you are able to do, as employers have the right to reject you if you are not qualified for the job. If you have a choice, work for a company with a large diverse workforce, as there will be less likelihood of discrimination and it will be easier to obtain life and health insurance.

I have not experienced barriers in the workforce. In most cases, my coworkers did not know that I had childhood cancer, unless I told them. I am not ashamed of it, but I also don't want to announce it unless it makes a difference to the work I do. People at work who know I am a cancer survivor have been nothing but lovely to me about it.

When applying for jobs, I do typically mention my childhood cancer history, but I only when it is applicable. If the application asks for a personal statement, I usually mention it. If asked about dealing with a challenge or why I want to go into healthcare, I talk about my experience with cancer. It tends to really resonate with my interviewers. By not overly expressing my experience, I show that I am more than just a cancer survivor. But it does show I have experienced difficulties and am resilient when faced with a challenge.

I always struggle to answer the question on applications "Do you have a disability?" One of the disabilities listed is cancer, but I'm cured, so do I check "yes" or "no"? I'm still trying to navigate how I want to go about some of those things in my life.

Unless you have specific mental or physical limitations that affect your ability to perform certain types of work, your cancer history should have no bearing on your qualifications for the job. An employer who is covered by anti-discrimination laws such as the Americans with Disabilities Act (ADA) cannot refuse to hire you simply because you are a cancer survivor. Some employers are covered by neither federal nor state laws and therefore could discriminate against someone because of a cancer history. Knowing your rights and preparing strategies for your job interview can make the difference between getting hired or being rejected. The following are suggestions on how to conduct yourself in a job interview on the website for Cancer Nation (formerly National Coalition for Cancer Survivorship): https://canceradvocacy.org

- ***Do not volunteer information about your cancer history.*** Employers have the right only to determine if you are capable of performing the job. They do *not* have the right to ask about personal or confidential information during an interview.

- Under the ADA, employers cannot ask about medical history, require you to take a medical exam, or ask for medical records unless they have made a job offer.

- ***Do not lie on a job application or during an interview.*** You can be fired later if your dishonesty is uncovered. Instead, answer only the specific questions asked. Try to steer the conversation toward your current ability to do the job, rather than explaining your past.

Job discrimination

Job discrimination can spell economic catastrophe for cancer survivors because most health insurance is obtained from employment. Under federal law and many state laws, an employer who is covered by the relevant law cannot treat a survivor differently from other employees because of a history of cancer except in certain circumstances involving health, life, and disability insurance. A guide to U.S. disability rights laws can be found at www.ada.gov/cguide.htm.

Americans with disabilities act

The ADA prohibits many types of job discrimination by employers, employment agencies, state and local governments, and labor unions. In addition, most states have laws that prohibit discrimination based on disabilities, although what these laws cover varies widely. The ADA prohibits discrimination based on actual disability, perceived disability, or history of a disability. Any employer with 15 or more workers is covered by the ADA.

The ADA requires that:

- Employers cannot make medical inquiries of an applicant, unless one of the following situations applies:
  - Applicant has a visible disability, such as amputation.
  - Applicant has voluntarily disclosed cancer history.
- Such questions are limited to asking the applicant to describe or demonstrate how he would perform essential job functions. Medical inquiries are allowed after a job offer has been made or during a pre-employment medical exam.
- Employers provide *reasonable accommodations*, unless it causes undue hardship. An accommodation is a change in duties or work hours to help employees during or after cancer treatment. An employer *is not required* to make these changes if the changes are very costly, disruptive, or unsafe.
- Employers cannot discriminate because of family illness. For instance, if an employee has a child who has cancer, the employer cannot treat the employee differently thinking that the employee might miss work or file expensive health insurance claims.
- If employers offer healthcare, they must offer healthcare fairly to all employees. However, employers are not required to provide health insurance.

In Canada, the Canadian Human Rights Act provides essentially the same rights as the ADA. The act is administered by the Canadian Human Rights Commission. See Resources at the end of the chapter.

The Federal Rehabilitation Act

The *Federal Rehabilitation Act* bans public employers and private employers that receive public funds from discriminating on the basis of disability. The following employees are not covered by the ADA, but are governed by the Rehabilitation Act:

- Employees of the executive branch of the federal government (Section 501 of the Rehabilitation Act)

- Employees of employers who receive federal contracts and have fewer than 15 workers (Section 503 of the Rehabilitation Act)
- Employees of employers who receive federal financial assistance and have fewer than 15 workers (Section 504 of the Rehabilitation Act)

If you are a federal employee (Section 501), you must file a claim within 30 days of the job action against you. If you are an employee whose employer has a federal contract (Section 503), you must file a complaint within 180 days with your local office of the U.S. Department of Labor, Office of Federal Contract Compliance Programs. If your employer receives federal funds (Section 504), you have up to 180 days to file a complaint with the federal agency that provided funds to your employer, or you can file a law-suit in a federal court.

The federal Rehabilitation Act is enforced by the Civil Rights Division of the US Department of Justice. See Resources under Civil Rights Division for website and contact information.

Family and Medical Leave Act

The Family and Medical Leave Act (FMLA) is a federal law that entitles eligible employees of covered employers to take unpaid, job-protected leave for specified family and medical reasons with continuation of group health insurance coverage under the same terms and conditions as if the employee had not taken leave. Reasons for leave include: caring for a seriously ill child caring for another family member who is seriously ill, when employee is unable to work because of his/her own medical condition, or birth or adoption of a child or foster care placement. An employee must have worked 25 hours per week for 1 year to be covered. Some states offer paid family leave. For more details about those eligible and conditions, see Resources at the end of the chapter for website of *Office of Disability Employment Policy (ODEP)*.

The FMLA conditions:

- Applies to employers with 50+ employees within a 75-mile radius.
- Applies to employees who have been employed for 12 months and worked 1250 hours in a 12-month period

- Provides *12* weeks of unpaid leave during any 12-month period to care for serious illness of self, spouse, child, or parent. In certain instances, the employee may take intermittent leave, such as reducing normal work hours.
- Requires employers to continue to provide benefits, including health insurance, during the leave period.
- Allows leave when a health condition renders an employee unable to perform the functions of the position.
- Requires employees to make reasonable efforts to schedule leave so as *not* to disrupt the workplace.
- Requires employers to return employee to the same or equivalent job position upon return from the leave. Some benefits, such as seniority, need not accrue during periods of unpaid FMLA leave.
- Requires employees to give 30-day notice of the need to take FMLA leave when the need is foreseeable.
- Any qualifying exigency arising out of the fact that the employee's spouse, son, daughter, or parent is a covered military member on "covered active duty;"
- Twenty-six work weeks of leave during a single 12-month period to care for a covered servicemember with a serious injury or illness if the eligible employee is the servicemember's spouse, son, daughter, parent, or next of kin (military caregiver leave).
- You have up to 2 years to file an FMLA complaint or a lawsuit.

FMLA is enforced by complaints to the Employment Standards Administration, Wage and Hour Division, U.S. Department of Labor, or by private lawsuit. For more information and contact information, see *Resources* at the end of the chapter.

State laws regarding discrimination

The District of Columbia and almost all states have laws banning discrimination against people with disabilities. The type of protection varies from state to state. For information about your state laws, contact the state agency that enforces employment rights, the local bar association, the National Coalition for Cancer Survivorship, or your state chapter of the American Cancer Society. To file a complaint under state law, contact your state civil rights or human rights commission. See Website: https://www.eeoc.gov, Search, *filing charge discrimination*

Changing jobs

Survivors are often reluctant to change jobs because of fear of losing insurance for themselves and their families. A cancer history requires lifelong medical surveillance that may be impossible to finance without insurance. Survivors often stay in unsatisfying jobs that offer health insurance because they cannot risk losing health insurance if they take a better job. This is sometimes called *job lock*. Parents of young survivors also face the same dilemma. There will be a bigger safety net under the Patient Protection and Affordable Care Act (ACA). Despite many of the positive impacts on insurability and healthcare among childhood cancer survivors, the ACA has not provided health care affordability as it was planned (Fiala, 2021). Still, staying in a job with better coverage may continue to be a real issue.

Armed services, police and fire department personnel

Some survivors of childhood cancer may want to enlist in the Armed Services including the Reserve Officers' Training Corps (ROTC), the Reserves, or the service academies or work for a police or fire department. Applications from survivors for the Armed Services are considered on a case-by-case basis, and you may be eligible for a medical waiver to obtain admission.

Applicants are asked to provide information about their disease, treatment, and current health status. The recruiter should also be given the results from a recent medical examination and articles from the latest medical literature. If you are granted a waiver, you must still meet the physical requirements for the position sought.

Childhood cancer survivors interested in applying for training or jobs in police and fire departments will need to check their local department's standards for physical requirements. Generally, one's current physical condition is what matters, and employers cannot ask about health history until they have made a conditional job offer.

ADVOCACY

Cancer is a life-transforming experience. After treatment ends, many survivors want to contribute or give back to the cancer community. No matter what your education, experience, or time restrictions, there is much you can contribute to others if you choose to advocate.

Survivors and their families have the potential to effect individual, institutional, and social change. Advocacy means using the things learned from your personal experience and joining with other survivors to help change the laws and healthcare rights/regulations to provide you or other survivors what you need to live the healthiest life possible. Sometimes this consists of educating health professionals, politicians, or society at large. It can mean setting up a peer support network, whether it consists of two survivors who meet for coffee once a week or an organization with thousands of members. It can take a little time or become a focal point of your life.

It is hard for our daughter to fathom the reality and responsibility of being a cancer survivor. She was diagnosed at just three years old. As her parents, we have tried to take on as much as we can so as to not burden her as she continues her cancer journey. Even when treatment is over, though, it is never fully "over." Our journey was never easy, but we are forever grateful that our daughter is in remission.

We now feel that we have a responsibility to educate people about the facts of childhood cancer. It isn't that rare, but people sometimes do not understand much about it or don't want to think about it because it is such an unpleasant topic. Whether it is spreading the word that childhood cancer research is underfunded, volunteering at an event, or educating people about childhood cancer, we strive to give back as well as educate others. Our advice to all going through this awful journey - know you are not alone, everyone's journey is different, and never, ever give up hope.

I had acute lymphoblastic leukemia and was treated from the age of four to six years, from 2004 to 2006. My treatment began at the same time that *Alex's Lemonade Stand Foundation* was establishing itself as an official 501(c)(3) non-profit. I visited multiple lemonade stands during my treatment, and have felt very connected to the foundation over the years having supported many fundraisers. I always stop when I see a lemonade stand and am happy to support such an important mission.

We are now grateful for every tiny thing in life. We also cherish our precious time together, as we have stood at the edge, looked over, and seen how life could be without our beloved daughter. We always set aside time for family dinners, family events, and simply talking with each other. We also realize how vital it is to advocate for children with cancer -- whether it is giving back to all of the organizations that helped us survive, volunteering, or spreading the word that childhood cancer is not rare and that research is severely underfunded.

I want to express my appreciation for *Alex's Lemonade Stand Foundation*. ALSF stands for everything I stand for. As a survivor, it really helps to know that there are non-profit organizations like ALSF whose sole motivation is to help cancer patients, cancer survivors, and their families and make treatments safer. It is reassuring to know that there are organizations who don't care about the money aspect and just care about helping people.

Individual advocacy

Individual advocacy means being able to stick up for yourself in order to get what you need for the rest of your life. You need to learn how to work within the system to get the best healthcare, an appropriate education, and a job without discrimination based on your cancer history.

Obtain detailed medical records of your cancer treatment. The first step in being the best advocate for you or your child, is to obtain the medical details of your/your child's cancer history and treatment, and educate yourself about the risks and possible late-effects to expect from that type of treatment, continuous tests and monitoring that is necessary, and where to access these resources.

Unfortunately, I am one of many survivors who has to deal with long-term severe and permanent medical effects. During the time leading up to my diagnosis at age 9 until today, my parents allowed me to give my opinions and advocate for myself. I am extremely fortunate and thankful and urge any parent whose child is facing challenges similar to mine to do the same. Having to make decisions that would impact me not just in the moment but my whole life really forced me to grow up. Some may see this as tragic, but having that autonomy and self-awareness at a young age has been critical for my self-advocacy and my medical journey as a teenager and young adult.

Because knowledge and studies regarding late-effects of treatment and cancer survivorship are growing daily, you should be seen at least yearly by a healthcare provider (preferably in a survivorship clinic) who keeps updated on the latest studies, research and information or by a provider who is in close communication with a survivorship expert. You should remain active in your follow-up care, especially since other symptoms may develop over time.

It can be a heavy load to be an advocate in the healthcare system, school, and community. However, much satisfaction can result. The following is a list of activities you and/or your family can do to advocate for improvements.

Advocacy Activities:

- Obtain copies of your records and/or treatment summary in order to advocate for your future healthcare.
- Work with the school to get your child an IEP or 504 Plan to get the best possible education.

It is helpful to have your own record of the types of treatments and/or surgeries and dates. Request a copy of your cancer treatment summary and medical history from your survivorship or treatment provider. See example of Cancer Treatment Summary by Children's Oncology Group:

Website: https://www.survivorshipguidelines.org

From the beginning, we've had to advocate for proper accommodations at school for my daughter. When anyone sees brain tumor, they assume so many things; other times teachers see she had cancer so long ago that they assume everything is okay. She has also had to learn to advocate for herself. And since this has been her entire life—she's pretty good at it. She's taken the lead on researching services at college—and I hope she continues to be the fierce self-advocate she has been in high school.

- Register with the office for students with disabilities at the college or university.
- Challenge rules that restrict the options of survivors.
- Volunteer to staff a local organization's cancer information line.
- Start a support group in your community or hospital.
- Talk to local civic groups about your experience.
- Write letters to newspapers, magazines, or politicians about survivorship issues.
- Share your experience with the media or legislatures to help shape public opinion or policies about cancer.
- Become a counselor at a camp for children with cancer.
- Offer to be a support person for newly diagnosed families.
- Join or start committees to effect changes at your hospital.
- Donate to groups that lobby for survivors.
- Help fundraise to start or sustain a comprehensive follow-up clinic.
- Participate in follow-up studies that may be available through a comprehensive follow-up clinic. Information from these studies can have impact through publications, media attention, and public policy change.
- Tell your friends and family your feelings about your cancer journey.

Advocacy is not for everyone. Sometimes survivors just want to carry on with their lives. Over time, you may have greater or lesser interest in your cancer history.

Group advocacy and networking

Networking with other survivors and advocating for change will help survivors following in your footsteps. *Group advocacy* can be very effective in encouraging and creating change at the community, state, or national levels. Issues that can be addressed are national funding (e.g., increased monies needed for late effects research), institutional funding (e.g., starting and supporting comprehensive follow-up clinics), political changes (e.g., improving anti-discrimination laws), federal and state programs (e.g., improving insurance options for survivors), and hundreds of others.

Group advocacy opportunities. The following are some of the ways for groups to effect changes.

- Start an online support group.
- Organize a conference at a treating facility to educate caregivers about survivorship issues.
- Lobby an institution to provide comprehensive services for survivors.
- Attend local, state, or national gatherings of survivors.
- Encourage family and friends to create or join committees that work for survivor issues.

REFERENCES

Fiala MA. (2021) Disparities in health care affordability among childhood cancer survivors persist following the Affordable Care Act. Pediatr Blood Cancer. (2021) Dec;68(12): e29370. doi: 10.1002/pbc.29370. Epub 2021 Oct 9. PMID: 34626446.

Long-Term Follow-Up Guidelines for Survivors of Childhood, Adolescent, and Young Adult Cancers, **Version 6.0 (October 2023)** http://www.survivorshipguidelines.org/

Mariotto B, et al. (2009). Long-term survivors of childhood cancers in the United States. *Cancer Epidemiol Biomarkers Prev*, 18(4): 1033–40.

Wolfson J, Ruccione K, Reaman GH. Health care reform 2010: expected favorable impact on childhood cancer patients and survivors. Cancer J. 2010 Nov-Dec;16(6):554-62. doi: 10.1097/PPO.0b013e3181feee83. PMID: 21131785.

Weiner SL, et al. (2010). Pediatric cancer: advocacy, insurance, education, and employment. In *Principles and Practice of Pediatric Oncology*, 1441–1450. In Pizzo PA and Poplack DG, (Eds.), Philadelphia, PA: Lippincott, Williams & Wilkins. Philadelphia, PA.

RESOURCES

Website: ccgresources.org

All resources and references mentioned in this book are available on
the website and will be routinely reviewed and updated.

Alex's Lemonade Stand Foundation

Website: www.alexslemonade.org

Search, *childhood cancer families*

Alex's Lemonade Stand Foundation (ALSF) is changing the lives
of children with cancer by funding impactful research, raising
awareness, supporting families, and empowering everyone to help
cure childhood cancer. ALSF offers many programs and tools to
help families navigate the challenges of childhood cancer.

Federal Social Security Administration (SSA)

Phone: 1-800-772-1213 (TTY 1-800-325-0778)

To find your local office:

Website: https://www.ssa.gov/locator

Help obtaining adequate insurance

Website: https://triagecancer.org

Search, *state laws*

**Passport for Care, Survivor Care Plans by Children's
Oncology Group (V6, Nov 2023)**

Website: https://cancersurvivor.passportforcare.org

Survivors and family can find online updated tailored long-term
care plans which should be reviewed with their oncologist or
health care provider.

DISABILITIES AND EDUCATION

Administration of Community Living (ACL)

The Administration for Community Living was created around
the fundamental principle that older adults and people of all ages
with disabilities should be able to live where they choose, with
the people they choose, and with the ability to participate fully in
their communities.

Website: https://acl.gov/

Locate your state agencies:

Website: https://dial.acl.gov/home

Advocacy Institute
   Website: https://www.advocacyinstitute.org/
   To file a complaint if you feel your home state is denying or an
   inadequate response for rehabilitative services/accommodations.
   Also find **IDEA** (Individuals with Disabilities Education Act)

American Childhood Cancer Organization
   Website: www.acco.org
   Search for: *IEP, Education issues,*
   For free download of book: *Educating the Child With Cancer,
   A Guide for Parents and Teachers, 3rd ed.* Edited by Ruth I.
   Hoffman, MPH; ACCO books and resources: Search, *Digital
   library*

American Disabilities Act
   Website: https://www.ada.gov/resources/
   Search, *Disability rights guide*
   Phone: (800) 514-0301

Cancer Nation (formerly the *National Coalition for Cancer
Survivorship*)
   Website: https://canceradvocacy.org
   Founded by and for cancer survivors, our mission is to offer
   resources and guidelines for navigating survivorship and to advo-
   cate for quality cancer care for all people touched by cancer.

Center for Parent Information & Resources (CPIR)
   Website: https://www.parentcenterhub.org
   The central hub of valuable information and products specifically
   designed for the network of Parent Centers serving families of
   children with disabilities.

Civil Rights Division, US Department of Justice
   Website: https://www.justice.gov/contact-us
   Search, *File a complaint*
   Phone: (202) 514-2000

Disability Rights Legal Center
   Website: https://www.thedrlc.org

Disabled Adult Child (DAC)
   Website: https://www.ssa.gov/benefits/disability
   Find your local office, call for an appointment:

Website: https://www.ssa.gov/locator
Phone: 1-800-772-1213 (TTY 1-800-325-0778)

FastWeb – college scholarships
Website: www.fastweb.com
An internet site that matches individual students with eligibility requirement for more than 1.3 million scholarships. It also contains a college directory of more than 4,000 schools with information about admissions, financial aid, and other topics.

Federal Student Aid Program
Website: https://studentaid.gov

Individuals with Disabilities Education Act (IDEA), US Department of Education
Website: https://sites.ed.gov/idea
Information and resources on infants, toddlers, children and youth with disabilities. Also access to Office of Special Education and Rehabilitation Services (OSERS) and Office of Special Education Programs (OSEP)

Learning Disabilities Association of America
Website: https://ldaamerica.org
When visiting colleges, ask to speak with Disabled Student Office

Northwestern Mutual Foundation College scholarships
To apply: https://news.northwesternmutual.com/
Program that offers college scholarships to survivors of childhood cancer opportunity to continue their education and pursue college dreams. Twenty-five $5,000 undergraduate awards given each academic year and renewable up to one year or until a bachelor's degree is earned which ever occurs earlier.

EMPLOYMENT RIGHTS AND BENEFITS
Employee Benefits Security Administration, US Department of Labor
Website: www.dol.gov/agencies/ebsa
Agency that enforces laws related to COBRA, ERISA and parts of HIPAA and ensures that disabled are entitled to receive healthcare. Phone: (866) 444-3272

Employee Retirement Income Security Act (ERISA)
U.S. Department of Labor, Washington, DC 20210
  Website: https://www.dol.gov
  Search, *retirement or workplace protection for individuals impacted by cancer*
  Phone: (866) 487-2365

Equal Employment Opportunity Commission (EEOC)
  www.hhs.gov/answers/medicare-and-medicaid
  call your state insurance department or commissioner
  Phone: (800) 669-4000
  To file a job discrimination lawsuit, all laws enforced by EEOC, except for the Equal Pay Act, require you to file a Charge of Discrimination with us
  https://www.eeoc.gov/filing-charge-discrimination

Family and Medical Leave Act
  Website: https://www.dol.gov/agencies/odep
  Search for: *employment-laws, medical and disability related leave*

Health Insurance Portability and Accountability Act of 1996 (HIPAA)
  Website: https://www.hhs.gov/hipaa
  This law allows individuals to change to a new job without losing coverage if they have been insured for at least 12 months.

Job Accommodation Network
  Website: www.askjan.org

Office of Disability Employment Policy,
US Department of Labor
  Website: https://www.dol.gov/agencies/odep
  For information about various work programs for disabled, including *Competitive Integrated Employment (CEI)*

Rehabilitation Services Administration,
US Department of Education, Office of Commissioner
  Office of Special Education and Rehabilitation Services
  Website: https://rsa.ed.gov
  400 Maryland Avenue SW, Washington, DC 20202-7100

HEALTH INSURANCE AND FINANCIAL ASSISTANCE

Free or low-cost medicine programs in the United States
Website: https://www.needymeds.org

Find your local SSA office:
Website: https://www.ssa.gov/locator/

Help obtaining adequate insurance
Website: https://triagecancer.org
Search, *state laws*

Medicaid
Website: https://triagecancer.org/state-laws/Medicaid
Find local SSA office https://www.ssa.gov/locator
Website: https://triagecancer.org/medicaid-cancer

Supplemental Security Income (SSI)
Website: http://www.triagehealth.org
Search: *quick guides, ssi*
Website: www.ssa.gov/apply/ssi
or call 1-800-772-1213

Savings Account for SSI recipients ABLE (Achieving a Better Life Experience)
Special savings account which allows SSI recipients to save above the $2,000 dollar earning limit and stay eligible for SSI and other benefits.
Website: https://www.ablenrc.org
Website: https://www.ssa.gov/benefits/disability

Canadian Healthcare Coverage
Website: www.canada.ca/en/health-canada.html
Search for: *cancer survivors, disability benefits*, or *health-related video gallery*
Email: hcinfo.infosc@canada.ca
Phone: 613-957-2991 or Toll free: 1-866-225-0709

Canadian Human Rights Commission
Website: www.chrc-ccdp.gc.ca
Search. *Resources, Forms*
Phone: (613) 995-1151

GLOSSARY

advocacy, using your personal experiences as a cancer survivor and joining with other survivors to help change the laws and health-care rights/regulations to provide you and other survivors what you need to live the healthiest and most satisfying life possible

504 Plan, special educational accommodations outlined in Section 504 of the Federal Rehabilitation Act (1973) to address the needs of children who do not meet the full criteria of "disabled"

Americans with Disabilities Act, federal law that prohibits many types of job discrimination by employers, employment agencies, state and local governments, and labor unions based on an individual's actual disability, perceived disability, or history of a disability. In addition, most states have laws that prohibit discrimination based on disabilities, although what these laws cover varies widely. Any employer with 15 or more workers is covered by the ADA

Family and Medical Leave Act (FMLA), protects the job security of workers in large companies who must take a leave of absence to care for a seriously ill child, medical leave when the employee is unable to work due to his/her own medical condition, or for the birth or placement of a child for adoption or foster care

Comprehensive Omnibus Budget Reconciliation Act (COBRA), a federal law that requires public and private companies employing more than 20 workers to provide continuation of group coverage for 18 months to employees if they quit, are fired, or work reduced hours

Canada Health Act ensures coverage for all Canadian citizens and non-citizens who require medically necessary (as defined by provincial and territorial health insurance plans) hospital and doctors' services

cancer predisposition syndromes (CPS), a group of inherited genetic disorders that increase an individual's risk of developing certain types of cancer. These syndromes are caused by mutations in specific genes, which can be passed down through generations, leading to a higher likelihood of cancer occurrence in affected families.

age of majority, the age at which a person is granted by law the rights and responsibilities of an adult; full age

comprehensive health insurance plans (CHIPs), insurance plans offered by the majority of states to individuals at high risk because of their physical condition or medical history

Employee Retirement and Income Security Act (ERISA), a federal law that prohibits employers from discriminating against an employee for the purpose of preventing the employee from collecting benefits under an employee benefit plan

job coach, a person who helps those with disabilities adjust to a new workplace, learn work skills and rules/regulations, and how to handle workplace environment and stress

fundamental justice, the term used in Canadian legal system that means the same as *due process* in the US legal that insures all citizens are entitled to the same treatment by law

group health insurance policy, a policy that provides lower rates because of the large pool of employees, these policies offered by large corporations or government agencies

General Educational Development (GED), a high school equivalency program by which a student receives a GED diploma by passing 4 subject areas tests in language arts, math, social studies and science. Passing these four tests demonstrates the student has the same knowledge as a student attending 4 years of high school.

group health insurance policy, policy that provide lower rates because of the large pool of employees, these policies offered by large corporations or government agencies

Health Insurance Marketplace Exchange, health plan shopping and enrollment services through websites by which families or individuals can compare policies online and buy individual health insurance plans

Health Insurance Portability and Accountability Act of 1996 (HIPAA) also known as the *Kennedy-Kassebaum law*, allows individuals to change to a new job without losing coverage if they have been insured for at least 12 months

independent mediator or hearing officer, a third party to settle disagreements between parents and school representative

individual education plan (IEP), a special educational plan for a physically or cognitively disabled child that is agreed upon between parents and the school system to assure that the student will be taught the same things as other students: reading, writing, mathematics, science, history, and other preparation for college or vocational training. The plan is in writing and approved/signed by both the parents and the educators and specifically states what, how and when the student will be taught and all specialized services—such as small classes, home schooling, speech therapy, physical therapy, counseling, and instruction by special education teachers.

IEP diploma, a high school diploma that demonstrates the student has completed all of the objectives set out in his IEP for graduation

job lock, survivors feeling trapped in a job and not changing jobs for fear of losing healthcare benefits for themselves and families

job coach, a person who helps a person learn work skills, rules/regulations, and how to handle workplace stresses. In some cases, the job coach may accompany the survivor on the job for a period of time or only make periodic visits to see how the survivor is getting along and resolve any problems.

late effects, physical, psychological or social problems/issues that arise after treatment and cure of cancer as a result of the treatment received and can be immediate or develop/occur years after treatment completed

limited conservatorship, a court proceeding where a judge gives a responsible person, called a (limited conservator), certain rights to care for another adult who has a developmental disability. A limited conservatorship is specifically tailored to the individual's developmental disability and grants only specific powers to the conservator, preserving as many rights for the conservatee as possible.

Medicaid, a joint federal/state insurance program that covers approximately 36 million individuals, including children, the aged, blind, and/or disabled, and people who are eligible to receive federally assisted income maintenance payments like Supplemental Security Income (SSI). The federal government administers the program through the Department of Health and Human Services. Each state has an agency that administers Medicaid in that state (sometimes called the Department of Social Services or the Department of Public Welfare)

Patient Protection and Affordable Care Act (ACA) of 2010, is a comprehensive health care reform law enacted in March 2010 designed to achieve near universal, affordable health coverage. The law's provisions create premium and cost-sharing subsidies, give new rules for the health insurance industry, create a new system for buying health insurance plans, and protect survivors from detrimental insurance industry practices, such as denying coverage due to a preexisting health condition.

pro bono, free legal aid

sheltered workshop*,* jobs that are in segregated facilities where disabled people go to work for very low sub-minimum wages (e.g., sorting recyclables, light assembly work) and are meant to be temporary workplaces that prepare them for finding and working regular jobs

survivorship program or clinic, a program designed to provide long-term, multidisciplinary follow-up of successfully treated patients at the original treatment center or by a team of healthcare professionals who are familiar with the potential late effects of treatment for childhood cancer. Teams include a nurse coordinator, pediatric oncologist, nurse practitioner, social worker, and psychologist. The team has a close working relationship with specialists such as cardiologists, endocrinologists, orthopedic surgeons, and other specialists whose services are needed by some survivors.

survivorship, the point in life when your cancer treatment ends and the journey into the future begins

survivorship visits*,* annual or more frequent visits to your team of healthcare professionals that are familiar with your medical history and cancer treatment and potential late effects of treatment and help monitor your health and well-being and help with any issues/concerns you might have

supported placement employment*,* provides people with severe disabilities the appropriate, ongoing support necessary for success in a competitive work environment. These are jobs within the community such as grocery clerks, office helpers, and factory workers. Often the survivor works with a *job coach* for a period of time.

special education advocate*,* person with special training and expertise in helping to get appropriate education services for children with special needs and who attends all meetings and give advice about legally mandated services and how to obtain them

transition-to-work services, services or training that help adults with disabilities transition from school into the job force such as teaching skills needed for interviews, filling out applications, money management etc.

5
Staying Healthy

LISA BASHORE, PhD, APRN, CPNP-PC, CPON

Science is organized knowledge. Wisdom is organized life.
— *Immanuel Kant*

HEALTHY HABITS OR WHAT we call *lifestyle choices* including regular medical care can keep you healthy and potentially decrease the impact or even prevent you from developing late effects of cancer treatment. Adult cancers are often linked to *lifestyle choices*, and you have control over lifestyles choices you make that keep you healthy. The most important ones include:

- Eat a healthy diet
- Engage in physical activity (exercise)
- Maintain a healthy body weight (not too thin or overweight)
- Do not smoke or vape
- Avoid alcohol
- Attend all recommended follow-up healthcare examinations and testing
- Update childhood vaccines missed during treatment or re-immunizations needed after radiation or chemotherapy according to Centers for Disease Control guidelines (www.cdc.gov/vaccines); including Human Papillomavirus (HPV) vaccine to avoid related cancers to HPV (www.cdc.gov/hpv).

Getting regular healthcare exams from your physician who knows your cancer history and receiving early treatment for any *late-effects of your cancer* is crucial to maintaining your health.

Other choices not related to cancer risk but help keep one healthy and safe are: wearing bike or motorcycle helmets, wearing seat belts, calling a cab (or other paid driver) instead of getting into a car with a drunk driver, not texting while driving, and practicing safe sex (abstain from sex or use condoms).

Some aspects of life you may have little or no control (such as the genes you inherited from your parents), but healthy life-style choices are under your control. This chapter focuses on health-protective choices such as medical follow-up, diet, and exercise and *health-risk behaviors* such as overexposure to sun, smoking, drinking alcohol, and exposure to sexually-transmitted illnesses.

HEALTHCARE FOLLOW-UP AND TESTING

With the increasing numbers of long-term childhood cancer survivors today, it is apparent that young survivors often face medical and psychosocial late effects from years of treatment and the importance of long-term follow-up. Many institutions now have long-term follow-up or survivorship-focused clinics to provide a multidisciplinary team to follow-up and support survivors throughout their life.

Doctors, researchers, nurse practitioners, and psychologists are learning more about the late effects from treatment for childhood cancer, although there are still many unknown areas. Recommendations for your follow-up care will change continuously as more is learned about late effects. It is very important to keep in touch with a center that specializes in follow-up care.

Request copy of your cancer treatment summary and medical records

The first step to ensure you receive good follow-up care is to request from the oncologist or clinical nurse practitioner who treated you a written summary of your treatment and the complications that occurred during treatment. This permanent record will provide all future healthcare providers with your complete health history and cancer treatment in order to work with you to maximize your health. Download a copy of Comprehensive Cancer Treatment form used by the Children's Oncology Group (see Resources for website) and have your cancer treatment team fill out all the information that includes: the name of the disease, date of diagnosis, all treatments and surgeries, place of treatments, total dosages of drugs, amounts of radiation, and necessary follow-up.

Survivors should keep copies of their medical records in their possession. Most hospitals have *electronic medical records (EMR)* systems and you can gain access to your treatment summary. However, request a paper copy of your treatment summary before you leave that institution or at your first survivorship visit. It is very important to keep your own copy of your treatment summary and medical record (including all scans/MRIs) in your possession. Gaining access to your records at institutions years after treatment for cancer can be difficult, especially if you relocate to another medical institution, **so request copies soon after treatment.**

Choose a healthcare provider and schedule yearly follow-up visits

The second step is to pick a healthcare provider. Refer to the information in *Chapter 1, Survivorship*, which will help you to select an appropriate healthcare provider. You should regularly schedule and attend follow-up care visits, usually yearly, unless other symptoms or problems occur.

A few different medical effects have continued to impact me during the 15 years since treatment ended. I have dealt with paralyzed toes, heart issues, and memory problems. A former athlete and someone who tries to stay in relatively good shape, I have been advised to lift no more than 50 pounds when training so as to not strain my heart too much.

I have already experienced some late medical effects of treatment. That has been hard and discouraging because I want to be done with being sick; somehow though it creeps back into my life even though I've finished treatment. It's both mentally and physically challenging. Something that has helped me is to be open with doctors and continue to get checked routinely to ensure the best possible health outcomes.

Yearly medical care should include the following:

- Physical examination
- Complete blood count (CBC)
- Kidney and liver function test
- Recommended immunizations (chemotherapy and radiation can render prior immunizations ineffective, so ask your health care provider to update any vaccines recommended by the CDC guidelines (see Resources for website).
- Manual breast examination for women
- Testicular examination for men
- Screening tests (e.g., mammogram, stool check) as recommended by your healthcare provider based on your unique treatment history

Other medical tests you will need for follow-up depend on the treatment you received for your cancer. You and your healthcare provider can refer to an important resource: the *Children's Oncology Group Long-Term Follow-Up Guidelines for Survivors of Childhood, Adolescent, and Young Adult Cancers* (V 6.0, 2023) (see Resources for website). This resource allows you/your healthcare team to check your specific type of treatment and determine which tests may be necessary in the future. Your provider and healthcare team can help interpret this information. The Guidelines also contain patient-focused education.

Lifelong long-term survivorship-focused follow up visits

You can protect your good health by getting regular examinations from health providers experienced or educated in treating the late-effects of childhood cancer. These experts can inform you of your risk of potential late-effects and what you might expect in years to come. They will inform you of appropriate tests to ensure early detection and intervention if a late effect occurs. Delayed effects from treatment occur in only some survivors and range from mild to severe to even life-threatening. Many of these effects are easy to detect and treat, but may occur many years after treatment, so you need lifelong long-term survivorship-focused follow up visits.

Many survivors do not receive follow-up care from experts in the late-effects of childhood cancer. This information is vital to your future health and well-being. When you leave home to work or attend college, you will begin to make your own medical decisions and you need to be informed. You may not know the specific type of treatments you received or what medical surveillance you need to check for possible late-effects. You may think the chances of developing problems or late-effects are so slight that you just don't want to think about it. You should consult an expert and educate yourself about the type of cancer treatments you had and what to expect from possible late-effects.

See *Chapter 1 Survivorship*, the section, *How to create your own follow-up healthcare team*, for guidelines to help you select a health care provider in your area who is knowledgeable of survivorship and possible late effects, willing to review your treatment history, and develop your follow-up plan of care for regular visits and any recommended screenings/tests. *Passport for Care* (see Resources for website) is another useful resource to use with your healthcare provider to develop your follow-up care.

Many survivors (or their parents) take an active role in their own follow-up care. They search out follow-up programs in nearby or distant cities and travel to get the care they need. Today telehealth video or phone appointments are often available making it easy to chat with experts regarding any late-effects that develop.

> Since I'm an adult now, I have to contact my doctors myself instead of asking my parents to do it for me. It can be a bit intimidating to keep track of my records and information, but I know that my parents are still here to support me (even if they won't do things for me anymore).

Consulting an expert regarding late-effects after childhood cancer can help with the following information:

- Help with transitions from treatment to post-treatment and from child to adult care
- Screening and health promotion to help prevent and manage late effects
- Education and information needed to maintain health

HEALTHY DIET

The typical American diet contains more meat and processed (already prepared and sealed) foods, but few fruits and vegetables (plant-based foods). Eating a healthier diet can cut your risk of cancer and provide other benefits, such as more energy and lower weight. While genetics and the environment play a role, you control the rest. Eating a diet rich in fruits and vegetables and other plant-based foods that are low in fat, salt, and sugar is a good general health practice and may even prevent other cancers.

> In terms of my diet, I try to eat relatively healthy. I don't think my diet is overwhelmingly healthy, but I don't go overboard with junk food either. I think it is important to stay healthy as a cancer survivor.
>
> ———
>
> I am an extremely picky eater. I hardly eat any fruits or vegetables, eat very few snack foods, and drink mainly water. I think the pickiness is half from throwing up so much during chemo and half a symptom of my anxiety. I haven't been diagnosed with ARFID (avoidant-restrictive food intake disorder), but I think my anxiety functions the same way. It's very embarrassing to be an adult and a picky eater, so I've started to see a nutritionist. My issue is that I will actually get sick if I try eating something I don't like, so I am working with my nutritionist to try and introduce new, healthy food options and find ways to like foods that I have had issues with in the past. I don't over eat, but I would like to add healthier options to the list of foods.
>
> ———
>
> We definitely eat a lot healthier as a result of cancer. We limit our sugar intake and seek out healthy options. Fortunately, Mom is an incredible cook, and we hardly eat any fast food.

A healthy diet includes small portions of meat, fish, poultry, whole eggs (use egg whites or egg substitutes) and dairy products. Most of your meals should be made up of:

- Fruits and vegetables
- Whole grains
- Tubers such as potatoes, turnips, and sweet potatoes
- Legumes such as peas, beans (especially black beans), and lentils

Cancer prevention is not the only benefit of a healthy diet. Eating an abundance of fruits, vegetables, and grains may protect against stroke, high blood pressure, diabetes, and heart disease. Fiber from legumes and grains may help keep your cholesterol low and antioxidants contained in plants help prevent cataracts and other eye diseases.

If you are overweight or underweight, consider consulting a nutritionist. Most hospitals have a registered dietitian on staff, or you can ask to meet with one through your healthcare provider or follow-up clinic. If you combine the visit with an appointment in the hospital, your insurance may be more likely to cover the costs. If you are looking for a dietitian on your own, ask about credentials (usually a master's degree) and experience. Beware of anyone who tries to sell nutritional products during a consultation; you do not always know what is in them, and they may not be safe for you especially if they interfere with other medications you take.

Obesity is a possible late-effect from treatment for childhood cancer. To learn more about this, see *Chapter 18, Muscles and Bones*.

IMPORTANCE OF REGULAR EXERCISE

Many childhood cancer survivors are not engaging in physical activity levels at the recommended requirements for many reasons including fatigue, pain, and limitations in physical functioning. Regular daily exercise is very important for survivors' daily routine and helps you maintain overall health. It helps your heart work efficiently, helps your muscles and bones stay stronger, and keeps your brain more alert. It can also reduce depression. Briskly walking for 30 minutes a day can make remarkable changes in your health (Figure 5-1).

If you are at risk for heart problems or have physical limitations, exercise can make a big difference in your long-term health. Including physical activities into your life can help you stay healthier as well as feel better. One way to start exercising more is to use a pedometer or Fitbit tracker (devices that you strap on your leg, wrist, waistband, or access on a smartphone that measure distance you walk/jog/swim each day). This is a way to track how many steps you take every day; then you can set reasonable goals to increase the number

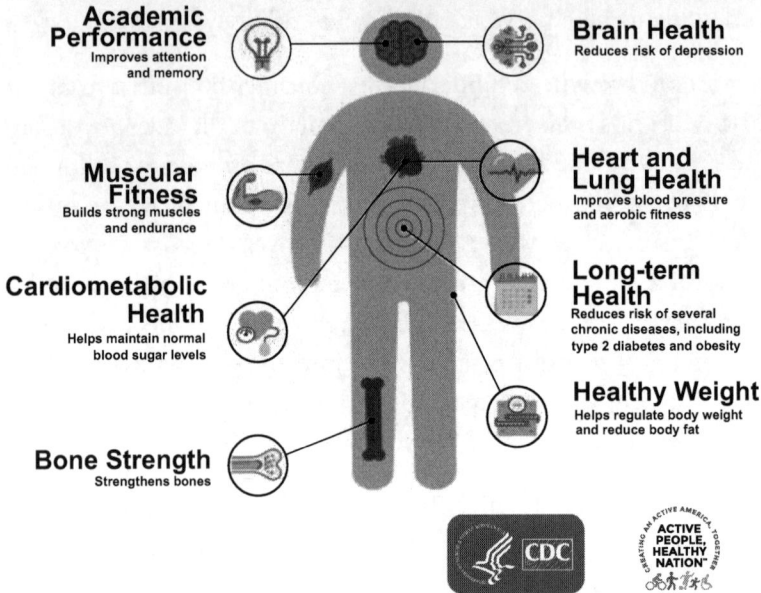

Health Benefits of Physical Activity

FOR CHILDREN

Academic Performance
Improves attention and memory

Brain Health
Reduces risk of depression

Muscular Fitness
Builds strong muscles and endurance

Heart and Lung Health
Improves blood pressure and aerobic fitness

Cardiometabolic Health
Helps maintain normal blood sugar levels

Long-term Health
Reduces risk of several chronic diseases, including type 2 diabetes and obesity

Healthy Weight
Helps regulate body weight and reduce body fat

Bone Strength
Strengthens bones

CDC

ACTIVE PEOPLE, HEALTHY NATION™

Source: Physical Activity Guide line for Americans, 2nd edition
To learn more, visit https//www.cdc.gov/physicalactivity/basics/adults/health-benefits-of-physical-activity-for-children.html   October 2021

FIGURE 5-1. Health benefits of physical activity for children. *Source*: Physical Activity Guidelines for Americans, 2nd edition, CDC; https://www.cdc.gov/physical-activity-basics/health-benefits/children.html

of steps each day. Before starting an exercise program, check with a healthcare provider experienced in follow-up for survivors of childhood cancer.

When choosing exercises, choose ones you enjoy. You are much more likely to stick with something fun. Exercising with a friend also helps make the time pass quickly and more enjoyable.

---

* The use/publication of figures/images in this book taken from the CDC website does not indicate endorsement or accuracy of content presented in this book by the CDC or US government. These images are considered in public domain and can be used for educational purposes in electronic and print media. Click the links below images which directs you to specific CDC webpages for more information.

For a year, I went through this whole health journey. I was working out all the time, I was all-in, and then I received an autoimmune disease diagnosis. Now that I am coming out of the depression, I realize the importance of taking care of myself. I really enjoy being active and need to incorporate working-out into my life again.

I tend to take care of my body about the same as anyone else would. I do at least one active thing a day, whether it is a walk, weightlifting, or some sort of sport; staying active is a part of my daily routine.

As a mother of a cancer survivor, I saw what my child went through and vowed if she survived and flourished, I would finally work on myself. During her treatment, I didn't care about myself. I was overweight, having heart issues, depressed, and my diabetes was out of control. One day during chemotherapy, I had to step out of the hospital room due to my heart palpitations. I told myself then and there that if our daughter survived this, I would get healthy not only to be there for her future, but to do it for ME. Three years later, I kept that promise. I lost 110 pounds and no longer take medicine for my diabetes. I work out, eat healthily, and am a much happier person. My cancer kid motivated me to keep going. She helped me realize that I need to stay healthy myself so I can always be there for my daughters. I think to myself, "Our daughter survived cancer as a child. My family survived the worst time of our lives. I can do hard things. I can keep going. I can make myself better. I can be healthy and be THERE for my daughters in all aspects of life."

RISKY BEHAVIORS

Cancer causes some young people to reprioritize their values. During their cancer treatment, they may have spent months or years avoiding crowds, forcing themselves to eat when they weren't hungry, and fighting for their lives. Some survivors lost friends to the disease and view engaging in risky behaviors as taking a chance with something very precious—one's life. Others may feel like they spent too much time being sick and separated from normal living and thus more inclined to engage in detrimental behaviors such as smoking (vaping), and excessive drinking or marijuana use.

Some people are cautious by nature and others are adventurous. Survivors of childhood cancer sometimes change their attitudes toward taking risks after treatment ends and begin to engage in risky behaviors and habits such as smoking (vaping), drinking alcohol, not exercising regularly, not eating healthy, and overall, not taking care of their health. This is taking a huge risk for their future health and well-being. The use of alcohol, tobacco, and marijuana can have lasting effects for childhood cancer survivors (Capelli C, Miller KA, Ritt-Olson A et al. 2021).

I am a cautious person. I don't take risks. I have had to work through my anxiety to be able to get things done. I didn't get my driver's license until I was 22 years old. I still have stress dreams about running through red lights or crashing my car, but I get up and drive every day because I know that it's a safe thing for me to do, and I wouldn't be doing something if it wasn't OK.

I prioritized doing things that made me feel alive —not the best things for my health. I was doing whatever made me feel good. I am a stallion in my brain trapped in a sick person's body. I used substances for a while during/after college. Not only was I going through cancer, but my whole family was going through it, so I was just living on the wild side.

I am definitely more likely to take risks. I have learned very early on in my life that life is short, and I am definitely more willing to go on adventures, especially trips. I think living in the moment is so important, and I try to always say "yes" to everything at least once. I may not like everything I try, but I won't know how I feel until I try it.

Risk of smoking/vaping

Smoking (which may include vaping) remains the most preventable cause of mortality in the United States. Smoking negatively affects all body organs including the heart, lungs, head and neck, and sexual function to name several. Engaging in smoking/vaping or the use of mood-altering drugs like marijuana may place survivors at increased risk for serious health problems, such as cancer and heart disease because of the treatments they received (https://www.cancer.org). See Resources for specific website.

Almost half a million people in the United States die each year from tobacco-related illnesses such as cancer of the lung, mouth, neck, esophagus, bladder, and pancreas. Another 16 million live with serious illness caused by smoking (https://www.cdc.gov/tobacco/index.html). Many adults no longer smoke or chew tobacco-containing products because of health warnings on packages, increased awareness of the dangers, and increased costs associated with these risk-taking behaviors.

One component of good follow-up care is education about the effects of tobacco use. Part of the discussion should focus on your increased risks of developing cancer after using tobacco. For instance, if you were treated with the drugs bleomycin, carmustine (BCNU), or lomustine (CCNU) and/or had chest radiation, you have an increased risk of lung problems. It is very dangerous to smoke if your lungs might already be damaged from these drugs or radiation. Smoking/vaping (including marijuana) and taking pills are also sometimes used as a self-medication for depression. If you think depression may be the reason you smoke, you need to get information, and seek treatment for the underlying depression from a licensed health provider.

Survivors of childhood cancer should not smoke or vape because of their risk of cardiac problems, premature emphysema, lung fibrosis (scarring), and increased risk for second cancers. But many survivors do smoke. This is not surprising that survivors smoke, given that more than a million adolescents and pre-adolescents start smoking every year (https://www.cancer.org/cancer).

E-cigarettes and other similar vaping devices

This is a quote of facts regarding e-cigarettes and other vaping devices from the American Cancer Society's research and study:

E-cigarettes and other types of 'vaping' devices are still fairly new, and more research is needed over a longer period of time to know what the long-term health effects may be. Research on these devices is complicated by the fact that many different devices are being sold, and many different chemicals can be used in them.

The most important points to know are that the long-term effects of e-cigarettes are still unknown, and all tobacco products, including e-cigarettes, can pose health risks to the user. For example, e-cigarettes can irritate the lungs and can have negative effects on the heart.

Learn about the dangers of smoking at the American Cancer Society website: www.cancer.org/cancer/risk-prevention/tobacco Search, *Health Risks of Smoking.*

If you don't smoke or vape, don't start. If you smoke or vape, try to stop.

By smoking/vaping, you may be causing more damage to your body than all of the surgeries, radiation, and chemotherapy you had to treat your cancer. The one thing you can do that will make the biggest difference in your health is to *stop smoking (including vaping)*. See Figure 5-2. Ask for help from your follow-up clinic or a healthcare provider.

You can find motivation and tips about how to stop smoking at www.smokefree.gov and in Resources at the end of this chapter. It is very important to remember that no matter how long you have smoked, you can always improve your health by stopping.

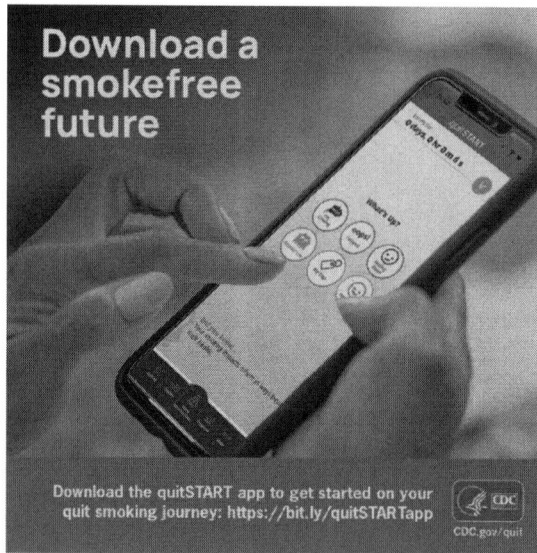

FIGURE 5-2. Download the quitSTART app to get started on your quit smoking journey. It can help you create a quit plan, find tips to help you quit smoking, manage cravings, and more! Website: https://bit.ly/quitSTARTapp

I don't smoke anything--cigarettes, weed, vapes, etc. It bothers me when people do, because I had friends who couldn't breathe at the end of their lives, and it seems so unfair. I will never smoke, and it would be a big red flag for a future friend or partner.

I don't drink alcohol. Health reasons are part of that, because I know that heart and liver health are affected by alcohol. I also just don't really like the taste of alcohol, in any form. I have a weird theory that I link the smell of alcohol to the hospital and the alcohol wipes before blood draws, so maybe that makes a difference. A big part is that I'm freaked out by the idea of being drunk and not being "in control" of my body. I think being a patient and not getting a say in what happens to your body had a big impact on me, so I'm scared at the thought of not being fully in control of what I do or say.

(Continued)

(Continued)

As a teenager and college student, I was involved with the smoking and drinking lifestyle for a while. It is something I am not proud of, but after doing research and getting advice from doctors, I have stopped smoking (vaping). It does feel like a weight lifted off my shoulders, knowing I am doing something to help myself and my overall health.

As an adult, I don't think my childhood cancer impacted my experience with alcohol at all. When I drink with friends that did not have cancer, I do not find that they are overly cautious around me or that I have issues "keeping up" with them. I'm just like any regular person, and cancer hasn't impacted this part of my life at all.

Risk of excessive alcohol

When used in moderation (one drink or less a day), alcohol can be part of a healthy life. Many adults enjoy a glass of wine with meals or with friends. However, alcohol is often abused causing both physical and emotional problems to survivors and their families.

Alcohol is a depressant that affects the central nervous system. Just two beers or drinks can impair coordination and thinking. Excessive drinking can cause liver damage and increase your risk of mouth and liver cancer. This number of drinks can also cause high blood pressure, stroke, decreased fertility, and miscarriages in women. If you drink at all while pregnant, your baby can be harmed. Drinking beer produces the same results as drinking wine or liquor. One beer contains the same amount of alcohol as a glass of wine or a shot (ounce) of hard liquor. *Binge drinking* (periods of excessive drinking followed by periods of no drinking, for example, drinking excessively only on weekends) is just as dangerous to your body as daily, heavy drinking. Binge drinking is especially prevalent in high schools and on college campuses. Rather than being swayed by peer pressure to engage in drinking parties or activities, avoid them altogether or think of strategies ahead of time to avoid excessive drinking. You could drink a soft drink at parties instead of alcohol or sip one weak to lower-containing alcoholic drink throughout the entire evening.

Although a daily glass of wine may slightly lower the risk of heart disease, there are better ways to accomplish this such as regular exercise, eating less fat, and maintaining a normal weight. Survivors of childhood cancer may already have damaged organs side-effects of radiation or chemotherapy treatments. Excessive alcohol can increase that damage. In addition, if you are infected with the hepatitis C virus, you should not drink any alcohol.

To get help for problem drinking, join Alcoholics Anonymous® (to find a meeting near you visit www.aa.org) and talk with your healthcare provider.

Sexually transmitted illnesses

As with all adolescents and young adults, cancer survivors should be counseled about safe sexual practices. Despite the many sexual messages in our culture, most adolescents are not well informed about the facts. Many survivors think, erroneously, that if they are infertile, there is no reason to use condoms. However, there are many diseases, some potentially fatal (e.g., hepatitis C, Acquired Immune Deficiency Syndrome [AIDS])) and some life-altering (e.g., genital herpes, genital warts, gonorrhea) that can be transmitted through sexual activity. Condoms can help prevent transmission of these diseases. Sexually transmitted illnesses can also reduce fertility.

> I always use sunscreen whenever outside. I certainly don't want to deal with something as preventable as skin cancer due to sun exposure. I take care of my skin and apply sunscreen when needed. I take this very seriously and believe everyone should, not just cancer survivors.
>
> ---
>
> I am very careful about sun exposure. I'm already very pale, so I would have used sunscreen even without my cancer history, but I'm especially diligent because I know the risks. I use SPF 50+ and reapply at least every 2 hours. I normally do get burned at least once a year, because I do burn so easily, but I've only had a handful of severe burns in my life.

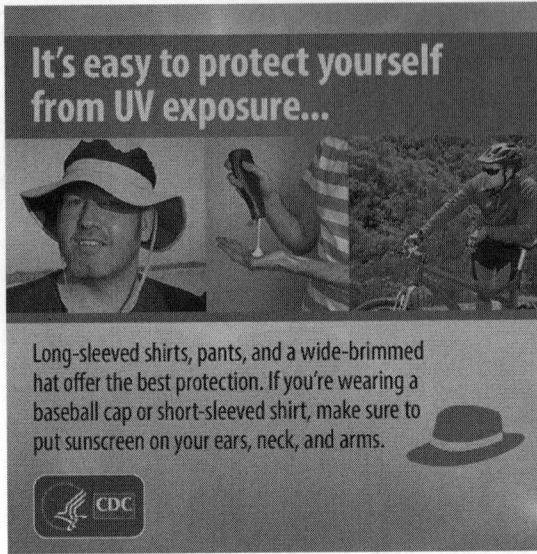

FIGURE 5-3. Use sunscreen of at least 30 SPF to protect yourself from damaging UV rays. *Source*: https://www.cdc.gov/cancer/features/skin-cancer.html

Sun exposure can cause skin cancer and cataracts

Skin cancer is very common, but the likelihood of getting it is somewhat under your control. Most skin cancers are caused by exposure to the sun. A lifetime of tans and burns increases your cancer risk and can also cause wrinkles and brown spots on your skin.

Hazards of overexposure to the sun include:

- **Skin cancer.** The risk of skin cancer increases the more your skin is exposed to sunlight or UV (ultraviolet) light from sun lamps, especially in areas that have been exposed to radiation. Most skin cancers can be removed, but many can be life-threatening if not diagnosed and treated early.
- **Sunburns.** These can occur to both skin and eyes.
- **Premature skin aging.** Years of overexposure to the sun can result in dry, wrinkled, and leathery skin.

---

*The use/publication of figures/images in this book taken from the CDC website does not indicate endorsement or accuracy of content presented in this book by the CDC or US government. These images are considered in public domain and can be used for educational purposes in electronic and print media. Click the links below images which directs you to specific CDC webpages for more information.

- **Cataracts.** The risk of developing cataracts is increased by long-term exposure to the sun's UVB (ultraviolet B) rays.

Skin cancer and sun protection

Those at highest risk for damage from the sun are people with fair skin, blond or red hair, and blue eyes. However, anyone can be damaged by too much exposure to the sun or to the lights used in tanning beds or booths. In addition, any skin that has been irradiated is at risk for developing skin cancer. You can prevent these problems by:

- Limiting the amount of time you are in the sun, especially during the middle of the day. The sun's rays are strongest between 10 am and 2 pm. If your shadow is shorter than you are, seek shade. Sun exposure at high altitudes and in places near the equator increases your exposure to harmful rays.
- Wearing sunscreen with an SPF (sun protective factor) of 30 or higher (American Academy of Dermatology, https://www.aad.org/media/stats-sunscreen). It should be applied at least 30 minutes before going outdoors and reapplied every 2 hours regularly throughout the day. (See Figure 5-3) Sunscreen must be worn on cool or cloudy days, especially if you are around snow, sand or water that reflect the sun's rays. If you have acne, use an alcohol-based and non-waterproof product.
- Covering your skin (especially areas that have been irradiated) with clothing, sunglasses, or hats
- Avoiding tanning beds or tanning booths which use ultraviolet A light that damages the skin.
- Some medicines, foods, and cosmetics may increase your sensitivity to sunlight.
- When you use sunscreen, you may not absorb enough vitamin D. It is a good idea to make sure you take a vitamin D supplement based on a registered dietitian consultation.

Monitor irradiated areas of skin and moles

Routinely check any areas of skin that were irradiated and ask someone else to check areas you can't see well, such as on your back. If you have numerous moles, see a dermatologist on a regular basis to monitor for any signs of possible cancer. If you develop any of the following symptoms, bring them immediately to the attention of your healthcare provider:

- A bump or mole that has different colors rather than being a uniform color
- A bump or mole that changes size or bleeds
- A bump or mole that is red or sore
- Any freckling or color changes in the skin

NURTURING YOUR BODY, MIND AND SPIRIT

The mind and body are intertwined. Many survivors were raised to be tough through treatment, to soldier on through difficult and painful experiences. Not releasing strong emotions can cause all sorts of physical and psychological (emotional) problems. It's simply not healthy to try to stuff uncomfortable feelings deep inside and not talk about it. As one survivor remarked, "It's like not taking the trash out. Pretty soon it starts to pile up and stink."

Survivors like other individuals need to identify stress, anxiety, and depression and get help if necessary. Many survivors use exercise, counseling, and mind-body activities to reduce their stress. Realizing one needs help and seeking help takes great courage and strength.

Some survivors find that writing about their feelings is very helpful, while others talk to loved ones, get comfort from their faith, or give back to the cancer community. Many start or join support groups for survivors of cancer. Certain periods of life after cancer are more difficult than others. Survivors are sometimes surprised when intense feelings surface years after treatment ends.

Although cancer may alter the lives of young survivors and their families, accepting what they went through and expressing their feelings about it allows them to move forward. Parts may be better and parts may be worse. It is certainly not what anyone in the family expected or wanted. But how one manages the future is the important thing. Finding meaning and purpose in the new, altered life and trying to live life to the fullest can bring satisfaction and fulfillment.

When finding ways to de-stress and care for myself, I find that reading, movies, writing, being active, and connecting with others are incredibly helpful. Reading and watching movies allow me to shut my brain off and just relax and enjoy the content in front of me. Before I go to bed, I put my phone away and read a chapter of a book to relax my eyes after staring at screens all day. I have recently taken up journaling which really helps center me and keep me focused throughout the day. I am a naturally active person, and find exercise especially cardio or lifting weights is a great way to focus on one activity and forget about all the other stressors in life. Lastly, I love spending time with my friends and loved ones. I think it is incredibly important to have a strong social life because my friends always allow me to be my truest self when I am around them.

I go to doctors and get bloodwork done annually to make sure I am still doing okay. I put more effort into avoiding things that could potentially cause cancer, and I put extra effort into trying to exercise and eat healthy. Reading books about cancer helped me to connect with my experience, and I have done a lot of journaling and writing over the years. Whenever possible, I try to connect with other survivors.

Our daughter developed many fears from cancer treatment. After treatment, we went as a family to a couple of retreats that were life-changing. They helped our daughter face these fears and try to conquer them. We strive to try new things and go on adventures, as there was a time we didn't think we would be able to do any of these things as a complete family again. Our daughter still works constantly on her mental health, but she also tries everything once because she knows some people do not get opportunities to begin again or to continue in the gift of life.

Now as a 26-year-old, I still regularly talk to my therapist and take prescribed medication for my anxiety and depression. Although a constant work-in-progress, I have made great improvements to my mental health and wellbeing. I now have the professional and personal support I need to continue this progress and to lean on if/when things get more severe. My parents, too, have made great strides in their respect understanding of

(Continued)

(Continued)

mental illness and are great supporters of the work I continue to do on my mental health.

I have felt it is pretty easy to network with other childhood cancer survivors. There are Facebook groups and online forums that are easily accessible. Additionally, the network I have from knowing people through treatment has been extraordinarily steady, and the people I have forged a bond with are some of my best friends today. Staying involved in things like camps for kids with cancer or other events where I can help as a survivor has led me to some incredible people who have made an impact on my life. From my experience, this brotherhood/sisterhood of survivors is a strong one, and the support system is truly second to none.

Participating with *Alex's Lemonade Stand Foundation*, raising funds and awareness for kids with cancer, I met loads of like-minded people who had been through similar experiences or were intimately connected with the cause in some other way. I'm fortunate now to have a career in nonprofit fundraising for cancer and found my way back to *Alex's Lemonade Stand* as a full-time employee. I couldn't be happier. As an adult, coworkers and employers also become a part of your support network.

Lastly, my parents were and continue to be my greatest support and champions. They have stuck by my side through it all, and I know they always will.

REFERENCES

American Cancer Society, www.cancer.org, https://www.cancer.org/cancer/risk-prevention/tobacco/health-risks-of-tobacco.html

Bradley KA, et al. (1998). Medical risks for women who drink alcohol. *Journal of General Internal Medicine,* 13(9): 627–39.

Capelli C, Miller KA, Ritt-Olson A, et al. (2021), Binge drinking, tobacco, and marijuana use among young adult childhood cancer survivors: a longitudinal study. *Journal of Pediatric Oncology Nursing, 38*(5), 285-294. https://doi.org/10.1177/10434542211011036

Children's Oncology Group Long-Term Follow-Up Guidelines for Survivors of Childhood, Adolescent, and Young Adult Cancers (version 6.0 October 2023). (COG LTFU Guidelines) www.survivorshipguidelines.org

Centers for Disease Control and Prevention (CDC) Website: www.cdc.gov/physical-activity/

Hollen PJ, Hobbie WL, et al. (2007). Substance use risk behaviors and decision-making skills among cancer-surviving adolescents. *J Pediatr Oncol Nurs*, 24(5): 264–73.

Stolley MR, et al. (2010) Diet and physical activity in childhood cancer survivors: a review of the literature. *Ann Behav Med*, 39(3): 232–49.

Tobacco Use: Targeting the nation's leading killer at a glance (2011) Retrieved April 21, 2012, from https://stacks.cdc.gov/view/cdc/5527

Wasserman AL, et al. (1987) The psychological status of survivors of childhood/adolescent Hodgkin's disease. *American Journal of Diseases of Children*, 141: 626–31

RESOURCES

Website: ccgresources.org

All resources and references mentioned in this book are available on the website and will be routinely reviewed and updated.

Children's Oncology Group (V6, 2023). *Long-Term Follow-Up Guidelines for Survivors of Childhood, Adolescent, and Young Adult Cancers*

Website: www.survivorshipguidelines.org

How to use this resource

This is a resource for healthcare professionals who provide ongoing care to survivors of pediatric malignancies. Healthcare professionals who do not regularly care for survivors of pediatric malignancies are encouraged to consult with a pediatric oncology long-term follow-up center if questions or concerns arise when reviewing or using these guidelines. Survivors who choose to review guidelines are strongly encouraged to do this with the assistance of a healthcare professional about long-term follow-up care for survivors of childhood, adolescent, and young adult cancers. The screening recommendations in these guidelines are appropriate for *asymptomatic* survivors of childhood, adolescent, or young adult cancer presenting for routine exposure -based medical follow-up. For survivors presenting with signs and symptoms suggesting illness or organ dysfunction, more extensive evaluations are needed, as clinically indicated.

For survivors:

Download a copy of *Summary of Cancer Treatment (Abbreviated or Comprehensive Health Links (Appendix II)* access

patient education materials on a variety of subjects listed alphabetically (ie. *bleomycin alert, breast cancer, chronic pain, dental
health, eye health, mental health, precocious puberty*)

**Passport for Care, Survivor Care Plans by Children's Oncology
Group (V6, Nov 2023)**
Website: https://cancersurvivor.passportforcare.org
Survivors and family can find online updated tailored
long-term care plans which should be reviewed with
their oncologist or health care provider.

Alcoholics Anonymous (AA)
Website: www.aa.org

American Academy of Dermatology - sunscreen sun protection
Website: https://www.aad.org/media/stats-sunscreen

American Cancer Society
Website: www.cancer.org
Search, *risk prevention, tobacco, health risks of smoking/vaping*
https://www.cancer.org/cancer/risk-prevention/tobacco/

**Centers for Disease Control and Prevention (CDC) Smoking/
vaping**
U.S. Department of Health
Website: www.cdc.gov/tobacco/site.html
Website: www.smokefree.gov
(tips on how to quit/live chats)
Website: https://bit.ly/quitSTARTapp

**Centers for Disease Control and Prevention (CDC) Skin can-
cer/sun protection**
Website: https://www.cdc.gov/skin-cancer/
Videos: https://www.youtube.com/watch?v=QrZRlNdfEz4

**Centers for Disease Control (CDC) – Vaccination/immuniza-
tion recommendations (2025)**
Website: www.cdc.gov/vaccines
Human Papillovirus (HPV) vaccine
Website: www.cdc.gov/hpv

Centers for Disease Control (CDC) – Physical activity/exercise
Website: www.cdc.gov/physical-activity/

CDC photos

FIGURE 5-1. Health benefits of physical activity for children. *Source*: Physical Activity Guidelines for Americans, 2nd edition, CDC; https://www.cdc.gov/physical-activity-basics/health-benefits/children.html

FIGURE 5-2. Download the quitSTART app to get started on your quit smoking journey. It can help you create a quit plan, find tips to help you quit smoking, manage cravings, and more! https://bit.ly/quitSTARTapp

FIGURE 5-3. Use sunscreen of at least 30 SPF to protect yourself from damaging UV rays. *Source*: CDC, https://www.cdc.gov/skin-cancer/sun-safety/

GLOSSARY

Fitbit® tracker or pedometer, a device that one straps on your leg, wrist, waistband, or access on a smartphone that measure distance you walk/jog/swim each day

health-risk behaviors, life-style choices and behaviors that put one's health at risk such as overexposure to sun, smoking, drinking alcohol, and exposure to sexually-transmitted illnesses

binge drinking, periods of excessive drinking followed by periods of no drinking, for example, drinking excessively only on weekends

6

Genetic Testing and Childhood Cancer

LIRON D. GROSSMANN, MD AND JOHN M. MARIS, MD

Science is organized knowledge. Wisdom is organized life.
– Immanuel Kant

GENETICS IS THE SCIENCE or study of the body's cells (genes, DNA, and chromosomes) and how genes are passed from parents to their offspring (called *heredity*). Genetic testing is an emerging and evolving area in childhood cancer. As a survivor of childhood cancer, it is important to understand how genetics played a role in diagnosis and treatment. Future monitoring of you or your child's health should include a conversation around genetics for yourself and any future children. It could also have an impact on immediate family members like parents and siblings. This chapter will help you to understand some of the terms, testing, surveillance practices around genetics. Talking with a genetic counselor or oncologist will help you determine testing or monitoring options based on specific cancer diagnosis. (See Health of Offspring and Genetics Counseling and Testing in *Chapter 3, Relationships*)

PRECISION MEDICINE IN PEDIATRIC CANCER

The field of pediatric oncology has led the way in individualizing cancer care based on genetics testing and the use of diagnostic, prognostic, and therapeutic biomarkers. We are starting to move away from a standard approach for any specific cancer type to the practice of precision medicine and individualized therapeutic approach based on biomarkers.

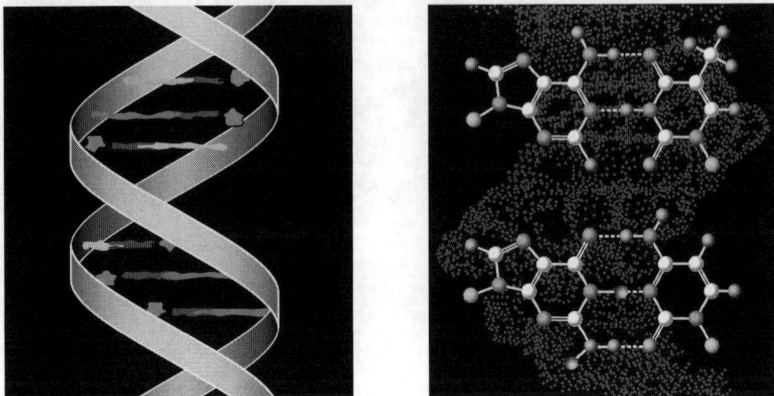

FIGURE 6-1. DNA molecules (©*Alex's Lemonade Stand Foundation, 2025*)

Childhood cancer is not one disease but instead multiple different entities. What makes most of these different entities childhood cancer is they are thought to be malignancies occurring due to changes in normal human developmental programs. Pediatric cancers differ from each other not only by the tissue in which they appear, but also how aggressive they are, likelihood to respond to different types of drugs, and risk of cancer recurrence. For example, certain types of cancers tend to have a poor response to conventional chemotherapy, but other cancers are exquisitely sensitive. Researchers have found that certain types of leukemias that are resistant to chemotherapy harbor a genetic abnormality termed the *Philadelphia chromosome*. This subgroup responds better to a different class of drugs which can be given in the form of a pill and when combined with chemotherapy is often considered as curative therapy. This approach of tailoring therapy according to the genetic and molecular characteristics of the cancer is called *precision medicine*.

Precision medicine and genetics hold the promise of changing the way cancer is diagnosed, treated, and monitored. While we still have a long way to go, advancements have been rapid and produced a major positive impact on the field of childhood cancer.

At the heart of precision medicine is the idea of *biomarkers*—measurable biological identifiers that can predict medical phenomena such as how aggressively a cancer grows/behaves. In this chapter, we introduce key concepts in *biomarker testing* that are relevant to pediatric cancer. We hope that after reading this chapter, you will become more familiar and comfortable with the basic terminology that is becoming part of the routine practice of pediatric oncology.

THE HUMAN GENOME AND CANCER

To better understand the terms throughout this chapter, we provide a brief overview of *the human genome*. More comprehensive background can be found in the reference section.

The genetic information in our cells is coded by the DNA molecule (**Figure 6-1**), which is composed of four chemical building blocks, abbreviated by the letters A, C, G and T. Each cell contains two copies of each building block, one copy inherited from the mother and one from the father. This creates a three-billion letter DNA strand. The DNA molecules making up the strand are packaged into 23 pairs of very long pieces called *chromosomes*. Each of the 46 chromosomes contains genes, which are stretches of letters within the DNA that encode the instructions to make proteins. The DNA regions that do not contain genes are called *non-coding regions*. There are approximately 20,000 genes in the human genome, however, not all of them are active in every cell at any given time. Many factors determine whether a gene will be active or not in a particular cell, and whether its corresponding protein will be produced. For example, some non-coding regions control gene activity and can turn a gene on or off. In addition, a chemical modification around a gene or within it, called *methylation*, can alter the gene activity.

Once a gene becomes active its DNA letters are copied to another molecule called RNA in a process named *transcription*. Levels of RNA molecules from a given gene can be measured and indicate how active the gene is. Each RNA molecule is then further translated into a *protein* which is the main building block of cells.

Cancer cells arise from normal cells by modifying the structure and/or number of genes that control cell growth, cell death, ability to spread to other parts of the body, and other important processes that give the cancer cells survival advantage and makes them hard to destroy. The modified genes and their products, namely RNA and proteins, can be used as biomarkers in pediatric cancer as described below. Many of the genes involved in childhood cancer control the normal process of fetal development which make them quite distinct from adult cancers.

WHAT IS BIOMARKER TESTING?

A *biomarker* is a characteristic of the body that can be measured as an indicator of a normal or abnormal biological process. There are several types of biomarkers including *molecular, radiographic*, and *physiologic*. For example, blood glucose (sugar) is a molecular biomarker, tumor size is a radiographic biomarker, and blood pressure is a physiologic biomarker.

Molecular biomarkers play a major role in precision medicine and in pediatric cancer in particular. Since cancer cells modify DNA and as a result their RNA and proteins, both the DNA and its products can be used as biomarkers to help identify individuals at risk of developing cancer, help define the type of cancer, help understand the mechanism by which it arose, determine how aggressive it is, and predict how likely the response to certain classes of drugs. Molecular biomarkers are also used in cancer research, mainly in drug development, as discussed below.

Categories of biomarkers in cancer medicine

Biomarkers are routinely used in clinical practice in the following important ways:

- to help identify people genetically predisposed to a type of cancer,
- to help in diagnosis,
- to guide therapy,
- to monitor response to therapy,
- to guide drug dosing,
- in post-treatment surveillance (monitoring),
- to aid in cancer research and new drug development.

These seven categories are explained below. The categories are not mutually exclusive, and a biomarker can fall into multiple categories depending on the context it is used.

Indicator of cancer predisposition

Although the majority of cancers arise spontaneously, several genetic mutations can be inherited and increase the risk of developing cancer. For example, individuals carrying a mutated retinoblastoma (*RB1*) gene are at increased risk of developing retinoblastoma, a type of cancer arising in the retina of the eye at a very young age. Children with a family history of retinoblastoma can be tested for the presence of a *RB1* mutation and should obtain frequent eye screening that enables earlier detection of this cancer. In this case, *RB1* is used as a biomarker for cancer predisposition. Many other cancer predisposition gene mutations have been discovered over the past decades.

Biomarkers help in diagnosis

The gold standard for diagnosing cancer is by observation of malignant cells under the microscope which is performed by a *pathologist*, a medical doctor with specialized training in identifying abnormal cells and cell activity. Pathologists look at the size, shape, and number of cells to help determine whether a cell is cancerous and identify the type of cancer. In addition, the cells are stained for different types of proteins that are specific to the suspected cancer. This process allows the pathologist to increase the accuracy of the diagnosis.

Neuroblastoma is a pediatric cancer of the peripheral nervous system that expresses a protein called PHOX2B. This protein is not found in healthy tissues after birth and can be used as a specific biomarker for the diagnosis of neuroblastoma.

Occasionally, the origin and type of tumor can be difficult to determine only from the way the cells appear under the microscope. In these situations, testing for specific genes known to be altered can aid in diagnosing the type of cancer. For example, a class of pediatric tumors, called *NTRK*-fusion positive tumors, are characterized by an alteration in one of three genes in the *Neurotrophic Tyrosine*

Receptor Kinase (NTRK) family. The DNA coding for this gene is fused to another DNA molecule and form a fusion gene. This group of tumors can appear almost anywhere in the body, and it is therefore difficult to make a diagnosis based solely on the cellular appearance. In this case, the *NTRK* gene is used as a diagnostic marker and also as a biomarker for very specific treatments designed to "turn off" these unusually "turned on" fusion genes that instruct a cell to continue to grow (see below).

Biomarkers that guide therapy

Biomarkers can also help clinicians choose the appropriate therapy for a child's cancer (Table 6-2). For example, as described above, *NTRK*-fusion cancers are treated with drugs that were developed to inhibit the protein which is the product of the fusion *NTRK*-gene. One such drug is called *Larotrectinib* and allows for a more effective and less toxic treatment for this group of cancers. Here, the *NTRK*-fusion gene serves as a biomarker to guide therapy.

The Philadelphia chromosome that was described earlier is another example of a biomarker used to guide therapy. Currently, clinicians routinely test for the presence of the BCR-ABL1 fusion gene (the medical term for the Philadelphia chromosome) in patients with acute lymphoblastic leukemia. A positive test warrants the incorporation of drugs that inhibit the action of the fusion protein. Other examples of biomarkers used to guide therapy include the same fusion protein *BCR-ABL1* in chronic myeloid leukemia (CML) and mutated *BRAF* in pediatric brain tumors called gliomas. Both of these cancers can be targeted with drugs known to inhibit the corresponding abnormal gene product.

A large clinical effort to use various genetic biomarkers to guide therapy is exemplified by the Molecular Analysis for Therapy Choice (MATCH) trial. This is a clinical trial in which patients with cancer are assigned to receive a treatment tailored to the genetic characteristics of their type of cancer. A sample of the patient's tumor is then subjected to genetic analysis (see below) and if a genetic change matches a drug being used in the trial, the patient may receive the treatment with that drug if eligible. In this case, the genetic changes of the cancer are biomarkers that guide specific drug therapy. Finally, genetic analysis of pediatric tumors may identify mutations that match to an FDA-approved drug for the same mutation found in adult cancers. Clinicians may recommend "off label" drug treatment for children when a clinical trial is not available.

Prognostic marker

A *prognostic marker* is a biomarker used to predict the course of disease, also known as *prognosis*. The products of certain genes (e.g. RNA and proteins mentioned above) and the quantity in tumors can be used as a biomarker to determine how aggressive the tumor is. For example, the gene *MYCN* is amplified in a subset of neuroblastomas. That is, the cancer cells have multiple DNA copies, usually hundreds, of the gene *MYCN* instead of the normal two copies. The presence of *MYCN* amplification in neuroblastoma tends to require more intense therapy. Prognostic biomarkers are used to stratify patients in clinical trials and/or assign appropriate treatment.

Biomarkers that monitor response to therapy

Biomarkers can be used to determine if a patient responds to therapy. In acute lymphoblastic and other leukemias, a bone marrow aspirate and biopsy are performed during treatment to measure a set of cell surface markers present on the leukemic cells collectively known as *minimal residual disease* (MRD). The absence of MRD suggests that therapy was successful in eliminating the cancer cells. In solid cancers, technology now allows detection of genetic mutations in blood samples or from the fluid removed from a spinal tap, also called *liquid biopsies.* The detection of circulating tumor DNA (ctDNA) is increasingly being used to monitor response to therapy and also to detect gene mutation-drug matches, especially when performing a tumor biopsy might be dangerous to the patient.

Biomarkers that guide drug dosing

Certain genes in our DNA are responsible for the way our body responds to drugs. Changes in these gene can result in accumulation of several drugs in the body and lead to side effects. Measuring the presence of the changes in these genes can help your healthcare provider/oncologist decrease the dose of a drug and prevent accumulation. Such genes are considered biomarkers for drug dosing. For example, an enzyme called *thiopurine methyltransferase* (TPMT) is required for metabolizing the drug *mercaptopurine* used in leukemia therapy. High levels of mercaptopurine result in decreased white blood cells leading to increased susceptibility of infections. Individuals with DNA changes in the gene coding for TPMT are unable to metabolize mercaptopurine appropriately and need dose reduction of this drug. In this case, the gene TPMT is considered a biomarker for drug dosing.

Biomarkers in post-treatment surveillance

Following completion of cancer therapy, patients usually undergo routine surveillance studies, such as magnetic resonance imaging (MRI) or positron emission tomography (PET) scans, to ensure that the cancer does not recur. These studies can only detect tumors that are large enough to be seen by the naked eye.

The emerging group of biomarkers mentioned above called ctDNA or liquid biopsies are based on the DNA content of cancer cells that are released into the bloodstream. Levels of cancer cell-free DNA can be monitored before, during, and after therapy and be used to detect disease recurrence earlier than current imaging methods.

BIOMARKERS IN CANCER RESEARCH AND DRUG DEVELOPMENT

Cancer researchers use biomarkers routinely during drug development. The process of drug development is long and complex, including multiple steps before a drug is approved to treat human patients. It may take a decade or more from the start of the process until the drug is approved and costs around 1 billion dollars. Unfortunately, approximately 5% of drugs developed make it to the final stage of FDA approval (https://www.fda.gov/).

While detailed discussion of drug development is beyond the scope of this chapter, we briefly review the main steps and provide examples of biomarkers used throughout the process.

Preclinical laboratory studies

Drug development starts with *target* identification in the laboratory. The target, usually a protein, should play an important and unique role in the cancer cell life. Biomarkers can help identify *molecular pathways*, that is, a group of genes that acts together and contributes to the development or maintenance of a specific cancer. By narrowing down the list of genes of interest, the process of identifying potential targets becomes more efficient and biologically sound.

Once a target is identified, thousands of compounds are typically screened for potential drug candidates against the target. Biomarkers can aid in selecting the most promising compound (known as *lead compound*) and gain insight into its mechanism of action.

The lead compound then undergoes a battery of laboratory tests. Biomarkers can help to assess the safety and efficacy of the drug, to understand the drug mechanism of action and aid in dose selection.

An example of a preclinical tool that can be used to predict response to therapy is called the *Avatar* system. In this system, a small piece of a patient's tumor is injected into a mouse lacking an immune system, also known as *patient-derived xenograft* (PDX). The tumor is allowed to grow in the mouse and subsequently re-injected into multiple mice. These PDXs have become a major tool for testing candidates' drugs as they reflect the genetics of patient tumors seen in the clinic. While this in *vivo* approach is promising, it should be noted that the process of establishing a PDX is long, expensive, and does not always mimic the tumor heterogeneity in the human cancer. Some investigators are attempting to establish Avatar systems to individualize drug selection, but this remains unproven and very much a subject of ongoing research studies.

A faster and cheaper way to perform drug testing is to use cell cultures (in *vitro*). In this approach cancer cells from patients are grown in a plastic plate to which drugs are added and tested for efficacy. The main drawback of this approach is that cancer cells do not grow in the artificial conditions of cell cultures which include oxygen levels, nutrients and exposure to plastic. Another difference is that cancer cells in the body are typically surrounded by normal cells termed a *microenvironment*. Despite these limitations, cell culture studies can be a useful screen and provide valuable information.

Clinical research steps

The steps following preclinical or laboratory studies are known collectively as *clinical research*. The main purpose of clinical research is to test safety and efficacy of the selected drug in humans.

Phase 1 of clinical trial is aimed at assessing the safety of the drug in humans and also collect data on the appropriate dosing. It typically consists of a relatively small number patients, especially in childhood cancer where many drugs have already been studied in adult trials. Approximately 70% of drugs tested in **Phase 1 trial** move to the **Phase 2 clinical trial** in which the efficacy and side effects of the drug are evaluated. About 33% of Phase 2 trials move to the Phase 3 trial (https://www.fda.gov/). The goal of **Phase 3 trials** is to test the efficacy of the drug and compare it to current therapies for the specific type of cancer. These studies enroll several hundreds to thousands of patients and can continue for many years. Phase 3 trials also provide new safety data about the drug that was not detected in previous phases. Roughly 25 to 30% of the drugs that enter Phase 3 trials are approved by the FDA for marketing and move to Phase 4 trial or a post-market safety monitoring phase.

Biomarkers play an important role in clinical trials and help select patients for enrollment into clinical trials, stratify patients into a subgroup of treatment, guide dose selection, help in assessment of safety and evaluation of drug efficacy, and help to monitor side effects. For example, the presence of *NTRK*-fusion gene can be a biomarker for selection of patients into a clinical trial that tests the efficacy of *Larotrectinib* in *NTRK-fusion positive tumors*. The levels of liver enzymes (aminotransferase) are typically used as safety biomarkers for drugs that can cause liver injury, such as Larotrectinib. The presence of *NTRK*-fusion gene in cell-free DNA blood samples can be used as biomarkers for response to therapy.

TYPES OF BIOMARKER TESTING

In this section we describe in more detail the types of tests used to measure cancer biomarkers in the clinical setting. The *ideal biomarker* is one that is always positive for a specific type of cancer but negative for all others, allows for treating that type of cancer, and is low cost, and fast to identify in a test. It is important to note that similar to other tests in medicine, no such perfect test exists.

Biochemical testing

This type of testing measures the level of a biomarker, usually a protein, that is secreted by the tumor cells into the blood or other body fluids such as urine or cerebral spinal fluid. The healthcare provider/oncologist orders the test and the appropriate sample is collected from the patient. Testing for the majority of biochemical biomarkers does not require insurance approval. The result of the test is reported as a number and is interpreted as abnormal if outside of the normal range of expected values. For example, the protein alpha-fetoprotein (AFP) is usually secreted by a pediatric liver tumor called *hepatoblastoma*. High levels of this protein can be used to aid in diagnosis, prognosis, and response to therapy.

Another example of a biochemical biomarker is urine catecholamines. These molecules are secreted by the sympathetic nervous systems and can be detected in the urine. High levels of these molecules aid in the diagnosis, response to therapy, and prediction of relapse in neuroblastoma. See Table 6-1 for biochemical biomarkers used in pediatric cancers and Table 6-2 lists the genetic biomarkers used in pediatric cancers.

Immunohistochemical staining

Immunohistochemical staining (IHC) testing uses antibodies to detect biomarkers, usually proteins, that are inside or on the surface of cancer cells in a tissue on microscope slides. The cancer tissue is taken via biopsy or surgical removal, prepared (either frozen or paraffin embedded) and stained using an antibody directed at the protein of interest. The pathologist then confirms the presence or absence of the protein under the microscope.

The protein PHOX2B, which was discussed above in the context of diagnostic biomarkers, is detected using IHC staining. Additional diagnostic biomarkers detected by IHC staining include myogenin for rhabdomyosarcoma, CD99 for Ewing sarcoma, CD19 for B acute lymphoblastic leukemia and others.

Table 6-1. Biochemical biomarkers used in pediatric cancers

Biochemical biomarker	Type of biomarker	Type of pediatric cancer
AFP	Diagnosis, response to therapy, post-treatment surveillance	hepatoblastoma, GCT
LDH	Response to therapy, post-treatment surveillance	GCT, non-Hodgkin lymphoma, osteosarcoma
bHCG	Diagnosis, response to therapy, post-treatment surveillance	GCT
ESR	Response to therapy	Hodgkin lymphoma
Uric acid	Diagnosis of tumor lysis syndrome, guide therapy, response to therapy	ALL, AML
Urine catecholamines	Diagnosis, post-treatment surveillance	neuroblastoma

ALL, acute lymphoblastic leukemia, AML, acute myeloid leukemia, GCT, germ cell tumors

Genetic testing

Genetic testing is based on methods that measure changes in the DNA. The changes can be in the number or structure of chromosomes, genes and/or non-coding regions. The broader definition of genetic testing also encompasses changes in the number or structure of RNA molecules which are derived from DNA. Types of genetic tests can be broadly classified as *sequencing-based methods* and *non-sequencing-based methods*. Described below are the most common types of genetic testing encountered in pediatric cancer with examples for each type of test.

Non-sequencing based methods

Cancer cells usually change the size, number, and shape of chromosomes. The methods below differ not only by the way they detect

Table 6-2. Genetic biomarkers used in pediatric cancers

Genetic biomarker	Type of test	Type of biomarker	Type of pediatric cancer
hyperdiploid, hypodiploid	Karyotype	Prognostic	ALL
BCR-ABL	FISH	Diagnostic, guide therapy	CML, ALL
MYCN	FISH	Diagnostic, prognostic	neuroblastoma, medulloblastoma
ESWR1-FLI1	FISH	Diagnostic	Ewing sarcoma
FOXO1-PAX3	FISH	Diagnostic, prognostic	alveolar rhabdomyosarcoma
1p loss, 11q loss, 17q gain	SNP array	Prognostic	neuroblastoma
1p and 16q loss, 1q gain	SNP array	Prognostic	Wilms tumor
FLT3	DNA sequencing	Prognostic, Guide therapy	AML
BRAF	DNA sequencing	Guide therapy	LGG, LCH, melanoma
ALK	DNA sequencing	Guide therapy	neuroblastoma, IMT
NTRK-fusion	RNA sequencing	Diagnostic, guide therapy	NTRK-fusion positive cancers

ALL, acute lymphoblastic leukemia; AML, acute myeloid leukemia; CML, chronic myeloid leukemia; LGG, low grade glioma; LCH, Langerhans cell histiocytosis; IMT, inflammatory myofibroblastic tumor; NTRK, Neurotrophic Tyrosine Receptor Kinase (NTRK)
q = the long arm of the chromosome
p = the short arm of the chromosome

chromosomal changes, but also but the minimal size of the change that can be detected.

Karyotype. This test produces an image of the cancer cells' chromosomes and allows the detection of large chromosomal abnormalities. It requires growing the cancer cells in culture and typically takes 1 to 2 weeks to result.

Karyotyping is used as a prognostic biomarker in acute lymphoblastic leukemia. Specifically, patients with leukemia cells showing low number of chromosomes (less than 40 chromosomes on karyotype, also called *hypodiploid*) tend to be harder to treat than patients with high number of chromosomes (*hyperdiploid*).

Fluorescence in situ hybridization (FISH). This test uses a fluorescent probe that binds to specific regions of chromosomes and can detect regions where part of the chromosome is amplified, deleted, or fused to another chromosome (an aberration referred to as *chromosomal translocation*). This test can detect smaller changes than karyotype, is low cost and takes approximately 1 to 2 days for results. The disadvantage of this test is that it requires prior knowledge of the changed region in the DNA.

FISH is used to detect biomarkers in many types of childhood cancers including acute lymphoblastic leukemia, acute myeloid leukemia, neuroblastoma, Ewing sarcoma, rhabdomyosarcoma, neuroblastoma, and others (See Table 6-2).

Single Nucleotide Polymorphism Microarray (SNP array). Occasionally, only small regions of the chromosome are amplified or lost and the orientation of the DNA letters can be inverted. Such changes cannot be detected using Karyotype or FISH. In such cases, a SNP array can help detect biomarkers by analyzing tumor DNA with hundreds of thousands of DNA *polymorphisms* or spelling changes in DNA that vary based on race and ethnicity. This allows for the detection of gains or losses of chromosomal regions without any prior knowledge of where these exist. SNP arrays are used to detect prognostic biomarkers in neuroblastoma and Wilms' tumor.

Sequencing-based methods

Sequencing is the process of determining the sequence of letters of a DNA or RNA molecule. DNA and RNA sequencing technologies continue to evolve to allow for faster, cheaper, and more accurate results.

The traditional sequencing method referred to as *Sanger sequencing* or *First Generation Sequencing* is clinically used to determine the sequence of a single gene. First Generation Sequencing is accurate but time consuming. Next Generation Sequencing (NGS) is a technology that allows the sequencing of many genes or all of the gene in parallel. The following are sequencing-based genetic tests and their use in pediatric cancer.

Single gene test. This test is used to detect a change in a gene that is known to be modified in a type of cancer and for which a targeted therapy exists. For example, the gene *ALK* is mutated in approximately 15-25% of neuroblastomas. The presence of an *ALK* mutation may warrant the addition of an ALK-inhibitor to a treatment, and this is currently be tested in clinical trials. With the evolution of NGS, single gene testing is largely being replaced by NGS multi-gent strategies.

Targeted genetic panel. This test relies on NGS technology and is performed on a set of genes that are known to contribute to a specific type of cancer of a group of cancers. The number of genes included in a panel varies depending on the type of cancer and laboratory that performs the test, but typically is in the range of several hundred.

Germline testing. Most cancers are _not_ inherited. However, well described cancer predisposition syndromes exist and offer an opportunity for biomarker testing. A *liquid biopsy* is a sequenced-based genetic testing that is performed on normal tissue, most often on blood or saliva, to detect a change in a gene or other regions in the DNA that affect all the cells of the body and could give rise to cancer.

Your oncologist may decide to order germline testing if other family members had cancer at a young age, if the cancer originates on both sides of the body (for example, in both eyes or both kidneys), and/ or if your child has concerning features on physical exam. With the increased use of NGS on tumor tissue, it is now not uncommon to uncover a potentially concerning genetic predisposition mutation even if no family history exists. This typically leads to a referral to a genetic counselor for a discussion of the test result, potential confirmation testing, and further counseling as to what this means for the patient and family members.

Various tests ordered for you/your family

Depending on the type of cancer your oncologist suspects, he/she may choose to order single gene or a genetic panel test and recommend testing other family members. However, there are occasions when neither a single gene nor genetic panel testing reveal the cause of familial cancer. In these situations, your oncologist may decide to test all the genes or the entire genome.

Whole exome sequencing (WES). Each gene is composed of DNA regions that are protein coding, called *exons*, and non-protein-coding regions, called *introns*. WES is a NGS test which sequences all the genes, which comprise approximately 1% to 5% of the genome.

Whole genome sequencing (WGS). Remember that most of the genome contains sequences that do not code for protein. Growing evidence suggests that the non-coding regions of DNA play an important role in cancer development and maintenance. When WES testing does not discover the etiology of cancer, your oncologist/geneticist may recommend WGS testing. Currently this is very rarely pursued, but may be ordered with increasing frequency as we understand more about the noncoding genome.

RNA sequencing. this test provides the sequences of the genes that are active in the cancer. Remember that the DNA of active genes is copied into RNA molecules. These molecules can be sequenced (by converting them to a DNA molecule and using DNA sequencing technologies) and reveal a group of genes that act in concert in a particular type of cancer, called a *gene signature*. While still uncommon in pediatric cancers, the use of signatures to classify cancer types and predict outcome is becoming more clinically useful in adult cancers. In pediatric cancers, the use of RNA sequencing is mostly reserved for detecting gene fusions. The advantages of using RNA sequencing over FISH for the detection of gene fusion is that RNA sequencing does not require knowing both partners of the fusion and it can detect novel fusions. *NTRK*-fusion positive cancers are diagnosed using RNA sequencing.

PRACTICAL ISSUES TO KNOW BEFORE TESTING

Informed consent

Typically, the healthcare provider ordering the test would be your oncologist. However, in some institutions your oncologist may refer you to a geneticist who will order the test.

Prior to collecting a sample for genetic testing, the ordering healthcare provider will ask you to sign a document that gives patient consent to perform the test known as *informed consent*. This document states that the test is voluntary and that the patient or patient's parent if the child is under 18 fully understands and agrees to the test. Your healthcare provider should discuss the risks, benefits, and limitations of the test prior to signing the consent form.

Turnaround time for results

Turnaround time for results depend on the laboratory where the test is performed. Typically, single gene testing can take up to a week for results, whereas most current NGS assays take 2 to 4 weeks for results.

Tissue banking

You may elect to store the cancer tissue of your child for the purpose of basic science and clinical research. *Tissue banks* are repositories that collect and store biological samples and associated clinical data. Importantly, some clinical trials require that your child's tumor tissue be collected and stored in a central biobank. You will also be asked to sign a consent to allow a local or remote biobank to collect and store your child's sample. The name of your child will remain undisclosed.

Interpreting the results

The ordering provider/oncologist should deliver and explain the results of the genetic testing. It is important to know that the results of genetic testing are not always straightforward, especially sequencing-based methods. For example, the sequence of a gene of interest may reveal a change from the normal sequence, but it does not necessarily mean that the change (often termed *variant*) causes a change in the function of the gene resulting in cancer.

In addition, when performing WES or WGS, unexpected secondary findings for which the test was not initially indicated may be found. For example, a WES test may reveal a change in a gene that causes heart disease. A thorough discussion with your oncologist prior to undergoing the test should include any potential secondary results, their significance and future actions that would need to be taken.

REFERENCES/RESOURCES

Website: ccgresources.org
All resources and references mentioned in this book are available on the website and will be routinely reviewed and updated.

Children's Oncology Group. (V6, 2023). *Long-Term Follow-Up Guidelines for Survivors of Childhood, Adolescent, and Young Adult Cancers*
Website: www.survivorshipguidelines.org

Clinical trials
Website: https://clinicaltrials.gov
Search, *nci-match*

Drug development
Website: https://www.fda.gov
Search: *drug development approval process, patient focused drug development guidance series*

Genetic testing in cancer
Website: https://www.cancer.gov
Search: *genetics, genetic testing, causes and preventions*

Genetic panels
Website: https://www.chop.edu
Search, *cancer-panels*

NTRK-fusion positive cancers
Website: https://www.bayer.com
Search: *trk-fusion-cancer*

US Food and Drug Administration (FDA)
Website: https://www.fda.gov/
Search: *patients/drug-development-process, step-3 clinical research*

National Cancer Institute–Children's Oncology Group; Pediatric MATCH Trial (revised June 2023)
Website: https://www.cancer.gov
Search: *clinical trials, nci supported, nci match*

NCI-COG Pediatric MATCH (Molecular Analysis for Therapy Choice), also known as *Pediatric MATCH*, is an international pediatric precision medicine cancer treatment trial that explores whether targeted therapies can be effective for children, adolescents and young adults with solid tumors that harbor specific gene mutations. *Pediatric MATCH* is a phase 2 trial that investigates different study drugs, each targeting a defined set of gene mutations, in order to match patients with therapies aimed at the molecular abnormalities in his or her tumor.

The Children's Oncology Group (COG), a National Cancer Institute supported clinical trials group, is the world's largest organization devoted exclusively to childhood and adolescent cancer research. The COG unites more than 10,000 experts in childhood cancer at more than 200 leading children's hospitals, universities, and cancer centers across North America, Australia, and New Zealand in the fight against childhood cancer.

Today, more than 90% of 16,000 children and adolescents diagnosed with cancer each year in the United States are cared for at Children's Oncology Group member institutions. COG's unparalleled collaborative efforts provide the information and support needed to answer important clinical questions in the fight against cancer.

The Children's Oncology Group has nearly 100 active clinical trials open at any given time. These trials include front-line treatment for many types of childhood cancers, studies aimed at determining the underlying biology of these diseases, and trials involving new and emerging treatments, supportive care, and survivorship. The Children's Oncology Group research has turned children's cancer from a virtually incurable disease 50 years ago to one with a combined 5-year survival rate of 80% today. Our goal is to cure all children and adolescents with cancer, reduce the short and long-term complications of cancer treatments, and determine the causes and find ways to prevent childhood cancer.

GLOSSARY

biomarker (tumor marker), a measurable biological identifier that can predict medical phenomena such as how aggressively a cancer grows. There are several types of biomarkers including *molecular, radiographic*, and *physiologic*.

biomarker testing, a method to search for genes, proteins, and other substances (called biomarkers or tumor markers) that can provide information about cancer. Each person's cancer has a unique pattern of biomarkers. Some biomarkers affect how certain cancer treatments work.

chromosomes, a threadlike structure of nucleic acids and protein found in the nucleus of most living cells, carrying genetic information in the form of genes

clinical research, medical research that involves enrolling volunteers to take part in studies (*clinical trials)* that monitor an individual's progress during and after cancer treatment. The main purpose of clinical research is to test safety and efficacy of a selected drug. These studies help doctors and researchers learn more about specific diseases and find new medications or treatments to improve health care for people in the future.

gene signature or gene expression signature, a single or combined group of genes in a cell with a uniquely characteristic pattern of gene expression that demonstrates an altered or unaltered biological process or medical condition or disease

genetic testing, to examine one's DNA, the chemical database that carries instructions for your body's functions. Such testing can reveal changes (mutations) in genes that may cause illness or disease.

germline testing, sequenced-based genetic testing that is performed on a normal tissue, most often on blood or saliva, to detect a change in a gene or other regions in the DNA that affect all the cells of the body and could give rise to cancer

human genome, the entire set of DNA instructions found in a cell. In humans, the genome consists of 23 pairs of chromosomes located in the cell's nucleus.

ideal biomarker, An "ideal" biomarker includes *all* of the following 4 characteristics: 1) shows positive result for a specific type of cancer and negative result for all others (*cancer-specific*); 2) allows for treatment of that specific cancer; 3) is low cost to test; and 4) rapid results from the test.

karyotyping, a test that produces an image of the cancer cells' chromosomes and allows the detection of large chromosomal abnormalities. It requires growing the cancer cells in culture and typically takes 1 to 2 weeks to result.

liquid biopsy or ctDNA, blood samples or fluids removed from a spinal tap used to detect genetic mutations in solid cancers

informed consent, a document that must be signed by a patient or parent if the child is under age 18 giving consent to perform any genetic testing including collecting all samples for the genetic testing. Before signing this informed consent, patient and family must be informed of risks, benefits and limitations of the test. If patient results are to be included in a clinical trial, the patient or parent must agree to the results to be included in the specific study and any future follow-up required.

minimal residual disease (MRD), a small number of cancer cells left in the body after treatment which have the potential to come back and cause relapse

Molecular Analysis for Therapy Choice (MATCH), Trial is an international pediatric precision medicine cancer treatment trial that explores whether targeted therapies can be effective for children, adolescents, and young adults with solid tumors that harbor specific gene mutations. Pediatric MATCH is a phase 2 trial that investigates different study drugs, each targeting a defined set of gene mutations, in order to match patients with therapies aimed at the molecular abnormalities in his or her tumor

molecular pathways, a group of genes that act together and contribute to the development or maintenance of a specific cancer

Philadelphia chromosome, a defect in chromosome 22 of leukemia cancer cells where part of the chromosome is amplified, deleted or fused to another chromosome; scientific name is *BCR-ABL1* fusion gene

NTRK-fusion positive tumors/cancers, a group of pediatric tumors that can appear almost anywhere in the body, and therefore are difficult to make a diagnosis based solely on the cellular appearance

non-coding regions, DNA regions that do not contain genes

prognostic marker, a biomarker that helps predict the course of the disease and outcome

pathologist, a medical doctor with specialized training in identifying abnormal cells and cell activity

precision medicine, tailoring cancer therapy according to the genetic and molecular characteristics of the specific cancer by using genetics testing and molecular biomarkers

prognosis, a prediction of the probable course and outcome of the disease (how aggressive the tumor/cancer is) and the prospects of recovery

tissue banks, repositories that collect and store biological samples and associated clinical data

variant, a change in the normal sequencing of a gene

7
Diseases

JOANNE QUILLEN, MSN, APRN, PNP-BC

The world breaks everyone and afterward,
many are strong at the broken places.
— *Ernest Hemingway, A Farewell to Arms*

SURVIVORSHIP CONTINUES THROUGHOUT your life. Whether you develop any late effects from your treatment for childhood cancer depends on your disease, your age at diagnosis, your sex, the treatment received, genetic predisposition, and complications during treatment. For many cancers, treatment toxicity has lessened over the years; for others, eliminating the cancer came at a higher price with late effects that can affect future health and well-being.

This chapter is divided into sections of the following major cancers of childhood and adolescence (in alphabetical order), including brief description of the cancer, treatments, and possible late effects, including:

- Acute lymphoblastic leukemia (ALL)
- Acute myelogenous leukemia (AML)
- Brain tumors
- Ewing sarcoma
- Hodgkin lymphoma (formerly called Hodgkin's disease)
- Neuroblastoma
- Non-Hodgkin lymphoma (NHL)
- Osteosarcoma
- Rare cancers
- Retinoblastoma
- Rhabdomyosarcoma
- Wilms tumor

Because many diseases are now treated with stem cell transplants (which includes bone marrow, stem cell, and cord blood transplants), see Section on Stem Cell Transplantation late effects at the end of the chapter.

Long-Term Follow-Up Guidelines for Survivors of Childhood, Adolescent, and Young Adult Cancers, Version 6.0 (October 2023); http://www.survivorshipguidelines.org/) will help you better understand your risks based on the treatment you received and help you make choices that lessen your chances of developing a particular problem. For instance, if you are at increased risk for heart disease, you can decrease the full impact of this risk by eating a healthy diet, exercising regularly, and not smoking. You can also access *Passport for Care* online which allows survivors and family to find updated long-term care plans tailored to your specific treatment. This plan should be reviewed with your follow-up oncologist or health care provider when planning your specific long-term care. https://cancersurvivor.passportforcare.org

> Ask your oncologist or nurse practitioner provider to give you a copy of your detailed Cancer Treatment Summary to keep with your personal medical records at home. This is helpful if you move to a different town/city and need to find a new provider.

These Survivorship Guidelines will keep all medical caregivers updated on the follow-up necessary to maximize your health. Ask your oncologist or nurse practitioner to fill in a *Summary of Cancer Treatment* form from the website above or provide a treatment summary so you know which sections of the survivorship guidelines apply to you.

Adult survivors of childhood cancer are pioneers; researchers are still learning about effects of earlier treatments as survivors grow and age. The late effects from current protocols may not be completely understood for decades. At the time of diagnosis, it is not possible to predict all potential long-term effects. Even with known late effects, there is considerable variation from person to person. Just because it could happen does not mean it *will* happen for everyone.

Certain groups of children, adolescents, and young adult survivors are more at risk for side effects than others. Being aware of the possible late effects and getting thorough follow-up care will max-imize your chance for a long and healthy life and prepare you to talk over any questions or concerns with your healthcare provider. All of the statistics in the following sections are from the National Cancer Institute (NCI) website: www.cancer.gov (Search *child-hood cancers*).

Late medical effects are difficult because there is so much un-known. The fear around late effects is a regular issue, as there are so many possibilities to watch for. Maintaining a positive relationship with my current care team and having access to my cancer treatment medical records, as well as staying aware of new research, have been helpful in alleviating the burden.

My treatment took place from age 4 to 6. I made frequent visits to the hospital most of grade school for checkups. Immediately following treatment, we continued routine bloodwork and fol-low-up visits, which became increasingly less frequent. My care team continued to follow-up with me until I was 18, at which point I was finally phased out of hospital visits. A week after my 18th birthday, my mom and I took our last trip to the hospital and walked out knowing it was the last one. It felt like stepping over a threshold into a new era. Now, my current team of doctors still follow up with occasional bloodwork.

Both of our girls had 6 months of VEC chemotherapy and PRN laser/cryotherapy as treatment for retinoblastoma. They have both had chemotherapy injections into their eyes. Our oldest had 3 rounds of IAC. All of this to shrink and kill the tumors on their retinas and prevent them from spreading to the brain. One of our girls will only have peripheral vision in her left eye with close to normal vision in her right. The other will likely have nor-mal vision in both eyes.

Our oldest daughter donated her bone marrow to save her sister's life. The bone marrow transplant was the hardest part of treatment. That is saying something, because chemother-apy was beyond brutal itself. During recovery from the trans-plant, our daughter couldn't even get out of the hospital bed.

(Continued)

She developed sores that started on the inside of her mouth and went all the way through her digestive and genitourinary systems. Despite antinausea medication, she vomited constantly. She also had periodic accidents - explosive diarrhea, bedwetting. She developed rashes during every chemotherapy treatment that were itchy and uncomfortable. Four years later, our daughter still sees her oncologist every three months for bloodwork and checkup. She goes to the survivor clinic for screenings every four months. She sees a cardiologist every six months due to the effect that the harsh chemotherapy had on her heart.

ACUTE LYMPHOBLASTIC LEUKEMIA

Leukemia is the most common cancer in children under 20 years of age. Eighty percent of children and adolescents diagnosed with leukemia have acute lymphoblastic leukemia (also called Acute Lymphocytic Leukemia or ALL). Approximately 2500-3500 children and teens in the United States are diagnosed with ALL each year, and today approximately 90 percent of children younger than age 15 survive the disease (American Cancer Society, 2025, see Resources for website).

Childhood ALL is most commonly diagnosed in children between ages 2 and 5. In the United States, ALL is more common in Hispanic and white children than in other racial and ethnic groups, and boys have a slightly higher incidence than girls.

Description

ALL is a cancer that begins in the blood-forming tissues of the bone marrow—the spongy center of the bones that produces blood cells. In ALL, the bone marrow creates too many immature lymphocytes (a type of white blood cell) that cannot perform their normal function of fighting infection. As the bone marrow floods the bloodstream with these white blood cells, production of healthy white cells, red cells (which carry oxygen), and platelets (which form clots to stop bleeding) slows and stops. The blood carries the leukemic cells to organs such as the lungs, liver, spleen, kidneys, and testes. Leukemic cells can also cross the blood-brain barrier and invade the central nervous system (CNS)—made up of the brain and spinal cord.

Treatment

Treatment of childhood ALL is one of the major medical success stories of the last 3 decades. In the early 1960s, children with ALL usually lived for only a few months, but by 2010, about 90 percent of children younger than age 15 who receive optimal treatment survive. The appropriate treatment for each child with ALL is determined by an analysis of a multitude of clinical, biologic, and clinical features. Most childhood cancer treatment centers describe a child's risk of relapse using the terms of *standard risk, high risk,* or *very high risk*, and children with high-risk or very high-risk disease receive the most intensive therapy.

To determine the risk level, the following prognostic factors are considered:

- Initial white blood cell count
- Age at diagnosis
- Presence of CNS leukemia or testicular leukemia at diagnosis
- Presence or absence of chromosomal changes in the leukemic cells
- Response to treatment

Chemotherapy

The most common treatments for ALL are chemotherapy and CNS prophylaxis (i.e., chemotherapy and/intrathecal chemotherapy to the CNS to prevent the spread of cancer to the brain). For standard-risk patients, treatment is typically divided into three phases: induction, consolidation/intensification, and maintenance.

Induction is the most intensive phase of treatment because its purpose is to kill as many leukemia cells in the shortest amount of time possible. The majority of ALL induction programs include the following chemotherapy drugs: methotrexate, cytarabine (ARA-C), vincristine (Oncovin®), prednisone and/or dexamethasone (Decadron®), cyclophosphamide (Cytoxan®), asparaginase, and sometimes daunorubicin (Cerubidine®) or doxorubicin (Adriamycin®).

CNS treatment is an essential component of treatment for ALL. Because leukemia cells can hide in the brain and spinal cord, the CNS was a frequent site for relapse prior to the use of cranial radiation, high-dose systemic chemotherapy, or chemotherapy injected directly into the cerebrospinal fluid (called *intrathecal or IT*). Standard-risk patients usually receive several doses of intrathecal methotrexate or triple IT therapy—methotrexate, hydrocortisone, and ARA-C—to prevent the spread of leukemia to the CNS.

Consolidation/intensification phase of chemotherapy is begun after remission is achieved to destroy any remaining cancer cells. A combination of some of the following drugs is used: methotrexate, cyclophosphamide, cytarabine, mercaptopurine (6-MP, Purinethol'), asparaginase, prednisone, dexamethasone, vincristine, thioguanine, etoposide, and doxorubicin. A *delayed intensification phase* is administered prior to maintenance in current protocols.

Maintenance phase of chemotherapy consists of daily low-dose chemotherapy and continues for 2 to 3 years. The backbone of maintenance therapy in most protocols is daily mercaptopurine and weekly methotrexate. In addition, monthly doses of vincristine and prednisone (or dexamethasone) may be given. ALL protocols also include intrathecal methotrexate during maintenance.

Immunotherapy

Immunotherapy is cancer treatment that helps your own immune system fight cancer. One highly effective new form of immunotherapy is *chimeric antigen receptor (CAR) T-cell therapy* that can be used to treat children with relapsed/refractory acute lymphoblastic leukemia. This immunotherapy treatment specifically targets certain cancer cells of the body associated with leukemia treatment response. Treatment involves infusing new T-cells into the patient's blood that have been altered with a new gene receptor (chimeric antigen receptor) equipped to attack specific cancer cells and destroy them. This therapy is currently being studied for treatment of other types of cancer. Blinatumomab is an immune-based therapy given to many children with ALL and may improve survival, however long-term effects are not yet known. Survivors who have received these therapies should talk with their oncology provider about the potential for late effects which may result.

Radiation

For very high-risk patients, cranial radiation is sometimes needed to prevent the spread of leukemia to the CNS. Children who have leukemia in the cerebrospinal fluid at diagnosis require cranial and spinal radiation. Infants who are in the high-risk group are not given radiation to the brain, or it is delayed until they are older. Boys with disease in their testes are treated with testicular radiation.

Late effects of acute lymphoblastic leukemia

Children with standard-risk ALL often have few or no long-term effects. Children with high-risk ALL, or those who have relapsed and require more intensive treatment, sometimes pay a higher price. The following information briefly outlines some common and uncommon late effects from treatment. Remember that you may develop none, a few, or several of these problems in the months or years after treatment ends. Your individual risk depends on a number of different factors.

Learning disabilities. Treatment for childhood ALL may result in learning disabilities. Radiation and/or methotrexate can damage children's central nervous systems. The degree of damage depends on the dose of radiation, the child's age, and the child's sex, with younger female children more at risk than older children or teens. These cognitive difficulties can develop years after treatment ends. Typically, areas of difficulty are mathematics, memory, organization, planning, spatial relationships, problem solving, attention span, concentration skills, processing speed, and social skills. For more information, see *Chapter 9, Brain and Nerves*.

Growth. Radiation can affect growth. Children who receive 2400 centigray (cGy) or more of cranial radiation or spinal radiation often fail to grow to their potential height. Some children (most often girls) who receive 1800 cGy or more at an early age may also have shortened stature as adults. Radiation can cause early, delayed, or accelerated puberty. For more information, see *Chapter 10, Hormone-Producing Glands*.

Female fertility. Female fertility usually is not affected by treatment for leukemia unless a girl had spinal radiation that included the ovaries or had very high doses) of cyclophosphamide at a later age in adolescence. In the vast majority of cases, girls treated for leukemia exhibit normal sexual development and fertility. The chances of having a normal pregnancy and birth are the same as in the general population. For more information about growth, sexual development, and fertility, see *Chapter 10, Hormone-Producing Glands,* and *Chapter 3, Relationships.*

Male fertility. *Cyclophosphamide* causes a rapid decrease in sperm count in males who have entered puberty. Normal sperm production and motility generally return during maintenance or after treatment. Boys who go through puberty after leukemia treatment usually experience a normal puberty. However, boys who received very high doses of cyclophosphamide (more than 7.5 grams/m^2) and/or radiation to the testes should have testosterone levels and sperm count checked. Most males treated for leukemia with chemotherapy alone have normal growth, sexual development, and fertility. For more information about growth, sexual development, and fertility, see *Chapter 10, Hormone-Producing Glands,* and *Chapter 3, Relationships.*

Heart problems. Heart problems can occur months or years after treatment with anthracyclines (i.e., doxorubicin, idarubicin, or daunorubicin) or mitoxantrone. Symptoms include shortness of breath, fatigue, wheezing, anxiety, poor exercise tolerance, rapid heartbeat, and irregular heartbeat. The number of leukemia survivors who develop this late-effect is small, but regular checkups are crucial. Survivors who had standard risk leukemia rarely have any problems. Monitoring tests for heart late effects include echocardiograms, electrocardiograms (EKGs), Exercise Stress Test (EST), and Holter monitors. For more information, see *Chapter 13, Heart and Blood Vessels.*

Fatigue. After treatment for leukemia, most children resume normal activities at age-appropriate levels, but some children have persistent weakness and/or fatigue. Sometimes this can be from exposure to radiation to brain and/or chemotherapy which affects nerves (vincristine). For more information, see *Chapter 8, Fatigue.*

Obesity. A small number of survivors of ALL become overweight during or after treatment. An association has been noted between learning disabilities and obesity in ALL survivors—both effects are probably related to the effects of radiation on the brain. Some ALL survivors develop osteopenia or osteoporosis (low bone density). For more information, see *Chapter 18, Muscles and Bones.*

Dental problems. Dental abnormalities, such as failure of the teeth to develop, arrested root development, unusually small teeth, increased periodontal disease, and enamel abnormalities may occur after chemotherapy or radiation. For more information, see *Chapter 12, Head and Neck.*

Less common problems. Less common late effects include osteonecrosis (death of blood vessels that nourish bones) from methotrexate, high-dose steroids, especially dexamethasone; bladder problems (i.e., hemorrhagic cystitis and bladder fibrosis) from cyclophosphamide; hypothyroidism (from cranial radiation); cataracts (from cranial radiation); and secondary cancers (from cranial radiation).

See more information about the late effects from stem cell transplants (including bone marrow transplants) in section at the end of this chapter, *Stem Cell Transplantation Late Effects.*

ACUTE MYELOGENOUS LEUKEMIA

Acute myelogenous leukemia (also called acute myeloid leukemia, acute non-lymphocytic leukemia, or AML) is cancer of the granulocytes (a type of white blood cell). Approximately 15% of childhood leukemia diagnosis are AML in the United States each year. The incidence is highest in the first 2 years of life. Incidence rates gradually decrease until 9 years of age and then slowly increase during adolescence.

Description

AML is a cancer that begins in the blood-forming tissues of the bone marrow—the spongy center of the bones that produces blood cells. In AML, the bone marrow creates too many immature granulocytes (a type of white cell) that cannot perform their normal function of fighting infection. As the bone marrow floods the bloodstream with immature white cells, production of healthy white cells, red cells (which carry oxygen), and platelets (which form clots to stop bleeding) slows and stops. The blood carries the leukemic cells to organs such as the lungs, liver, spleen, and kidneys. The cancer can also cross the blood-brain barrier and invade the central nervous system (CNS)—made up of the brain and spinal cord.

AML is grouped into subtypes by the presence of genetic abnormalities in the leukemia cells. AML that doesn't fall into these categories is grouped into eight different subtypes of AML—M0 to M7—based on cell shape and chemical properties.

Treatment

Treatment for AML is intensive. Treatment is ordinarily divided into two or three phases: 1) induction (to attain remission), 2) stem cell transplantation or post-remission consolidation, and/or 3) post-remission intensification. Maintenance therapy is no longer used in most current protocols. Intrathecal (through a needle into the spine) chemotherapy is used to prevent leukemia in the CNS.

Chemotherapy

Chemotherapy for AML includes combinations of drugs. The chemotherapy drugs have changed over the years with new targeted therapy emerging. Discuss with your oncology provider/nurse the type of chemotherapy drugs to which you or your child was exposed. Intrathecal chemotherapy includes cytarabine, methotrexate, and hydrocortisone to treat or prevent leukemia in the CNS.

All types of AML except M3 (called promyelocytic leukemia or APML) are treated similarly. The inclusion of *all-trans retinoic acid* (ATRA) into M3 protocols has doubled the remission rates for this subtype of AML.

Stem cell transplantation

After obtaining a remission, treatment with additional chemotherapy or stem cell transplantation is necessary. See information about the late effects of stem cell transplants in section at the end of this chapter, *Stem Cell Transplantation Late effects.*

Late effects of treatment for acute myelogenous leukemia

Some children who were treated with chemotherapy alone have few or no long-term effects. Children who had stem cell transplants or children who relapsed and require more intensive treatment may experience more late effects. The following information briefly outlines some common and uncommon late effects from treatment. Remember that you may develop none, a few, or several of these problems in the months or years after treatment ends.

Heart problems. Heart problems can occur months or years after treatment with anthracyclines (i.e., doxorubicin, idarubicin, or daunorubicin), high-dose cyclophosphamide, and chest radiation. Symptoms include shortness of breath, fatigue, wheezing, anxiety, poor exercise tolerance, rapid heartbeat, and irregular heartbeat. The number of AML survivors who develop this late effect is small, but regular checkups are crucial. Survivors often have no symptoms, but problems may be found on cardiac tests such as echocardiograms, electrocardiograms (EKGs), Exercise Stress Test (EST) and Holter monitors. For more information, see *Chapter 13, Heart and Blood Vessels.*

Fatigue. After treatment for AML, most children resume normal activities at age-appropriate levels, but some children have fatigue. These children, usually those who have received cranial radiation and/or had stem cell transplants, may have long-term troubles with strength, coordination, and weakness. For more information, see *Chapter 8, Fatigue.*

Dental problems. Dental abnormalities such as failure of the teeth to develop, arrested root development, unusually small teeth, and enamel abnormalities occasionally occur after chemotherapy or radiation. For more information, see *Chapter 12, Head and Neck.*

Less common problems. Less common late effects include bladder problems (i.e., hemorrhagic cystitis and bladder fibrosis) from cyclophosphamide and osteonecrosis (death of blood vessels that nourish bones) from high-dose steroids. Children who receive cranial radiation have a small risk of developing a secondary cancer. Those treated with VP-16 have a slight chance of a second leukemia, which usually develops within 3 to 5 years after treatment. For more information, see *Chapter 20, Subsequent Malignancies*.

See information about the late effects of stem cell transplants in section at the end of this chapter, *Stem Cell Transplantation Late effects*.

BRAIN TUMORS

Primary brain tumors are the most common solid tumors occurring in children. Approximately 4,200 children are diagnosed with a brain tumor in the U.S each year. Seventy-two percent of children diagnosed with a brain tumor are younger than age 15. Because there are many different specific types of brain tumors, the number of children diagnosed with each type of tumor is small. The incidence of brain tumors is higher in males than females and higher among white children than black children.

Description

Brain tumors can be benign (noncancerous) or malignant (cancerous). Treatment of both benign and malignant brain tumors can result in numerous late effects. Most tumors are named for the type of cell from which the cancer originated and the location of the tumor in the brain. The most common pediatric brain tumors are astrocytoma, medulloblastoma, brain stem gliomas, ependymomas, and optic nerve gliomas:

- **Astrocytomas.** Astrocytomas are tumors that arise from star-shaped cells called astrocytes. Low-grade astrocytomas grow slowly, and many types have a favorable prognosis. High-grade astrocytomas grow quickly and are more difficult to treat.
- **Medulloblastomas.** Medulloblastomas are fast-growing, malignant tumors that are located in the cerebellum/posterior fossa (back of the brain). They are diagnosed most often in children between the ages of 4 and 8 and are more common in boys than girls.
- **Brain stem gliomas.** Brain stem gliomas are slow or fast-growing tumors that occur equally in both sexes and are most common in

children between the ages of 5 and 10.

- **Ependymomas.** Ependymomas are tumors that usually grow on the internal surfaces of the brain and spinal cord. Ependymomas in the brain occur most often in children younger than age 10; those of the spinal cord usually strike children older than age 12.

- **Optic nerve gliomas.** Optic nerve gliomas are tumors located along the optic nerves and the optic chiasm and connect the nerve to the eye. Sometimes the glioma may enter into the hypothalamus.

Treatment

Treatment for brain tumors usually is some combination of surgery, radiation, and chemotherapy. In some cases, stem cell transplantation is also used. If the tumor is benign, surgery may remove it completely. Whether the tumor is benign or malignant, its location in the brain usually determines how it is treated.

Surgery

Surgery has many uses in the treatment of brain cancers. It is used to get a sample of tissue to confirm the diagnosis, remove as much of the tumor as possible, or alleviate symptoms. For some brain tumors, surgery is used to place a shunt to drain fluid from the brain. There are some instances when surgery is *not* possible due to the location of the tumor and the damage that would be done to the child's ability to function by trying to remove it. After surgery for brain tumors, physicians classify, grade, and stage the tumor before deciding on what further treatment, if any, is necessary. Each step of this process is explained in the following list:

- **Classification.** A pathologist looks at a sample of the tumor under a microscope to determine the origin of the tumor cells. For instance, tumors that arise from glial cells in the brain are ependymomas, astrocytomas, and oligodendrogliomas.

- **Grading.** The pathologist estimates the degree of the malignancy by studying many different features of the tumor cells. Numbers are used to describe the aggressiveness of the tumor, with the higher numbers being the more aggressive. Aggressive means they will grow and spread if left untreated.

- **Staging.** Before surgery, the extent of the tumor spread is evaluated using scans. During surgery, the neurosurgeon decides whether the tumor can be completely removed (called resected) and whether other tumors are present. For most tumors, doctors recommend a lumbar puncture to check for cancer cells in the cerebrospinal fluid. The doctor will determine how many additional studies, if any, are needed after surgery to stage the tumor.

After the tumor has been classified, graded, and staged, the oncologist gives recommendations for treatment.

Radiation

Radiation therapy—directing high-energy x-rays at tissue—is frequently used for brain tumors. In most cases, the radiation is directed at the tumor itself, sparing surrounding healthy tissue as much as possible. For extremely malignant tumors, the entire cranium and sometimes the spine are irradiated to destroy any cancer cells that have broken off from the main tumor and lodged elsewhere.

To minimize damage to healthy brain cells, 3-dimensional conformal radiation therapy or charged-particle radiation therapy (such as proton beam therapy) are being used at many cancer treatment centers around the country. Research is on-going in studies of these new methods of radiation therapy and the acute and long-term effects in children. Studies have shown encouraging results with improved survival rates and decrease in incidence and severity of late effects. More research is needed to continue to observe long-term results and late effects of new methods of radiation such as proton beam therapy.

Radiation is generally given in many doses (called *fractions*) over a period of time. The length of radiation treatment and the amount of radiation given varies depending on the type of tumor, its location in the brain, and the child's age. Because of the critical brain growth that would be disrupted in young children, doctors try to postpone or avoid using radiation until children are at least 2-years-old.

Chemotherapy

Chemotherapy has variable effectiveness against brain tumors because the blood-brain barrier prevents many types of chemotherapy from penetrating brain tumors. In some cases, chemotherapy is used in very young children to slow the progression of their disease until radiation can be given with fewer long-term side effects. In other cases, chemotherapy is one of the front-line treatments used to cure disease.

Stem cell transplantation

Autologous bone marrow transplants and peripheral blood stem cell transplants have been used with increasing frequency to treat children with high-risk or relapsed brain tumors. See descriptions of the types of stem cell transplants and late effects in section at the end of this chapter, *Stem Cell Transplantation Late Effects*.

Late effects of treatment for brain tumor

This section briefly outlines some common and uncommon late effects from treatment. Remember that you may develop none, one, or several of these problems in the months or years after treatment ends.

The brain is the master of thoughts, emotions, and actions. All treatments for brain tumors can result in major effects on thinking and functioning. Following are brief descriptions of some of the more commonly known late effects after treatment for brain tumors. Of course, the specific treatment used (i.e., surgery, radiation, chemotherapy), the age of the child, and the location of the tumor determine the types of late effects that are likely to develop.

Learning disabilities. Both surgery and radiation can damage a child's CNS. When whole brain radiation is used, it can have profound effects on how well the brain functions. The amount of damage depends on the child's treatment, age, and sex, with younger female children more at risk than males and older children or teens. Learning disabilities can develop years after treatment ends, and social functioning is often impacted as well. For more information, see *Chapter 9, Brain and Nerves*.

Growth and hormonal problems. Radiation can also affect growth. Children who receive cranial radiation or spinal radiation may have problems with growing normally. Radiation can cause early or delayed puberty, thyroid problems, and other hormonal imbalances. For more information, see *Chapter 10, Hormone-Producing Glands.*

Hearing loss and kidney damage. Cisplatin can cause significant hearing loss and kidney damage. For more information, see *Chapter 11, Eyes and Ears,* and *Chapter 15, Kidneys, Bladder, and Genitals.*

Other late effects. Radiation to the head can also cause cataracts and secondary cancers. Common second tumor post radiation is a meningioma. For additional information, see *Chapter 11, Eyes and Ears* and *Chapter 20, Subsequent Malignancies.*

EWING SARCOMA

Ewing sarcoma gets its name from the physician who first described it in 1921, Dr. James Ewing. For many years it was believed that Ewing sarcoma occurred only in the bone; however, other tumors within soft tissues have since been found to be similar. These include extraosseous Ewing sarcoma (EES) and peripheral primitive neuroectodermal tumor (PNET). Together, these malignancies are called the Ewing sarcoma family of tumors (ESFT).

Each year in the United States, about 650-700 children and adolescents younger than age 20 are diagnosed with a bone tumor, of which only 200 are Ewings Sarcoma. Ewings sarcoma tumors may occur from ages 5 to 10. The peak incidence is between 10-15 years of age. Boys tend to be diagnosed with this disease more often than girls, and there is a much higher incidence in white children than children of other races. The treatment and late effects are similar for both types of tumors and are addressed together in this section.

Treatment

ESFT tumors usually require, multiagent induction chemotherapy followed by local treatment with surgery, definitive radiation, or a combination of surgery and radiation followed by additional chemotherapy.

Surgery

Before the development of limb-salvage surgery and newer radiation techniques, most children with extremity tumors had the affected limb amputated. Many children now are treated with state-of-the-art radiation therapy and/or have limb-salvage procedures that use autologous grafts, allografts, or endoprostheses. In some cases, orthopedic reconstruction is required after removal of the tumor.

Radiation

Radiation is needed to treat children diagnosed with ESFT tumors that cannot be completely removed. Some chest wall tumors are treated with whole-lung radiation.

The current guideline for radiation treatment for ESFT Tumors includes Involved Field Radiation with limited margin. Whole-lung radiation also was used in some studies to reduce the number of pulmonary relapses; however, this resulted in significant toxicity when combined with systemic chemotherapy. Currently, lung radiation is used only for some chest wall tumors.

Chemotherapy

In the 1960s before chemotherapy became a standard treatment against ESFT tumors, very few children survived. Chemotherapy improved the long-term survival rate and made it easier to remove the tumor by reducing the size before surgery. Treatment of Ewing sarcoma now includes chemotherapy for all children. This is necessary even for children with localized disease.

Late effects of Ewing sarcoma

This section briefly outlines some common and uncommon late effects from treatment. Remember that you may develop none, one, or several of these problems in the months or years after treatment ends.

Damage to soft tissues and bones. One of the most common and troublesome late effects from radiation treatment for ESFT tumors is damage to soft tissues and the underlying bones. If the leg of a young child gets high doses of radiation, it stops growing and will be shorter than the nonirradiated leg. Radiation around the arm or leg can result in fibrosis (meaning scarring), swelling, and poor function. Most of these changes happened with older radiation techniques.

Loss of function can also be minimized or prevented by a comprehensive physical therapy program during and after treatment. For more information, see *Chapter 18, Muscles and Bones*.

Heart problems. Heart problems can occur months or years after treatment with anthracyclines (i.e., doxorubicin, idarubicin, or daunorubicin) and/or chest radiation. Most ESFT tumor survivors receive a large amount of chemotherapy which may affect the heart. Symptoms include shortness of breath, fatigue, wheezing, anxiety, poor exercise tolerance, rapid heartbeat, and irregular heartbeat. Regular follow-up with oncology provider and cardiologist is crucial throughout life. Survivors may have no symptoms, but problems may be found on cardiac tests such as echocardiograms, electrocardiograms (EKGs), and Holter monitors. For more information, see *Chapter 13, Heart and Blood Vessels*.

Fertility. Abdominal radiation and high doses of cyclophosphamide and/or ifosfamide can affect fertility. For more information on fertility, see *Chapter 10, Hormone-Producing Glands*, and *Chapter 3, Relationships*.

Digestion. Abdominal radiation can also cause problems with digestion and absorption of food. For more information, see *Chapter 16, Liver, Stomach, and Intestines*.

Secondary cancers (*subsequent malignancy*). There is a small chance of developing a secondary cancer in the radiated area. For more information, see *Chapter 20, Subsequent Malignancies*.

HODGKIN LYMPHOMA

Hodgkin lymphoma (which used to be called Hodgkin's disease) accounts for 7 percent of all cancers in children in the United States. The disease, very rare in children younger than age 5, is most commonly diagnosed in 15- to 19-year-olds. It occurs more often in boys than girls in patients younger than age 10, although in adolescence, the incidence is slightly higher in females than males. Approximately 94 percent of children and adolescents treated today with the current methods (listed below) survive their disease.

Description

Hodgkin lymphoma, first described by Thomas Hodgkin in 1832, is a cancer of the lymph system. This system is made up of lymph vessels throughout the body that carry a clear liquid called lymph. Throughout this network are groups of small organs called lymph nodes that make and store lymphocytes—cells that fight infection. Lymph tissue is found throughout the body, so Hodgkin lymphoma can be found in almost any organ or tissue, such as the liver, bone marrow, or spleen.

Treatment

Treatment for Hodgkin lymphoma is *risk-based*, and usually involves multiagent chemotherapy with or without low-dose radiation. Risk is determined by the stage of the disease, symptoms, and/or the presence of bulky disease (i.e., a large mass).

The goal of treatment for Hodgkin lymphoma is to eliminate the disease with the smallest amount of long-term problems. The method of treatment is based on stage of the disease, the age of the child or teen, and possible long-term effects, called *risk-based treatment*.

Historically, children and adolescents diagnosed with Hodgkin lymphoma were treated first with surgery (i.e., removal of the spleen), chemotherapy, and high-dose radiation. Current treatment usually involves multiagent chemotherapy with or without low-dose radiation. Surgery is performed rarely, in certain cases.

Some clinical trials include stem cell transplantation for recurrent disease. The intensity and duration of chemotherapy and the location and amount of radiation are based on risk factors.

Radiation

Figure 7-1 shows the areas of the body that may be irradiated in children or adolescents with Hodgkin lymphoma. Typically, only one field is used for localized disease.

In the 1960s and 1970s, higher doses of radiation were given to children and teens. Survivors treated prior to the 1990s have very different late effects than those treated more recently. Researchers have

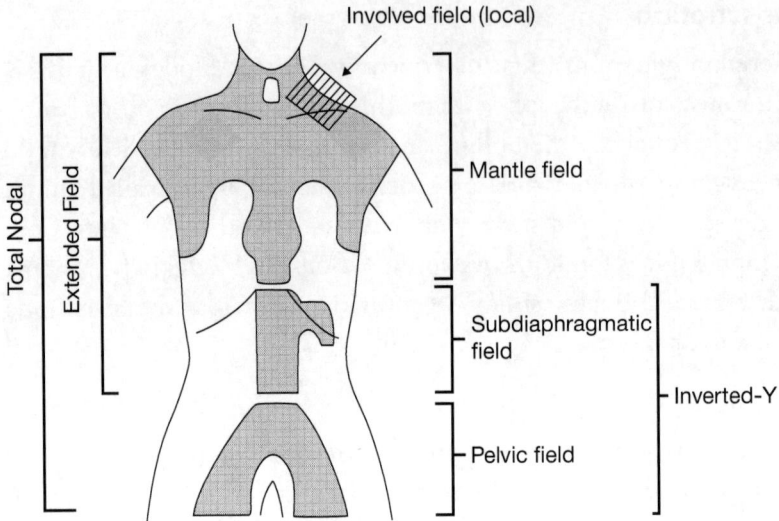

FIGURE 7-1. Radiation fields for Hodgkin lymphoma: local involved field, extended field, total nodal field (©*Alex's Lemonade Stand Foundation, 2025*)

worked diligently to fine-tune protocols to give children and adolescents only the amount of radiation treatment needed for cure and to minimize late effects. Today it is much more common to receive lower doses of radiation and Intensity Modulated Radiation Therapy and/or Proton Radiation than 20 years ago.

Chemotherapy

For decades the standard treatment for Hodgkins lymphoma was chemotherapy and consolidated radiation therapy. Today immunotherapy is being incorporated with some of the old chemotherapy drugs. Radiation is not always given but when it is, targeted treatment is the goal to limit healthy tissue exposure.

Today there are new drug studies directed at immunotherapy to reduce the long-term side effects of standard treatment. It is too early to comment now (2023) regarding results of these studies and whether this will become the new standard of treatment.

Late effects of treatment of Hodgkin Lymphoma

Much is known about possible late effects of treatment for Hodgkin lymphoma because so many children and adolescents survive the disease. Recent treatments have decreased the risk of serious late effects among Hodgkins' survivors. The following information briefly outlines some common and uncommon late effects from treatment. Remember that you may develop none, a few, or several of these problems in the months or years after treatment ends.

Obstructions and infections. Splenectomy is rarely performed today. Late complications after a splenectomy (surgery to remove the spleen) are adhesions and intestinal obstruction. In addition, bacterial sepsis (massive infection) occurs in some patients who had their spleen removed or irradiated. For more information, see *Chapter 17, Immune System.*

Growth. Radiation can also cause significant late effects in survivors. The growth may be slowed in prepubertal children who receive spinal radiation. Children who are past puberty are usually not as affected as younger children. For more information, see *Chapter 18, Muscles and Bones.*

Dry mouth and narrowed esophagus. If the jawbone is in the radiation field, malfunctioning salivary glands can cause dry mouth and tooth decay. Mantle radiation can also result in delayed or arrested tooth development. *Mantle radiation* is a technique used in 1970s to the 1990s which treated a large area of the neck, chest, armpits and mediastinum (area between the lungs) in order to cover all areas with cancer involvement (See Figure 7.1). Mantle radiation is rarely used today in current treatment.

Current treatment is *Involved Field Radiation Therapy (IFRT)* which delivers radiation to only those areas of the body involved by lymphoma and is more precise and limits exposure to healthy tissue. Another effect that can occur several years after radiation in chest/neck area is esophageal strictures (which is narrowing of the tube between the mouth and the stomach). Symptoms are difficulty swallowing or needing to drink liquid to help swallow solid food. For more information, see *Chapter 12, Head and Neck.*

Thyroid problems. Hypothyroidism in Hodgkin lymphoma survivors treated with neck/chest radiation is common. Other possible problems are thyroid nodules, hyperthyroidism, and thyroid cancer. For more information, see *Chapter 10, Hormone-Producing Glands.*

Osteonecrosis. Some patients who were irradiated and also received chemotherapy that included prednisone develop osteonecrosis (destruction of blood vessels that go to the bones). Osteonecrosis can develop during treatment, but it also can occur years after treatment ends. This condition weakens bones and increases the risk of fractures. For more information, see *Chapter 18, Muscles and Bones.*

Lung damage. Radiation to the chest can damage the lungs, especially in survivors who also received bleomycin. The extent of the injury depends on the total amount of radiation, the amount given each day (fraction size), and the amount of lung tissue in the radiation field. For more information, see *Chapter 14, Lungs.*

Heart problems. Chest radiation (especially in combination with doxorubicin) can affect how well the heart works. Children or adolescents who received chest/whole lung radiation are at risk for cardiac problems ranging from EKG changes (with no symptoms) to life-threatening pericarditis (which is inflammation of the pericardium, the sac surrounding the heart). Other injuries to the heart include underdevelopment of the blood vessels, coronary artery disease, thickening of the pericardium, valve damage, and accelerated atherosclerosis. Treatment with anthracyclines also increases the risk for heart problems. For more information, see *Chapter 13, Heart and Blood Vessels.*

Fertility. After pelvic radiation, sterility or changes in fertility can occur in girls. A young ovary can tolerate more radiation than can an older ovary. Girls whose ovaries are radiated during puberty or after are more at risk for ovarian problems, including infertility and early menopause.

In males, functioning of the testes may be affected by pelvic radiation. Pelvic radiation can cause temporary oligospermia (a decrease in the number of sperm) or azoospermia (no sperm). If the testes are not in the field of radiation, they are usually unaffected.

Chemotherapy can also affect fertility in males. Usually, hormone-producing cells of the testes function well after therapy, so boys continue to grow and have a normal puberty. For more information about fertility, see *Chapter 10, Hormone-Producing Glands,* and *Chapter 3, Relationships.*

Reynaud's syndrome. Reynaud's syndrome (when fingers and toes become icy, white, and plump when exposed to cold) is a rare late effect of patients treated with vinblastine (Velben') and bleomycin.

Secondary cancers (*subsequent malignancy*). One of the most serious late effects of treatment for Hodgkin lymphoma is *secondary cancers.* Some survivors develop either AML (acute myelogenous leukemia) or its precursor—pancytopenia myelodysplastic syndrome. The highest incidence of secondary leukemia is 5 to 10 years after treatment with chemotherapy. After 10 years, it is rarely seen. Solid tumors in the lungs, genitourinary tract, breasts, and thyroid sometimes occur after treatment of these areas with radiation. The risk of developing these cancers increases with time.

The risk of developing breast cancer after chest radiation for Hodgkin lymphoma has been estimated to be as high as 35 percent at 50 years of age, depending on radiation dose and age at diagnosis. The greatest risk of breast cancer appears to be in girls treated between the ages of 10 and 16. Thus, all female survivors of Hodgkin lymphoma should have routine mammograms starting 8 years after radiation or at age 25 (whichever occurs last) and have regular breast exams by their healthcare provider.

For more information, see *Chapter 20, Subsequent Malignancies.*

NEUROBLASTOMA

Neuroblastoma is cancer of the sympathetic nervous system—a network of nerves that carries messages from the brain to all parts of the body. Primary neuroblastoma is a solid, malignant tumor that usually first appears as a mass in the abdomen (most often in the adrenal glands) or near the spine.

Approximately 600 children are diagnosed with neuroblastoma each year in the United States. The average age at diagnosis is 2, and two-thirds of newly diagnosed children are younger than age 5. Neuroblastoma occurs slightly more often in boys than in girls. A very small number (1 to 2 percent) of children who are diagnosed with neuro-blastoma have a family history of the disease.

Treatment

Treatment of neuroblastoma is based on age, stage of disease, and biologic features and usually includes surgery, chemotherapy, and radiation. The International Neuroblastoma Staging System (INSS) categorizes neuroblastoma into six distinct stages. Most oncologists now also categorize patients into low-risk, intermediate-risk, or high-risk groups and tailor the treatments accordingly. See more details about risk groups at (Neuroblastoma Risk Groups | American Cancer Society | American Cancer Society).

Surgery

Surgery is used to treat virtually all neuroblastomas and has many important roles. It is used to establish the diagnosis, to obtain tumor tissue for examination, to stage the disease, and for second-look procedures. If the tumor is localized and appears to be removable, surgery is performed soon after diagnosis, before further therapy is begun. Most often immediate surgery is not possible and chemotherapy is used to shrink the tumor prior to surgery. Even after chemotherapy, surgical removal is often incomplete, and radiation is required to ensure that all tumor cells are destroyed.

The goals of initial surgeries are developed on an individual basis. Factors considered include tumor location, whether it can be removed, relationship to major blood vessels, and the child's prognosis. Lymph nodes in the area of the tumor usually are sampled to determine whether the disease has spread.

Chemotherapy

Chemotherapy is used to treat almost all children with neuroblastoma. Response rates have improved considerably by using combinations of chemotherapy drugs. The most commonly used chemotherapy drugs include cyclophosphamide (Cytoxan), carboplatin, cisplatin (Platinol'), doxorubicin (Adriamycin'), vincristine (Oncovin'), ifosfamide, etoposide (VP-16 or Vepesid'), and topotecan. For high-risk neuroblastoma, a combination of 13-cis-retinoic acid and GM-CSF is also used.

Radiation

Neuroblastoma is very sensitive to radiation. The primary goal of radiation is for local control of tumors that cannot be removed surgically, even after several courses of chemotherapy. Radiation can be used for symptomatic relief of painful bony lesions at any time.

In the past, patients with spinal cord compression were treated with radiation. Currently, chemotherapy is used instead, as it has proven to be just as effective with fewer side effects.

Stem cell transplantation

Since 2012, stem cell transplants (i.e., bone marrow, stem cell, cord blood) have been used with increasing frequency to treat children with high-risk or relapsed neuroblastoma. Various regimens are used to prepare the child for transplant.

See descriptions of the types of stem cell transplants and late effects in section at the end of this chapter, *Stem Cell Transplantation Late effects.*

Late effects of neuroblastoma treatment

This section briefly outlines some common and uncommon late effects from treatment. Remember that you may develop none, one, or several of these problems in the months or years after treatment ends.

Surgery for neuroblastoma results in complications in 5 to 25 percent of young patients. The highest rates occur after aggressive attempts to surgically remove abdominal tumors at diagnosis. Long-term effects from these surgeries may include adhesions, injuries to vessels to the kidneys resulting in kidney failure, and neurologic deficits. Surgeries after tumor shrinkage by chemotherapy have much lower complication rates. For more information, see *Chapter 16, Liver, Stomach, and Intestines.*

Heart problems. Heart problems can occur months or years after treatment with anthracyclines (i.e., doxorubicin, idarubicin, or daunorubicin) or chest radiation. Symptoms include shortness of breath, fatigue, wheezing, anxiety, poor exercise tolerance, rapid heartbeat, and irregular heartbeat. Survivors often have no symptoms, but problems may be found on cardiac tests such as echocardiograms, electrocardiograms (EKGs), and Holter monitors. For more information, see *Chapter 13, Heart and Blood Vessels*.

Hearing loss. Cisplatin can cause mild to profound hearing loss in some children. For more information, see *Chapter 11, Eyes and Ears*.

Secondary cancers. An uncommon side effect from treatment of neuroblastoma is developing secondary cancers. For more information, see *Chapter 20, Subsequent Malignancies*.

Opsoclonus-myoclonus syndrome. Patients with neuroblastoma and a syndrome called opsoclonus-myoclonus (also called dancing eyes-dancing feet) have an excellent response to treatment, but they tend to have severe long-term neurologic deficits, including cognitive and motor delays, language problems, and behavioral abnormalities. Although these are *not* treatment-related effects, they affect quality of life.

The possible long-term effects of stem cell transplants are listed at the end of this chapter in a section, *Stem cell Transplantation Late effects*.

NON-HODGKIN LYMPHOMA

Non-Hodgkin lymphoma (NHL) is the third most common childhood cancer (after leukemia and brain tumors). In the United States, approximately 800 children younger than age 20 are diagnosed with NHL in the United States every year. https://www.cancer.gov/types/lymphoma/hp/child-nhl-treatment-pdq#_536_toc

It is rare in very young children, and the incidence increases with age. There is an increased risk of NHL in children diagnosed with AIDS. Childhood NHL is more common in males than in females, and diagnosed slightly more in white children than black children.

The 5-year survival rate for children and adolescents with Stage I or II NHL is greater than 90%; and Stage III or IV 80-90%.).

Description

Lymphomas are cancers of the lymph system. This system is made up of lymph vessels throughout the body that carry a colorless liquid called lymph. Throughout this network, groups of small organs called lymph nodes make and store lymphocytes—cells that fight infection. Lymph tissue is found throughout the body, so NHL can be found in almost any organ or tissue, such as the liver, bone marrow, or spleen. Hodgkin and NHL are differentiated by cell type and require different treatments.

Although there are many different types of NHL, the three most common in children are lymphoblastic, small noncleaved cell lymphoma (Burkitt's and non-Burkitt's), and large cell lymphoma.

Treatment

Treatment for NHL is based on histology (meaning how the tissue and cells look under a microscope) and clinical stage. Several staging systems are used.

Radiation

In the past, radiation was given to most children with NHL, and its use significantly increased the toxicity of treatment. Currently, radiation is used only for tumors in the chest that cause trouble breathing, compression of major blood vessels, testicular tumors, or primary NHL of bone. The use of radiation in even these situations is in dispute in scientific circles. Many experts now believe radiation should be used only in exceptional circumstances for children or teens with NHL.

Chemotherapy

The mainstay of treatment for NHL is combination chemotherapy. There are new targeted chemotherapy drugs being incorporated into the treatment protocols with good results. It is too early to say the long-term effects of these drugs. We would recommend discussing the treatment protocol and drug effects with the treating physician/nurse practitioner/nurse.

Late effects of treatment for non-Hodgkin lymphoma

This section briefly outlines some common and uncommon late effects from treatment. Remember that you may develop none, one, or several of these problems in the months or years after treatment ends.

Children with stage I or II NHL may have few or no long-term effects. Children with stage III or IV NHL, or those who have relapsed and require more intensive treatment, sometimes experience more late effects.

Fertility. Female fertility usually is not affected by treatment for lymphoma unless the girl had spinal radiation that included the ovaries or had very high doses of cyclophosphamide. Teenage girls are more at risk than younger girls due to normal egg depletion as a girl ages. In the majority of cases, girls treated for lymphoma have normal growth, sexual development, and fertility. The chances of having a normal pregnancy and birth if fertility is not affected are the same as for the general population.

The use of methotrexate, vincristine, cyclophosphamide, and prednisone cause a rapid decrease in sperm count in male teens who have passed puberty. Normal sperm production and motility generally return after treatment. Boys treated for lymphoma before puberty usually experience a normal puberty. However, patients who received very high doses of cyclophosphamide (more than 7.5 grams/m^2) or radiation to the testes should have testosterone levels and sperm count checked. Most males treated with chemotherapy alone have normal growth, sexual development, and fertility. For more information about growth and fertility, see *Chapter 10, Hormone-Producing Glands*.

Heart problems. In a small number of survivors, heart problems can occur months or years after treatment with anthracyclines (i.e., doxorubicin, idarubicin, or daunorubicin) or chest radiation. Symptoms include shortness of breath, fatigue, wheezing, anxiety, poor exercise tolerance, rapid heartbeat, and irregular heartbeat. Survivors often have no symptoms, but problems may be found on cardiac tests such as echocardiograms, electrocardiograms (EKGs), and Holter monitors. For more information, see *Chapter 13, Heart and Blood Vessels.*

Learning disabilities. Cranial radiation, intrathecal methotrexate, and/or high-dose methotrexate may cause cognitive problems. Learning disabilities can develop years after treatment ends. Typically, problems develop in the areas of mathematics, spatial relationships, processing speed, problem solving, organization, planning, attention span, concentration skills, and social skills. For more information, see *Chapter 9, Brain and Nerves.*

Dental problems. Dental abnormalities can occur after chemotherapy or radiation to the jaw area. The most frequent problems are failure of the teeth to develop, arrested root development, unusually small teeth, and enamel abnormalities. For more information, see *Chapter 12, Head and Neck.*

Uncommon late effects. Extremely rare late effects include bladder problems (i.e., hemorrhagic cystitis and bladder fibrosis) from cyclophosphamide, osteonecrosis (death of blood vessels that nourish bones) from high-dose steroids, and second cancers.

OSTEOSARCOMA

Malignant bone tumors account for approximately 5 percent of all childhood cancers. Fifty-six percent of all bone tumors diagnosed are osteosarcoma, most of which occur during the adolescent growth spurt. Males are affected more than females, and more black children are diagnosed than are white children.

Description

Osteosarcoma is a primary malignant cancer of the bone. It typically occurs at the ends of the long bones, usually at the knee. Other, less common sites are the upper arm (close to the shoulder), the pelvis, and the skull.

Treatment

During the last 25 years, treatment for osteosarcoma has greatly improved. Today, the majority of young patients with a primary tumor in a limb and no metastases will survive. Advances in surgical techniques have also markedly improved the quality of life for survivors.

When osteosarcoma is diagnosed in a bone, more tests are performed to determine if the cancer has spread to other parts of the body. A biopsy is required to determine the type and stage of the tumor. Imaging studies that may be performed to check for metastases are magnetic resonance imaging (MRI), computed tomography (CT) of the chest, a bone scan, and sometimes a positron emission tomography (PET) scan.

There are two stages for osteosarcoma at diagnosis:

- **Localized,** tumors limited to the bone of origin
- **Metastatic,** tumors found in other parts of the body, including the lungs, other bones, or distant sites

Surgery

Surgery usually is performed after a period of chemotherapy. Successful surgical removal of the primary tumor most often consists of either limb-salvage surgery, *rotationplasty*, or amputation. A surgical procedure called a thoracotomy (i.e., opening the chest cavity) also is used when adolescents have metastases to the lungs.

Total removal of both gross and microscopic tumors is required to prevent recurrence. Factors that determine the choice of amputation or salvage therapy are tumor location, tumor size, presence of distant metastases, skeletal development, and patient preference. Whether or not the affected bone is broken at the time of diagnosis also affects the choice of treatment.

In up to 20 percent of osteosarcoma cases, areas of tumor develop inches away from the primary tumor. These areas, called *skip lesions*, can cause local recurrence in stumps after amputation. Prior to advances in CT and MRI techniques and radionuclide scanning, some surgeons removed the entire affected bone, resulting in disability and loss of function. Now a variety of methods are used to salvage limbs. Bones from cadavers (called *allografts*) or pieces of the patient's own bone (i.e., fibula or iliac crest) are used. Devices made from cobalt, chrome, or steel can be custom designed to replace the diseased bone. In some cases, the bone is removed and not replaced.

Radiation

Osteosarcoma usually does not respond well to radiation. Because of the risk of recurrence for tumors treated with radiation, it is used only in treating patients whose tumors cannot be completely removed surgically.

Chemotherapy

Chemotherapy is resumed after surgery has removed as much of the tumor as possible. A combination of some of the following drugs is used to treat osteosarcoma: doxorubicin (Adriamycin᷎), high-dose methotrexate, cisplatin (Platinol᷎), and cyclophosphamide (Cytoxan᷎). Ifosfamide (Ifex᷎), and/or etoposide, are sometimes used for children who relapse.

Late effects of treatment for osteosarcoma

This section briefly outlines some common and uncommon late effects from treatment. Remember that you may develop none, one, or several of these problems in the months or years after treatment ends.

Physical impairments. One of the universal late effects from treatment for osteosarcoma is coping with physical impairments from amputation or limb-salvage therapy. After limb-salvage therapy or fitting with a state-of-the-art prosthesis, many survivors are able to resume an active lifestyle, while others struggle to regain mobility. For more information, see *Chapter 18, Muscles and Bones.*

Heart problems. Heart problems can occur months or years after treatment with anthracyclines (i.e., doxorubicin, idarubicin, or daunorubicin) or chest radiation. Symptoms include shortness of breath, fatigue, wheezing, anxiety, poor exercise tolerance, rapid heart- beat, and irregular heartbeat. Survivors of Osteosarcoma are usually exposed to large amounts of chemotherapy which may affect the heart. Regular checkups are crucial. Survivors often have no symptoms, but problems may be found on cardiac tests such as echocardiograms, electrocardiograms (EKGs), Exercise Stress Test (EST) and Holter monitors. For more information, see *Chapter 13, Heart and Blood Vessels*.

Hearing loss. Cisplatin can result in mild to profound hearing loss in some children and teens. For more information, see *Chapter 10, Eyes and Ears*.

Learning disabilities. Treatment with high-dose methotrexate may result in cognitive problems. Learning disabilities can develop months or years after treatment ends. Typically, problems develop in the areas of mathematics, spatial relationships, problem solving, processing speed, organization, planning, attention span, concentration skills, and social skills. For more information, see *Chapter 9, Brain and Nerves*.

Fertility. Female fertility may be affected due to treatment for osteosarcoma with very high doses of cyclophosphamide (more than 7.5 grams per square meter [grams/m^2]) or ifosfamide (more than 60 grams/m^2). In the majority of cases, girls treated for osteosarcoma have normal growth, sexual development, and fertility. The chances of having a normal pregnancy and birth are the same as in the general population.

Cyclophosphamide can cause a rapid decrease in sperm count in male teens who have passed puberty. Normal sperm production and motility generally return after treatment. After osteosarcoma treatment, younger males usually experience a normal puberty. However, young men who received very high doses of cyclophosphamide— more than 7.5 grams/m^2) should have testosterone levels and sperm count checked. For more information about growth and fertility, see *Chapter 10, Hormone-Producing Glands*.

Second cancers (*subsequent malignancies*). A rare side effect from treatment of osteosarcoma is developing second cancers. For more information, see *Chapter 20, Subsequent Malignancies*.

RARE CANCERS

Very small numbers of children are diagnosed every year with one of the rare childhood cancers. Because so few doctors see these diseases, diagnosis may be difficult and treatment may not be standardized. The uncommon cancers covered in this section are chronic myelocytic leukemia, histiocytosis, liver tumors, and soft tissue sarcomas. Although these diseases are discussed here briefly, the late effects that might develop after cure are discussed in greater depth in the chapters about organ systems.

If your disease is not covered in this chapter, refer to the current (2023) Version 6 Children's Oncology Group's follow-up guidelines http://www.survivorshipguidelines.org. Locate the treatments you received and be informed about the tests you need to monitor your health.

Chronic myelocytic leukemia

Chronic myelocytic leukemia (also called chronic myelogenous leukemia or CML) accounts for less than 5 percent of all childhood leukemias. In CML, large numbers of cancerous mature granulocytes (a type of white blood cell) appear.

The two major forms of chronic myelocytic leukemia are adult CML, which occurs primarily in adolescents and adults, and juvenile myelomonocytic leukemia (also called juvenile CML), which occurs mostly in infants.

Adult chronic myelocytic leukemia (CML)

Adult CML is characterized by a large spleen and high white blood cell count (usually more than 100,000). In more than 90 percent of adolescents with adult CML, analysis of cells in the bone marrow shows a genetic abnormality called the *Philadelphia chromosome*. This chromosome contains a translocation (where genetic material has traded places) involving chromosomes 9 and 22, abbreviated t(9;22).

Chemotherapy. The goal of treatment for adult CML is to lower the white blood cell count and to reduce the size of the liver and spleen. The current treatment is imatinib mesylate (Gleevec`). Previously, hydroxyurea (Hydrea) or busulfan (Myleran) were used. In some cases, the biologic agent interferon alpha is given alone or in combination with hydroxyurea or cytarabine (ARA-C).

Radiation. Before chemotherapy was used to treat adult CML, radiation of the spleen was a common therapy. When clinical trials proved that radiation was inferior to chemotherapy in prolonging survival, it was used only to reduce the size of painful massive spleens in patients whose disease was resistant to chemotherapy.

Surgery. Removal of the spleen also was common practice in the past until clinical trials showed no improvement in prolonging the chronic phase or survival.

Stem cell transplantation (also known as *hematopoietic stem cell transplantation*). Although Gleevac and interferon alpha slow the progress of adult CML, the best hope for cure is stem cell transplant. The highest cure rates occur when the patient is transplanted during the chronic phase with marrow or stem cells from an identical twin, HLA-matched family member, or HLA-matched non-family member. See descriptions of the types of stem cell transplants and late effects in section at the end of this chapter, *Stem Cell Transplantation Late effects.*

Juvenile myelomonocytic leukemia

Juvenile myelomonocytic leukemia (also called juvenile CML or JMML) usually strikes children younger than age 5. Unlike the adult form of CML, juvenile CML does not have a chronic phase, and the cells usually do not contain the Philadelphia chromosome. This disease progresses rapidly.

Hematopoietic stem cell transplantation. As with adult CML, chemotherapy generally is not a successful treatment for juvenile CML, and stem cell transplantation is the best hope for a cure. However, chemotherapy is sometimes used while preparing for transplant. See descriptions of the types of stem cell transplants and their late effects at the end of this chapter, *Hematopoietic Stem Cell Transplantation.*

Histiocytosis

Histiocytosis is a poorly understood and frequently misdiagnosed disease. Patients can have a wide array of symptoms ranging from skin conditions to bone lesions. Approximately 1,200 new cases are diagnosed in the United States each year, but the true incidence is unknown because so many different types of doctors treat various aspects of the disease. It is common for children with histiocytosis to be seen by dermatologists, endocrinologists, and orthopedists, as well as oncologists.

Histiocytosis is a disease in which histiocytes (a cell of bone marrow origin) multiply and accumulate in various organs or bones in the body. Symptoms mimic other childhood illnesses or conditions, so the only way to obtain a definitive diagnosis is the thorough examination of a sample of affected tissue under an electron microscope.

Organs commonly damaged by the multiplying histiocytes are skin, bone, ears, lymph nodes, glands, lung, eye, liver, spleen, and bone marrow. Less frequently involved body parts are kidneys, jaw, thymus, thyroid, and intestines. Many of the lesions spontaneously heal with time. Diabetes insipidus is also commonly found at diagnosis.

There are three types of histiocytosis:

- **Langerhans' cell histiocytosis.** The most common type of histiocytosis, in which Langerhans' cells are found in lesions.
- **Class II histiocytosis.** A very rare disorder in which Langerhans' cells are not found in lesions. This is almost always a fatal disease, although stem transplantation is used experimentally to treat it.
- **Class III malignant histiocytosis.** A very rare malignant disorder best identified by lymph node biopsy. The disorder was previously always fatal, but new treatments are extending remissions significantly.

There are key differences in these three disorders in terms of diagnosis, treatment, and prognosis.

Langerhans' cell histiocytosis is poorly understood, and hence, numerous treatment methods have been tried over the years. The disease has been treated aggressively as an infection and just as aggressively with chemotherapy as a malignancy. Stem cell transplants are sometimes recommended for children with severe, unresponsive disease. Low-dose radiation is sometimes used for bone involvement, with doses ranging from 700 to 1,000 cGy.

Class II histiocytosis is treated with stem cell transplantation. See descriptions of the types of stem cell transplants and late effects in section at the end of this chapter, *Stem Cell Transplantation Late Effects.*

Children with *Class III malignant histiocytosis* are given induction therapy consisting of vincristine (Oncovin'), prednisone, cyclophosphamide (Cytoxan'), and doxorubicin (Adriamycin'). Maintenance drugs used are vincristine, cyclophosphamide, and doxorubicin.

Most survivors of histiocytosis have no long-term side effects from their treatment. For those who had numerous relapses of the disease or were treated with a stem cell transplant, the chances are higher of developing problems later in life.

Very rare late effects of treatment for histiocytosis:

Heart problems. Heart problems can occur months or years after treatment with high doses of anthracyclines (i.e., doxorubicin, idarubicin, or daunorubicin), high-dose cyclophosphamide, or chest radiation. Symptoms include shortness of breath, fatigue, wheezing, anxiety, poor exercise tolerance, rapid heartbeat, and irregular heartbeat. Survivors often have no symptoms, but problems may be found on cardiac tests such as echocardiograms, electrocardiograms (EKGs), and Holter monitors. For more information, see *Chapter 13, Heart and Blood Vessels.*

Hearing loss. Some children with Langerhans' cell histiocytosis develop hearing loss after years of chronic ear infections. For more information, see *Chapter 11, Eyes and Ears.*

Diabetes insipidus. If the disease infiltrated the pituitary gland, diabetes insipidus often develops.

Uncommon problems. Very rare late effects include bladder problems (i.e., hemorrhagic cystitis and bladder fibrosis) from cyclophosphamide, and damaged joints (from osteonecrosis—death of blood vessels that nourish bones) from high-dose steroids. For more information, see *Chapter 15, Kidneys, Bladder, and Genitals,* and *Chapter 18, Muscles and Bones.*

Liver tumors

Liver tumors comprise fewer than 5 percent of all childhood cancers. The two most common types of childhood liver cancer are hepatoblastoma and hepatocellular carcinoma. Eighty percent of childhood hepatoblastomas occur before age 3, whereas hepatocellular carcinoma has two common incidence peaks in children: from birth to age 4 and from ages 12 to 15.

Surgery. The primary goal of surgery is to remove as much of the tumor as possible. Generally, surgery occurs soon after diagnosis. In cases where the tumor is very large or if the disease has spread to other organs, chemotherapy sometimes is given before surgery.

Chemotherapy. Chemotherapy almost always is used to treat both types of liver cancer. Chemotherapy can be given systemically (i.e., injected into the bloodstream and reaching all parts of the body) or regionally (i.e., delivered directly to the liver). For hepatoblastoma, the most commonly used drugs are cisplatin (Platinol®), vincristine (Oncovin®), and fluorouracil (5-FU). Other drugs, such as doxorubicin (Adriamycin®), ifosfamide (Ifex®), carboplatin, and etoposide (VP- 16 or Vepesid®) have been used for more advanced stages of the disease. Initial treatment for hepatocellular carcinoma usually includes cisplatin and doxorubicin.

Possible late effects of treatment for liver cancers:

Heart problems. Heart problems can occur months or years after treatment with high doses of anthracyclines (i.e., doxorubicin, idarubicin, or daunorubicin), high-dose cyclophosphamide, or chest radiation. Symptoms include shortness of breath, fatigue, wheezing, anxiety, poor exercise tolerance, rapid heartbeat, and irregular heartbeat. Survivors often have no symptoms, but problems may be found on cardiac tests such as echocardiograms, electrocardiograms (EKGs), and Holter monitors. For more information, see *Chapter 13, Heart and Blood Vessels.*

Hearing loss. Cisplatin can result in mild to profound hearing loss in some children. For more information, see *Chapter 11, Eyes and Ears.*

Secondary cancers (*subsequent malignancies*). A rare side effect from treatment with etoposide is developing second cancers. For more information, see *Chapter 20, Subsequent Malignancies.*

Soft tissue sarcomas

Childhood soft tissue sarcoma is a disease in which cancer arises in the body's soft tissues. Soft tissues include muscles, tendons (which connect muscles to bones), fat, blood vessels, nerves, and synovia (tissues around joints). Forty-seven percent of all childhood soft tissue sarcomas have a histology (which is how the cells look under a microscope) that is different from rhabdomyosarcoma (discussed later in this chapter). These soft tissue sarcomas include the following:

- **Synovial sarcoma.** This is the most common non-rhabdomyosarcoma soft tissue sarcoma in childhood. Synovial sarcoma is found most often in older children and is very rarely diagnosed in children younger than age 10. The disease occurs most frequently in the lower extremities, most often in the thigh or knee area. The second most common sites are the upper extremities, followed by the head, neck, and trunk.

- **Fibrosarcoma.** This soft tissue sarcoma occurs most often in infants and children younger than age 5 and in children between ages 10 and 15. These tumors usually develop in the extremities, and the majority of children diagnosed have localized disease. Infants diagnosed with this disease tend to respond to treatment better than older children.

- **Malignant peripheral nerve sheath tumor** (also known as *neurofibrosarcoma or malignant schwannoma*). This is an aggressive malignancy that accounts for approximately 5 to 10 percent of all non-rhabdomyosarcoma soft tissue sarcomas of childhood. The disease often occurs in association with *neurofibromatosis*. The most common sites of origin are the extremities.

- **Malignant fibrous histiocytoma.** This form of soft tissue sarcoma most frequently occurs in the lower extremities and the trunk area. Other sites include the upper limbs, scalp, and kidneys.

The following are extremely rare forms of childhood soft tissue sarcomas. Young children with these diseases are generally treated on protocols based on those used for childhood rhabdomyosarcoma. Teens are usually treated on protocols similar to those used for adults with soft tissue sarcomas.

- **Leiomyosarcoma.** Leiomyosarcoma, which arises from smooth muscle, most often occurs in the gastrointestinal tract, especially the stomach.
- **Liposarcoma.** Liposarcoma arises in fatty tissue and is found most frequently in early adolescence. The most common sites of origin are the legs or trunk.
- **Hemangiopericytoma.** Hemangiopericytoma is a tumor of the blood and lymph vessels that occurs most frequently in infants.
- **Alveolar soft part sarcoma.** This rare soft tissue sarcoma, found most often in older children, arises from skeletal muscles of the extremities, head, and neck.

Treatment for non-rhabdomyosarcoma soft tissue sarcomas usually is surgery and sometimes radiation therapy. Chemotherapy may be used to shrink large tumors to make them operable. Although medical science has made advances in treating soft tissue sarcomas while reducing the side effects and long-term impact to the child, amputation is sometimes necessary. Limb-sparing procedures have made this less common.

Surgery. Surgery is the cornerstone of treatment for soft tissue sarcomas. The surgeon attempts to completely remove the mass with wide margins (i.e., removing a portion of the surrounding tissue) to ensure that no microscopic disease remains. This is often followed by

4000 to 5500 cGy of radiation. Investigational use of brachytherapy (which is implanting radioactive seeds for continuous low-level administration of radiation) is ongoing for children with rare soft tissue sarcomas. Another newer therapy used in current studies is *intraoperative electron radiation*. Radiation is directed at the site during surgery when the tumor and the surrounding areas are exposed.

Because these malignancies are so rare in children, treatment for non-rhabdomyosarcoma soft tissue sarcomas is based on experience with adults. However, children with non-rhabdomyosarcoma soft tissue sarcomas usually have a better outcome than adults with the same diseases.

Chemotherapy. The use of chemotherapy after surgery is controversial. Patients with tumors too large to remove or whose disease has spread may be treated with vincristine, dactinomycin, and cyclophosphamide.

RETINOBLASTOMA

Retinoblastoma is a malignant tumor of the retina in the eye. Approximately 300 children and adolescents younger than age 20 are diagnosed in the United States each year. Retinoblastoma usually is diagnosed in very young children and may be present at birth. Although it can occur at any age, 95 percent of cases are diagnosed before age 5. Children with more than one tumor or a tumor in both eyes (usually the hereditary form) tend to be diagnosed at a younger age than those with only one tumor and one eye involved (usually the non-hereditary form).

Treatment

Successful treatment of retinoblastoma depends largely on the size of the tumor and the extent of the disease. The staging system most widely used is the *Intraocular Retinoblastoma System*, which is based on tumor size, location, and presence of disease within the layers of the retina (called seeding). The Intraocular Retinoblastoma System sub-classifies the disease from 0-IV, with Stage 0 having a good outcome with treatment, and Stage IV retinoblastoma with metastases has a poor prognosis.

Chemotherapy

Historically, chemotherapy was thought to have limited usefulness in treating retinoblastoma. Chemotherapy has become the front-line treatment for selected groups of patients. Intraocular chemotherapy shrinks the tumors, which are then treated with cryotherapy and/or laser therapy. Drugs used in various combinations are vincristine (Oncovin®), etoposide (VP-16 or Vepesid®), and carboplatin (Paraplatin®).

Surgery and other therapies

There are several types of procedures used to treat retinoblastoma: enucleation, cryotherapy, and laser therapy. Decisions about the most appropriate treatment are made on an individual basis.

- Removal of the eye (called *enucleation*) is a simple operation that eliminates the need for repeated examinations under anesthesia required by more conservative therapies. This step is taken only when absolutely necessary. The enucleation procedure is done under general anesthesia. In addition to removing the eye, the surgeon removes a section of the optic nerve. An orbital implant is placed into the socket immediately after the eyeball is removed.

- *Cryotherapy*, sometimes called cryosurgery, is used to treat small primary tumors or new tumors that develop. Cryotherapy uses extreme cold applied by a small probe placed directly on the tumor. It is now often used in combination with chemotherapy and can also be used after radiation therapy.

- *Laser therapy*, which uses infrared wavelengths of light, is sometimes used to treat small tumors.

Radiation

Retinoblastoma is a radiosensitive tumor. Radiation is used to destroy local disease while attempting to maintain vision. The two methods of radiotherapy used to treat retinoblastoma are external beam radiation and radioactive plaques. Newer methods of delivering radiation are being used to try to reduce adverse long-term effects. These methods include *intensity-modulated radiation therapy, stereotactic radiation therapy*, and *proton-beam radiation therapy* (also called charged-particle radiation therapy). Radioactive plaque therapy (called *brachytherapy*) has been used in children with small, early-stage tumors and in those with recurrent disease who have previously been treated with radiation.

Late effects of retinoblastoma treatment

This section briefly outlines some common and uncommon late effects from treatments for retinoblastoma. Remember that you may develop none, one, or several of these problems in the months or years after treatment ends.

Bone growth. The most noticeable side effect of treatment for retinoblastoma is bone growth abnormalities around the eye, which develop after radiation to the orbit. Young children who have one or both eyes removed before age 3 may have an altered facial appearance when they mature due to the slowing of the growth of the orbit. After enucleation, a prosthesis needs to be placed and replaced periodically to foster orbital growth.

Dry eyes. A less common problem is decreased tear production, causing dry eyes and blurred vision. Some children who receive external beam radiation develop mild to severe keratitis sicca (inflammation of the cornea).

Loss of vision. Radiation can cause damage to the retina, resulting in loss of vision. If systemic chemotherapy also is given, the risk of damage increases. Radiation-induced cataracts may occur with any exposure to radiation in the area. In addition, vitreous leakage can occur near the edge of the tumor scar. For more information about these possible late effects, see *Chapter 11, Eyes and Ears*.

Secondary cancers (*subsequent malignancies*). Children with the genetic form of retinoblastoma have an increased rate of developing second cancers, especially sarcomas, lung cancer, skin cancers, and breast cancer. For more information, see *Chapter 20, Subsequent Malignancies*.

Risk of passing on to children. Survivors with the genetic form of retinoblastoma can pass the risk on to their children. Genetic counseling prior to pregnancy can help survivors sort out their options. For more information, see *Chapter 3, Relationships*.

RHABDOMYOSARCOMA

Rhabdomyosarcoma (RMS) is the most common childhood soft tissue sarcoma. Approximately 350 children are diagnosed with RMS in the United States each year. Two-thirds of these cases are diagnosed in children younger than age 5. The disease has a slightly higher incidence in males compared with females. Black children have a slightly higher incidence than white children.

Description

RMS is a malignant soft tissue tumor of primitive muscle cells called *rhabdomyoblasts.* Instead of maturing into muscle cells, the rhabdomyoblasts grow out of control. Because muscles are located throughout the body, the tumors can appear at numerous locations. The four sites where RMS is most commonly found are the head and neck, genitourinary tract, extremities, and chest and lungs.

Treatment

Treatment depends on the location of the tumor, whether it has spread, its *histology* (meaning how it looks under a microscope), and its molecular genetics. Prior to the 1950s, the only treatment for RMS was surgical removal of the tumor. Many tumors were not completely removable and up to 18 percent of children had metastatic disease at diagnosis. The addition of radiation in the 1950s and chemotherapy in the 1960s dramatically improved survival rates for children and teens with RMS.

Surgery

All children and teens with RMS have surgery, either to remove all or part of the primary tumor, or to perform a biopsy to reach a diagnosis. Surgery is used as early as possible in the course of treatment and is the quickest method to reduce the amount of the disease. However, complete removal may not be possible, particularly if the mass is located near vital blood vessels, if it deeply invades surrounding normal tissue, or if there are functional or cosmetic reasons for avoiding such a procedure.

During surgery the doctor removes as much of the tumor as possible and then samples surrounding tissues that are later examined by a pathologist. The pathologist determines whether the entire tumor has been removed or if some cells remain behind.

Second-look surgical procedures are sometimes performed after chemotherapy to remove any remaining residual disease and determine whether remission has been reached. This is especially important for choosing appropriate further treatment, such as the amount of radiation to be given. Approximately 10 percent of newly diagnosed children have tumors that can be completely removed. In most cases, residual disease is present. For this reason, chemotherapy is used in all treatment protocols, and radiation is used in most.

Chemotherapy

Chemotherapy is given to all children and teens with RMS to destroy any cancer not removed surgically. Giving several anticancer drugs in combination has markedly improved the survival rate for this disease. The most commonly used drugs include cyclophosphamide (Cytoxan®), vincristine (Oncovin®), ifosfamide (Ifex®), etoposide (VP-16 or Vepesid®), doxorubicin (Adriamycin®), and dactinomycin (Cosmegen®).

Radiation

Radiotherapy is an important tool used to treat children and adolescents with RMS. Generally, those with stages I and II disease do not receive radiation therapy if their tumors can be completely removed. However, the need for radiation also depends on the histology of the tumor. Current protocols give patients with residual disease 3000 to 5100 cGy of external beam radiation although, in the past, higher doses of radiation were given. New radiation methods such as *intensity-modulated radiation therapy* (IMRT), *fractionated stereotactic radiation therapy*, and *proton beam radiation* are sometimes used for patients with head and neck RMS.

Most often, radiation is given approximately 1 to 3 months after chemotherapy has begun. However, children with tumors in the skull, meninges, or spinal cord may start radiation therapy soon after diagnosis.

Investigational use of *brachytherapy* (i.e., implanting radioactive seeds for continuous low-level administration of radiation) is ongoing for children and teens with RMS, especially those with small tumors in critical areas such as the head, prostate, bladder, or vagina.

Late effects of treatment for rhabdomyosarcoma

This section briefly outlines some common and uncommon late effects from treatment. Remember that you may develop none, one, or several of these problems in the months or years after treatment ends.

Loss of tissue and scarring. One universal late effect from surgery for RMS is loss of tissue and a scar where the tumor was removed. In cases where the surgeon performed a radical lymph node dissection, lymphedema (i.e., backup of lymph in extremities) can result. For more information, see *Chapter 17, Immune System*.

Altered growth. The growing bodies of young children given high doses of radiation develop an altered appearance in the areas radiated, because growth is affected. Because RMS can appear in different areas of the body, refer to the chapters about those specific areas for detailed information about late effects. For instance, high doses of radiation to the orbit and surrounding tissues causes asymmetry in growth and development in the bones around the eye. One orbit will be smaller than the other. Cataracts and other side effects can also develop after radiation. For more information, see *Chapter 11, Eyes and Ears*.

Bladder and kidney problems. In the past, children with tumors in the genitourinary area had the bladder removed in the initial surgery. The resulting permanent ileal conduit (i.e., diversion of the flow of urine to a bag outside the body) could develop many complications over time. Current treatment is the bladder is only removed if the cancer remains after chemotherapy and radiation.

Radiation of the abdomen and/or pelvis can cause chronic nephritis (inflammation of the kidney) and a host of related kidney complications including fatigue, anemia, high blood pressure, hyperuricemia (excess uric acid in the blood), and gout. These problems can develop months or years after radiation treatment. Radiation of the abdomen can also cause fibrosis that obstructs the ureters. For more information about these problems, see *Chapter 15, Kidneys, Bladder, and Genitals.*

Problems after lymph node removal. Radical removal of the lymph nodes in the area of the testes or prostate can result in retrograde ejaculation or bowel obstruction. Problems with ejaculation and decreased sperm production are common in males who had RMS in or near the genitals. For more information, see *Chapter 10, Hormone-Producing Glands.*

Ovarian failure. Radiation to the abdomen can cause ovarian failure in some female survivors. For more information, see *Chapter 10,* Hormone-Producing Glands.

Curvature of the spine. Abdominal radiation at higher doses can also cause curvature of the back. For more information, see *Chapter 18, Muscles and Bones.*

Learning disabilities. Cranial radiation and intrathecal chemotherapy used to treat children with parameningeal RMS (in the membranes surrounding the spinal cord and brain) can cause cognitive problems. The severity of the damage depends on the child's treatment, age, and sex, with younger children being more at risk than older children or teens. Learning disabilities can develop years after treatment ends. Typically, problems develop in the areas of mathematics, memory, spatial relationships, problem solving, planning, processing speed, organization, attention span, concentration skills, and social skills. For more information, see *Chapter 9, Brain and Nerves.*

Heart problems. Heart problems can occur months or years after treatment with anthracyclines (i.e., doxorubicin, idarubicin, or daunorubicin), high-dose cyclophosphamide, or chest radiation. Symptoms include shortness of breath, fatigue, wheezing, anxiety, poor exercise tolerance, rapid heartbeat, and irregular heartbeat. Few survivors develop this late effect, but regular checkups are crucial. Survivors often have no symptoms, but problems may be found on cardiac tests such as echocardiograms, electrocardiograms (EKGs), and Holter monitors. For more information, see *Chapter 13, Heart and Blood Vessels*.

Uncommon late effects. Children and teens who receive radiation have a slight risk of developing a second cancer. Those treated with VP-16 have a small chance of developing a second leukemia within 3 to 5 years of treatment. For more information, see *Chapter 20, Subsequent Malignancies*.

WILMS TUMOR

Wilms tumor is a primary cancer of the kidney. It accounts for 5 to 6 percent of all childhood cancers in the United States—approximately 500 children are diagnosed each year. Wilms tumor occurs most commonly in children younger than age 5. Girls have a slightly higher incidence than boys. Blacks and whites have similar incidence rates, but Asians are much less likely to develop Wilms tumor. A small percentage of Wilms tumors are believed to be inherited. In cases where the disease is inherited, there is a higher incidence of bilateral disease.

Treatment

Choice of treatment depends on histology (i.e., how it looks under a microscope), extent of disease (called *stage*), size of the tumor, and age of the child.

Surgery

Children diagnosed with Wilms tumor usually have a surgical procedure called a *nephrectomy* (removal of a kidney) performed before any other therapy is started. Occasionally, if the diagnosis is questionable, a biopsy will be performed prior to the nephrectomy. After biopsy or surgery, the pathologist examines the nuclei of the cancer cells under a microscope. If the nuclei of some of the cells appear larger than normal or irregular in shape, it is called *anaplasia*. If there is a large amount of anaplasia scattered throughout the tumor, it is called diffuse anaplasia.

Tumor cells that are *not* anaplastic are called Wilms tumor of favorable histology. Ninety-five percent of children with Wilms tumor have favorable histology. Children with unfavorable histology require more intense treatment.

For the majority of children, the goals of surgery are to remove the tumor, prevent rupture of the tumor capsule, and provide tissue for examination and staging. During surgery, the kidney with the tumor is removed, the other kidney is examined (to diagnose the 5 percent of cases in which both kidneys have tumor cells), and lymph nodes in the region are biopsied.

Chemotherapy

All children diagnosed with Wilms tumor receive chemotherapy. There are several chemotherapy drugs that are effective against this type of cancer. The use of dactinomycin (Cosmegen®) and vincristine (Oncovin®) has dramatically increased survival rates. Children with early-stage disease are often treated with just these two drugs. For those who are diagnosed at more advanced stages, doxorubicin (Adriamycin®) and cyclophosphamide (Cytoxan®) may be added. In North America, only those children with bilateral Wilms tumor receive chemotherapy prior to surgery.

Radiation

In the past, all children with Wilms tumor received radiation, some at very high doses. But now, because of the risk of long-term complications from radiation therapy, the decision to use it to treat a child with Wilms is based largely on the stage and histology of the tumor.

Late effects of treatment for Wilms tumor

Some children with stage I or II disease have few or no long-term effects. Children with higher risk disease, or those who relapse and require more intensive treatment, sometimes experience more late effects. Approximately 40% of children diagnosed with Wilms tumor will have favorable staging and only receive two chemotherapy drugs with no late effects. Although, intestinal obstruction post-surgery may develop years later among all stages of Wilms' survivors.

Wilms tumors: common and uncommon late effects

Remember you may develop none, a few, or several of these problems in the months or years after treatment ends.

Growth problems. A child whose trunk is irradiated may have curvature of the spine and soft tissue underdevelopment in the radiated areas (most common in those treated prior to 1970). When lower doses of radiation are given to all or parts of the spine, up to 40 percent of survivors have reduced sitting heights (measured from the rump to the top of the head). This problem is more common in children who were younger than age 6 and in adolescents going through their growth spurt when irradiated. For more information, see *Chapter 18, Muscles and Bones.*

Heart problems. In some patients, heart problems can occur months or years after treatment with anthracyclines (i.e., doxorubicin, idarubicin, or daunorubicin), or chest radiation. Symptoms include shortness of breath, fatigue, wheezing, anxiety, poor exercise tolerance, rapid heartbeat, and irregular heartbeat. Survivors often have no symptoms, but problems may be found on cardiac tests such as echocardiograms, electrocardiograms (EKGs), Exercise Stress Test (EST) and Holter monitors. Abdominal radiation can cause damage to major blood vessels, including the aorta and renal vessels. For more information, see *Chapter 13, Heart and Blood Vessels.*

Fertility and pregnancy. Girls who had abdominal radiation can experience ovarian failure. Survivors who do become pregnant have a risk of delivering low birthweight babies, of impaired development of the fetus due to maternal scoliosis (curvature of the spine), or of reduced blood supply from damaged vessels. Offspring are not at risk of developing Wilms if the mother had the non-inherited form in only one kidney. Any young woman who had Wilms tumor should get genetic counseling to fully understand her particular situation, and, if pregnant, should be cared for by an obstetrician who specializes in high-risk pregnancies. This gives the best chance for a full-term pregnancy and a healthy baby. Children fathered by males treated for Wilms are just as healthy as children of fathers with no cancer history. For more information, see *Chapter 3, Relationships* and *Chapter 10, Hormone-Producing Glands.*

Newer technologies can sometimes help infertile couples have a baby. Fertility counseling and support for infertile couples allow them to explore their options and address their feelings about infertility. See *Chapter 3 Relationships,* section on Fertility.

Digestive problems. A very small number of survivors who were treated with flank or whole abdomen radiation develop chronic gastrointestinal disturbances. For more information, see *Chapter 16, Liver, Stomach, and Intestines.*

Secondary cancers *(subsequent malignancies).* Second cancers develop in a very small number of Wilms survivors. The most common—bone, breast, thyroid, leukemias, and lymphomas—are usually found in irradiated areas. For more information, see *Chapter 20, Subsequent Malignancies.*

HEMATOPOIETIC STEM CELL TRANSPLANTATION

Hematopoietic stem cell transplantation (also known as stem cell transplantation) which includes transplants of bone marrow, stem cell and cord blood is used to treat several types of childhood cancers. In these procedures, the child or teen is given high doses of chemotherapy and/or radiation to destroy all of the cancer in the body. During this process, the bone marrow is totally destroyed. Normal marrow or stem cells are then infused into the child's veins. The marrow or stem cells migrate to the cavities inside the bones where new, healthy blood cells are then produced.

Types of Stem Cell Transplants:

- **Allogeneic.** *Allogeneic transplants* are those in which donor bone marrow, stem cells, or cord blood is transplanted into the patient. The cells usually come from a sibling with a matching marrow type or a matched unrelated donor. In some cases, parents are used as donors. The risk of complications increases if the donor is mismatched or unrelated.

- **Syngeneic.** *Syngeneic bone marrow transplants (BMTS)* are those in which the donor is the patient's identical twin. Many late complications are avoided because the marrow is an identical match.
- **Autologous.** During an *autologous stem cell transplant*, the patient's own stem cells are extracted and cryopreserved (a type of freezing). The patient then undergoes radiation and chemotherapy, or high-dose chemotherapy alone. The frozen cells are thawed and infused into the child or teen intravenously.

The three sources of blood cell used for transplant are:

- **Bone marrow.** In a BMT, the donor's bone marrow is extracted from the hip bones. This is done in the operating room with the use of two large bore needles.
- **Peripheral blood stem cells.** For a peripheral blood stem cell transplant, the patient's or donor's stem cells (cells from which all other cells evolve) are harvested in a procedure called apheresis. Blood is removed through a catheter or vein in the arm and circulated through a machine that extracts the stem cells. The remaining blood is then returned to the patient or donor.
- **Umbilical cord blood.** Umbilical cord blood is a rich source of stem cells. In the 1990s, researchers began conducting transplants using the umbilical cord blood obtained during the birth of a sibling or from preserved unrelated donor cord blood.

Prior to the transplant, the patient's bone marrow is destroyed using high-dose chemotherapy with or without radiation. This portion of treatment is called conditioning. The purpose of the high doses of chemotherapy and radiation is to destroy all remaining cancer cells in the body, make room in the bones for the new bone marrow, and suppress the patient's immune system so it will accept the donor's marrow.

Conditioning regimens vary according to institution and protocol, and also depend on the medical condition and history of the child or teen. Typically, chemotherapy is given for 2 to 6 days, and radiation (if part of conditioning) is given in multiple small doses over several days. The drugs most commonly used during conditioning are cyclophosphamide (Cytoxan®), busulfan (Myleran®), etoposide (VP-16 or Vepesid®), thiotepa, and melphalan (Alkeran®).

The transplant itself consists of simply infusing the stem cells or marrow through a catheter or intravenously into the patient, just like a blood transfusion. The stem cells travel throughout the blood vessels, eventually filling the empty spaces in the long bones. Engraftment occurs when the new marrow begins to produce healthy white cells, red cells, and platelets—usually 1 to 4 weeks after transplantation.

Late effects of treatment with stem cell transplantation

This section briefly outlines some common and uncommon late effects from treatment with stem cell transplantation. Remember that you may develop none, one, or several of these problems in the months or years after treatment ends.

Graft-versus-host disease. Graft-versus-host disease (GVHD) is a frequent complication of allogeneic stem cell transplants. It does not occur with autologous or syngeneic transplants. In GVHD, the bone marrow provided by the donor (the graft) attacks the tissues and organs of the BMT child (the host). Approximately 30 to 50 percent of children and teens who have a related HLA-matched transplant develop some degree of GVHD. The incidence and severity of GVHD are increased for those children and teens who receive unrelated or mismatched marrow.

There are two types of GVHD: acute and chronic. Children and teens can develop one type, both types, or neither one. Acute GVHD usually occurs at the time of engraftment or shortly thereafter. Donor cells identify the patient's cells as different and attack the patient's skin, liver, stomach, or intestines. Acute GVHD is treated with cyclosporine, tacrolimus (Prograf), and steroids (i.e., prednisone, dexamethasone). Prolonged use of steroids to treat GVHD can cause osteonecrosis (death of the small blood vessels that feed bones). For detailed information about these late effects, see *Chapter 17, Liver, Stomach, and Intestines* and *Chapter 20, Skin, Breasts, and Hair*.

If chronic GVHD develops, it usually starts 100 or more days post-transplant. It primarily affects the skin (itchy rash, discoloration of the skin, tightening of the skin, hair loss with a dry flaky scalp, nail changes (dry and brittle), eyes (dry, light sensitive), mouth and esophagus (dry mouth, tooth decay, difficulty swallowing), intestines (diarrhea, cramping, weight loss), liver (jaundice), lungs (shortness of breath, wheezing, coughing), and joints (decreased mobility). Survivors with chronic GVHD can develop one, a few, or several of these problems. There are many medications, including tacrolimus (Prograf®), steroids, and mycophenolate (CellCept®) that can be used to treat chronic GVHD.

Cataracts. Numerous late effects can occur from *total body irradiation (TBI)* used during conditioning. Often, children and teens develop cataracts after transplant. If the TBI is given in one dose, the likelihood of developing cataracts is much higher than if TBI is given in smaller doses over several days (called fractionated). Currently, if radiation is used, it is given in fractionated doses. Decreased tear production is also common after transplant. For more information, see *Chapter 11, Eyes and Ears*.

Growth problems. Radiation can affect growth. Children who received prior cranial radiation, spinal radiation, or total body radiation should be monitored for learning disabilities, dental problems (e.g., facial bone and jaw growth, delayed development of permanent teeth, incomplete root development), and growth hormone deficiency resulting in delayed or decreased growth. Children and teens who receive TBI also may have a low thyroid function due to decreased production of thyroid hormone. For more information, see *Chapter 10, Hormone-Producing Glands*.

Problems with puberty. For the most part, children and teens who were given only cyclophosphamide during conditioning have normal sexual development. Children and teens who had TBI, however, may experience delayed puberty (the incidence is lower if the radiation was given in several small doses). All children and teens who received

TBI should be followed closely by a pediatric endocrinologist who can prescribe hormones to assist in normal pubertal development. Girls are more likely than boys to need hormonal replacement; boys usually produce testosterone but not sperm.

Fertility. Children and teens who received TBI usually—but not always— become sterile; that is, after puberty, girls will *not* be able to become pregnant, and boys will *not* be able to father children. The ability to have a normal sex life is not affected. Some children treated with cyclophosphamide but no radiation have remained fertile, and to date, all offspring have been normal. For more information, see *Chapter 10, Hormone-Producing Glands.*

Secondary cancers (*subsequent malignancies*). Children or teens who received a stem cell transplant have a small risk of developing a second cancer, particularly if TBI was used. For more information, see *Chapter 20, Subsequent Malignancies.*

TBI can also cause late effects to the lungs, heart, liver, and bowel. Any body system treated with radiation can be damaged, so survivors need follow-up for the rest of one's life.

RECOMMENDED FOLLOW-UP FOR SURVIVORS

Some tests are recommended to monitor your long-term health. By screening for problems that may occur, you can quickly identify and treat them.

Most survivors of childhood cancer should have yearly check-ups with their health-care provider or survivor clinic and the following tests/measurements every year:

- complete blood count
- liver function studies
- urinalysis
- measurements of blood pressure
- pulse and respirations
- height and weight

It is essential that all survivors have a *Summary of Cancer Treatment* form which captures their diagnosis, treatment exposures and recommended long term follow-up. See COG Survivorship Guidelines website in Resources and Click on : *Summary of Cancer Treatment (Comprehensive or Summary)*.

For comprehensive and up-to-date recommendations, refer to Long-Term Follow-Up Guidelines for Survivors of Childhood, Adolescent, and Young Adult Cancers, Version 6.0 (October 2023); http://www.survivorshipguidelines.org/

Recommendations are regularly updated as new information is learned about late effects, so survivors and their health-care providers should check these recommendations periodically.

REFERENCES

American Cancer Society, 2025
https://www.cancer.org/cancer/childhood-cancer
https://www.cancer.org/cancer/types/neuroblastoma

Baliga S, Yock TI. (2019) Proton beam therapy in pediatric oncology. *Curr Opin Pediatr*. 2019 Feb;31(1):28-34.

Dixon SB, Chen Y, Yasui Y, et al. (2020). Reduced Morbidity and Mortality in Survivors of Childhood Acute Lymphoblastic Leukemia: A Report from the Childhood Cancer Survivor Study. J. Clin Oncol. 38: 3418-3429. doi: 10.1200/JCO.20.00493. Epub 2020 Jul 24. PMID: 32706634; PMCID: PMC7527155

Children's Brain Tumor Foundation (CBTF), Website: https://cbtf.org

Hodgson D, Kieckmann K. et al. (2015) Implementation of contemporary radiation therapy planning concepts for pediatric Hodkin lymphoma: Guidelines from the International Lymphoma Radiation Oncology Group: Practical Radiation Oncology (2015) 5, 85-92

Hunger SP, Lu X, Devidas M, et al. (2012) Improved survival for children and adolescents with acute lymphoblastic leukemia between 1990 and 2005: a report from the children's oncology group. J Clin Oncol. 2012 May 10;30(14):1663-9. doi: 10.1200/JCO.2011.37.8018. Epub 2012 Mar 12. PMID: 22412151; PMCID: PMC3383113

Long-Term Follow-Up Guidelines for Survivors of Childhood, Adolescent, and Young Adult Cancers, Version 6.0 (October 2023) http://www.survivorshipguidelines.org

Louis DN, Perry A, Wesseling P, et al. The 2021 WHO Classification of Tumors of the Central Nervous System: a summary, *Neuro-Oncology*, Volume 23, Issue 8, August 2021, Pages 1231–1251, https://doi.org/10.1093/neuonc/noab106

Miller KD, Fidler-Benaoudia M, Keegan TH, et al. (2020) Cancer statistics for adolescents and young adults, 2020. CA Cancer J Clin 2020; 70:443–459.11.

Mulder RL, Hudson MM, Bhatia S, et al. (2020). Updated Breast Cancer Surveillance Recommendations for Female Survivors of Childhood, Adolescent, and Young Adult Cancer from the International Guideline Harmonization Group. J Clin Oncol 38: 4194-4207. doi: 10.1200/JCO.20.00562. Epub 2020 Sep 29. PMID: 33078972; PMCID: PMC7723685

Oeffinger KC, Stratton KL, Hudson MM et al. (2021). Impact of Risk-Adapted Therapy for Pediatric Hodgkin Lymphoma on Risk of long-Term Morbidity: A Report from the Childhood Cancer Survivor Study. J Clin Oncology 39: 2266-2275. doi: 10.1200/JCO.20.01186. Epub 2021 Feb 25. PMID: 33630659; PMCID: PMC826090615.

Pacenta HL, Laetsch TW, John S. CD19 CAR T Cells for the treatment of pediatric Pre-B Cell Acute Lymphoblastic Leukemia. Pediatric Drugs (2020) 22:1–11. doi.org/10.1007/s40272-019-00370-6

Reddy AT, Strother DR, Judkins AR, et al. (2020) Three-Dimensional Conformal Radiation for Atypical Teratoid/Rhabdoid Tumor: A Report from the Children's Oncology Group Trial ACNS0333. J Clin Oncol. 2020 Apr 10;38(11):1175-1185.: PMC7145589.

Ries LAG, Smith MA, Gurney JG, et al (eds). (1999) Cancer Incidence and Survival among Children and Adolescents: United States SEER Program 1975-1995, National Cancer Institute, SEER Program. NIH Pub. No. 99-4649. Bethesda, MD.

Weil BR, Murphy AJ, Liu Q, et al. (2023) Late Health Outcomes Among Survivors of Wilms Tumor Diagnosed Over Three Decades: A Report from the Childhood Cancer Survivor Study. J Clin Oncol. 2023 May 10;41(14):2638-2650. doi: 10.1200/JCO.22.02111. Epub 2023 Jan 24. PMID: 36693221; PMCID: PMC10414738.

RESOURCES

Website: ccgresources.org

All resources and references mentioned in this book are available on the website and will be routinely reviewed and updated.

American Cancer Society (ACS)

Website: www.cancer.org

Search, *childhood cancer, late effects, neuroblastoma*

Children's Brain Tumor Foundation (CBTF)

Website: https://cbtf.org/

CBTF supports survivors, parents, and siblings from diagnosis throughout the entire journey.

Children's Oncology Group (V6, 2023). *Long-Term Follow-Up Guidelines for Survivors of Childhood, Adolescent, and Young Adult Cancers*

Website: www.survivorshipguidelines.org

Passport for Care, Survivor Care Plans by Children's Oncology Group (V6, Nov 2023)

Website: https://cancersurvivor.passportforcare.org

Survivors and family can find online updated tailored long-term care plans which should be reviewed with their oncologist or health care provider.

National Cancer Institute (NIH)
https://www.cancer.gov
Search: *types of childhood/adolescent cancers*
For statistics: Search, *childhood cancer statistics*.

GLOSSARY

Acquired Immune Deficiency Syndrome (AIDS), a collection of symptoms caused by infection with the human immunodeficiency virus (HIV). HIV can be transmitted from person to person by coming into direct contact with certain body fluids from an infected person, such as blood (from a needle or syringe) or semen, rectal fluids, vaginal fluids, and from mother-to-child through breast milk.

acute lymphoblastic leukemia (ALL), (also called acute lymphocytic leukemia), a type of cancer of the blood and bone marrow — the spongy tissue inside bones where blood cells are made. It is the most common type of cancer in children, and treatments result in a good chance for a cure.

acute myelogenous leukemia (AML), (also called acute myeloid leukemia, acute non-lymphocytic leukemia), cancer of the blood and bone marrow — the spongy tissue inside bones where blood cells are made. It affects a group of white blood cells (called myeloid cells) which normally develop into mature blood cells such as red blood cells, white blood cells and platelets. The disease has rapid progression.

allogeneic stem cell transplant, using healthy blood stem cells from a donor to replace bone marrow that's not producing enough healthy blood cells. A donor may be a family member, often a sibling, an acquaintance or someone you don't know with a matching marrow type.

autologous stem cell transplant, using healthy blood stem cells from one's own body to replace bone marrow that's not working properly; healthy stem cells are extracted and cryopreserved (frozen) until ready for the transplant. Using cells from one's own body has the advantage of not having to worry about incompatibility between a donor's cells and the recipient's cells.

anaplasia, loss of structural and functional differentiation of normal cells

astrocytoma, a brain tumor that arises from star-shaped cells called astrocytes. Low-grade astrocytomas grow slowly, and many types have a favorable prognosis. High-grade astrocytomas grow quickly and are more difficult to treat.

benign, noncancerous

brachytherapy, a procedure used to treat certain types of cancer and other conditions that involves placing radioactive material inside or next to the area requiring treatment; sometimes called *internal radiation*

brain stem glioma, slow or fast-growing brain tumor that starts in the brain stem, which connects the brain to the spinal cord

CAR (chimeric antigen receptor) T-cell therapy, type of immunotherapy used to treat some blood cancers by infusing new T-cells into the patient's blood that have a new gene receptor (chimeric antigen receptor) equipped to attack cancer cells and kill them. This therapy is being studied for treatment of other types of cancer.

consolidation/intensification phase of chemotherapy, second phase of chemotherapy after remission is achieved to destroy any remaining cancer cells

cryotherapy, sometimes called cryosurgery, used to treat small primary tumors or new tumors that develop by applying extreme cold by a small probe placed directly on the tumor

dry eyes, a condition caused by decreased tear production and causes dry eyes and blurred vision

enucleation, removal of the eye

ependymoma, a tumor that usually grow on the internal surfaces of the brain and spinal cord.

Ewing sarcoma, a group of bone or soft tissue cancers that mostly affect children, teenagers and young adults, often developing during puberty when bones grow rapidly; typically appear in legs, arms and pelvis

granulocytes, a type of white blood cell

graft-versus-host disease (GVHD), a frequent complication of allogeneic stem cell transplants when the bone marrow provided by the donor (the graft) attacks the tissues and organs of the recipient host. GVHD does *not* occur when stem cells come from host's own body (autologous) or from an identical twin (*syngeneic*).

hematopoietic stem cell transplantation also known as *stem cell transplant*, (formerly called *bone marrow transplant*) a procedure that involves administering healthy stem cells (e.g., bone marrow, cord blood, or peripheral blood) to patients after the bone marrow has been destroyed by disease, chemotherapy (*chemo*), or radiation

histiocytosis, a disease in which histiocytes (cells in bone marrow) multiply and accumulate in various organs or bones in the body; diagnosis is by examination of a sample of affected tissue under an electron microscope

histology, how cells look under a microscope

Hodgkin lymphoma (formerly called Hodgkin's disease), a type of cancer that affects the lymphatic system which is part of the body's germ-fighting immune system. White blood cells called *lymphocytes* grow out of control, causing swollen lymph nodes and growths throughout the body. Advances in diagnosis and treatment have helped give people with this disease the chance for a full recovery.

induction, the most intense phase of chemotherapy with a goal of killing as many leukemia cells in the shortest amount of time

Involved Field Radiation Therapy (IFRT), radiation technique that delivers radiation to only those areas of the body involved with disease and is more precise and limits exposure to healthy tissue

maintenance phase of chemotherapy, the last phase of chemotherapy that consists of daily low-dose chemotherapy that continues for 2 to 3 years

malignant, cancerous cells that grow uncontrollably and spread locally and/or to distant sites in the body

neuroblastoma, a cancer that develops from immature nerve cells found in several areas of the body; most commonly in and around the adrenal glands but can also develop in other areas of the abdomen and in the chest, neck and near the spine. Infant form of neuroblastoma may go away on their own, while others may require multiple treatments.

non-Hodgkin lymphoma (NHL), a type of cancer that begins in the lymphatic system which is the body's germ/disease-fighting system; white blood cells called *lymphocytes* grow abnormally and can form tumors throughout the body; the lymphatic system includes the spleen, thymus, lymph nodes, and tonsils and adenoids.

Intensity-modulated radiation therapy, also called *IMRT*, is an advanced type of radiation therapy that uses powerful energy beams to kill cancer cells. The beams of radiation are carefully customized and shaped to match the shape of the cancer and can deliver a precisely controlled radiation dose as safely and efficiently as possible. The goal of IMRT is to deliver the correct dose of radiation to the target and minimize radiation outside of the target. This helps lower the risk of hurting nearby healthy tissue.

Intraocular Retinoblastoma Staging System, asub-classification system that divides intraocular retinoblastomas into 5 sub-goups based on tumor size, location, and presence of disease within the layers of the retina; stages from 0 to IV, Stage 0 having a good outcome with treatment, and Stage IV a poor prognosis of likelihood of the eye being saved using current treatment options

mantle radiation, a radiation technique used in 1970s to the 1990s to treat a large area of the neck, chest, armpits and mediastinum (area between the lungs) in order to cover all areas with cancer involvement; rarely used today in current treatment

medulloblastoma, a brain tumor that is fast-growing, malignant and located in the cerebellum/posterior fossa (back of the brain); diagnosed most often in children ages 4 to 8 and more common in boys

nephrectomy, surgical removal of a kidney

optic nerve gliomas, tumors located along the optic nerves and the optic chiasm and connect the nerve to the eye. Sometimes the glioma may enter into the hypothalamus.

osteosarcoma, (also called *osteogenic sarcoma*) is the most common type of cancer that starts in the bones. The cancer cells in these tumors look like early forms of bone cells that normally help make new bone tissue, but the bone tissue is not as strong as that in normal bones. Most osteosarcomas occur in children, teens, and young adults.

proton therapy, or proton beam therapy, a type of radiation treatment that uses a beam of protons to deliver radiation directly to the tumor. A proton beam conforms to the shape and depth of a tumor while sparing healthy tissues and organs. The advantage of proton therapy is that the physician can control where the proton releases the bulk of its cancer-fighting energy and deliver the most damage to the targeted tumor cells and less damage to surrounding organs and tissue in the rest of the body.

retinoblastoma, a malignant tumor of the retina in the eye that occurs in stages from 0-IV, with Stage 0 having a good outcome with treatment, and Stage IV retinoblastoma with metastases a poor prognosis

rhabdomyoblasts, primitive muscle cells

rhabdomyosarcoma (RMS), the most common childhood soft tissue sarcoma made up primitive muscle cells called *rhabdomyoblasts;* most commonly found in the head and neck, genitourinary tract, extremities, chest and lungs

second cancer, cancer that occurs after treatment (e.g. radiation and/ or chemotherapy) for a first (primary) cancer and is a new and different type of cancer, which usually arises in a different organ or tissue from the first (primary) cancer

subsequent malignancy (also referred to as, second cancer), cancer that occurs after treatment (e.g. radiation and/or chemotherapy) for a first (primary) cancer and is a new and different type of cancer, which usually arises in a different organ or tissue from the first (primary) cancer

stem cell transplantation, *also known as hematopoietic stem cell transplant*, procedure that involves administering healthy stem cells (e.g., bone marrow, cord blood, or peripheral blood) to patients after the bone marrow has been destroyed by disease, chemotherapy (*chemo*), or radiation

stereotactic radiation therapy, type of radiation therapy using 3D or 4D imaging and highly focused radiation beams that send high doses of radiation to the area to be treated resulting in the least amount of damage to the healthy tissues around the area; used to treat tumors in the lungs, spine, liver, neck, lymph nodes or other soft tissues

syngeneic bone marrow transplants (BMTS), bone marrow transplant in which the donor of the bone marrow is the patient's identical twin

total body irradiation (TBI), a type of radiation therapy that delivers radiation to the entire body; commonly used for the treatment of certain blood cancers before a bone marrow transplant

stages of cancer, the extent to which a cancer has progressed or grown; stage I through IV with stage I being the earliest stage of the cancer, and stage IV being the highest/worst stage

Wilms tumor, a primary cancer of the kidney that accounts for 5 to 6 percent of all childhood cancers in the United States most commonly in children younger than age 5. Approximately 500 children are diagnosed each year.

8
Fatigue .

LISA BASHORE, PhD, APRN, CPNP-PC, CPON

The patient is cured when he can again do the things he loves to do.
— *Stanley A. Herrings*

FATIGUE (EXCESS TIREDNESS) CAN be a side-effect among children and adolescents during active cancer treatment. For a small percentage of survivors, the profound tiredness lasts long after treatment ends. People with fatigue have little energy and feel emotionally, physically, and mentally exhausted. Fatigue may have an identifiable physical cause or may remain an elusive, yet life-altering late-effect of treatment. This chapter describes fatigue, the causes, the treatment, and the voices of survivors who live with and cope with chronic fatigue.

I don't deal with overwhelming fatigue, but I do certainly enjoy the occasional nap. As long as I get enough sleep the night before, I am typically good for the day unless I am incredibly active. If I stay up late or have to wake up early for a meeting or a workout, I am much more tired towards the middle of the day. I can typically fix it with a coffee, but if it persists, a nice nap never hurts.

My biggest struggle with fatigue is difficulty remembering or concentrating. Whenever I am really tired, my brain feels like mush. Combined with possible memory side-effects of my treatment, this is not the best recipe for success. Thankfully, this does not happen often and taking a five-minute break to recenter my mind helps significantly

(Continued)

(Continued)

I experience fatigue every day. I am fighting it every day. I just push past it. I don't focus on it until my body forces me to. That happens around once every three weeks. I am currently dealing with an autoimmune diagnosis which came from either the initial cancer or the treatment I received. I also have only one lung, so that contributes to the fatigue too. My right arm gets really tired, but the steroids are doing what they are supposed to do to help with it. We just do not know how long I will need to take them.

CONTRIBUTORS TO FATIGUE

During treatment, the effects of drugs, surgery, and radiation can sometimes combine to cause overwhelming fatigue. Survivors hope and expect that this frustrating condition will resolve when treatment ends. Most survivors are able to resume activities with normal energy levels. Others have occasional or constant exhaustion. Cancer-related fatigue is different from the tiredness one normally feels from daily activities. The differences for survivors are: it takes less activity to tire you out, is not completely relieved by sleep and rest, and can last a long time. This unexpected and unwelcome late-effect can cause physical, mental, emotional, and financial distress. At a time when you expect renewed energy and strength after treatment, you find that you cannot make it through the day.

More research is needed for a better understanding of how fatigue changes over time, what factors effect it, and what can be done to decrease it.

The first step in coping with fatigue is to understand that it can be a late-effect of treatment. The next step is to give your healthcare provider a specific description of how the fatigue affects your life so they can best help you and continue to assess your symptoms over time.

Most often, the cause of persistent fatigue is unknown. Fatigue can lessen over time, but it can take a long time. And while it lasts, fatigue can have a significant impact on every aspect of life.

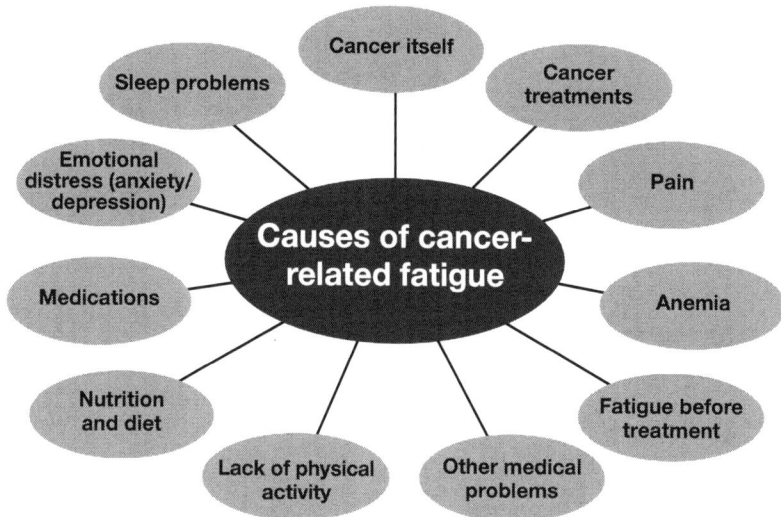

FIGURE 8-1. Causes of cancer-related fatigue. (©*Alex's Lemonade Stand Foundation, 2025*)

Fatigue usually does not occur by itself. More often, it occurs along with other symptoms (called *symptom clusters: pain, nausea, stress, sleep problems*). Stress can make fatigue worse. Many other factors can contribute to fatigue that persists long after treatment ends. See **Figure 8-1** Many causes of fatigue.

Other medical causes of fatigue:

- hormone imbalance (i.e., thyroid, testosterone, estrogen, growth hormone) (see *Chapter 10, Hormone-producing Glands*)
- gastrointestinal problems (see *Chapter 16, Liver, Stomach, Intestines*)
- liver dysfunction (see *Chapter 16, Liver, Stomach Intestines*)
- heart or lung disease (see *Chapter 13, Heart and Blood Vessels*)
- kidney disease (see *Chapter 15, Kidneys, Bladder, and Genitals*)
- anemia (low red blood cell count)
- mental/emotional illness (depression, anxiety, chronic stress) (see *Chapter 2, Emotions*)
- obesity (see *Chapter 5, Staying Healthy*)
- alcohol consumption/substance abuse

SIGNS AND SYMPTOMS OF CHRONIC FATIGUE

Chronic fatigue can interfere with all of the activities of daily life. It can come- and-go or be constant. Following are some of the signs and symptoms of fatigue:

- Whole body tiredness, weariness, or exhaustion even after sleep
- Mental and emotional exhaustion
- Difficulty concentrating, remembering, or completing tasks
- Confused thinking
- Decreased ability to work, do regular activities, or start new projects
- Decreased interest in enjoyable activities
- Feelings of sadness, frustration, or irritability
- Decreased sexual desire
- Spending more time resting or sleeping

Chronic fatigue is very hard on relationships with loved ones. You may not have the energy to go out with your spouse or significant other to have dinner or visit friends. Your interest in sex may disappear, or you may just be too tired even if you are interested. You may not have the energy to take your children to the park or play in the backyard. Your friends may not understand that you can look great but have no energy. Your fatigue may result in your inability to attend school or work. You may feel guilty or lazy. All of these worries—big and small—can take a toll.

Many children also suffer from fatigue long after treatment ends. Survivorship healthcare professionals have observed that children with cognitive changes, in particular, seem to have more fatigue. For helpful information on managing cancer side effects and fatigue, check these websites: Children's Oncology Group (V6, 2023). *Long-Term Follow-Up Guidelines for Survivors of Childhood, Adolescent, and Young Adult Cancers* (https://www.survivorshipguidelines.org/) and the American Cancer Society (www.cancer.org) and Search topics, *managing cancer side-effects and fatigue.*

SCREENING AND DETECTION

A thorough physical and psychological evaluation is needed to identify possible causes of fatigue and determine what may be treatable. It helps to keep a record/log of your pattern of fatigue prior to going to your healthcare provider. For example, note on your calendar hours spent working each day, how many naps you take, how long naps are, and how many hours sleep each night. Many survivors force themselves to go to work but feel absolutely exhausted by the afternoon. This is an important piece of information to share with your healthcare provider. This evaluation should be extensive to determine what is causing your fatigue, how long it has lasted, what makes it better or worse, medications you take, and how it is affecting your daily life.

Your chronic fatigue evaluation should include the following:
- Review of cancer history, treatment, and current health status
- Complete physical examination
- Fatigue history
- When it started, how long it has lasted, any changes
- Actions or events that make the fatigue better or worse
- Effect of fatigue on job, daily life, and relationships
- Assessment of contributing factors, such as:
  - Pain
  - Hormone levels (i.e., thyroid, testosterone, estrogen, growth hormone)
  - Current medications, including over-the-counter medicines and supplements
  - Emotions (e.g., depression and anxiety)
  - Sleep and napping habits
  - Level of physical activity
  - Nutrition history, including weight gain or loss and changes in appetite
  - Other health conditions that could affect fatigue

MEDICAL MANAGEMENT

Fatigue in long-term survivors of cancer can range from being a nuisance to being a disabling condition. For some survivors, the fatigue comes and goes. For others, energy and stamina are permanently reduced. Your healthcare provider can consult evidence-based guidelines specifically for cancer-related fatigue for ways to manage your fatigue.

Medical management can include pharmacologic/medications or non-pharmacologic interventions listed below:

- Enhancing activity level with exercise, physical therapy, or occupational therapy (See **Figure 8-2**. Health Benefits of Physical Activity – CDC recommendations)
- Consultation with a sleep expert to improve *sleep hygiene* (i.e., things you do to get a good night's rest)
- Counseling and support (individual or group) to help with emotions and stress management
- Consultation with a nutritionist about diet and supplements
- Medicines for pain, emotional distress, and anemia, if needed

Counseling

Sometimes there is no medical treatment for fatigue even when the cause is known such as a heart dysfunction. Many brain tumor survivors and some leukemia survivors treated with cranial radiation have fatigue from unknown causes. This exhaustion can affect a survivor's education, work life, and social life.

Counseling is needed for these survivors especially regarding how to receive special accommodations in the school system through an Individualized Education Program or Individualized Transition Plan (see *Chapter 4, Navigating the System*). Some options offered include attending school for half days, allowing more time to get from class-to-class, and participating in adaptive physical education.

When a survivor begins to plan for college or work, they need to know what special accommodations are available for the disabled as

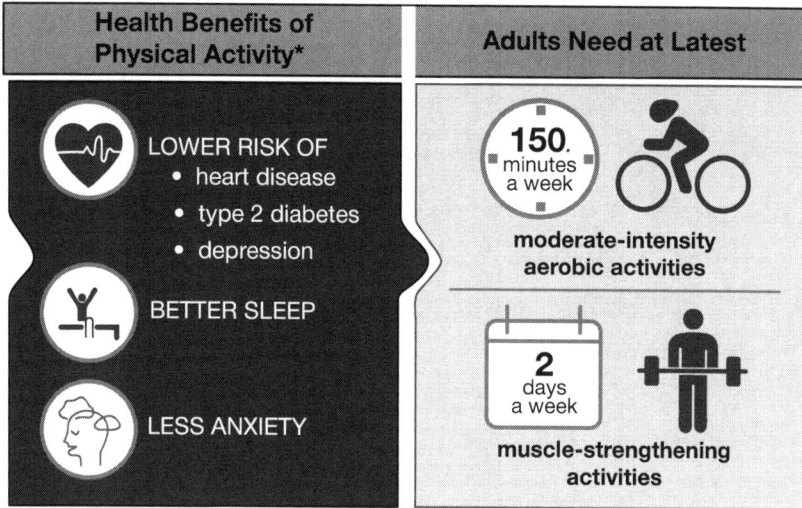

FIGURE 8-2. Health Benefits of Physical Activity.
*https://www.cdc.gov/physical-activity/php/public-health-strategy/

outlined by federal/state laws. See section on Education, *Chapter 4 Navigating the System*, which outlines application process and accommodations provided for disabled students in college or vocational-technical programs and section on Workplace which gives detail about filling out applications for jobs and insurance, and workplace accommodations.

Counseling for all survivors suffering from post-cancer fatigue can address several issues. Psychological distress that existed prior to cancer or resulted from cancer treatment may make fatigue worse. Resolution of these issues may improve your energy level. Therapists who specialize in this area can help you to devise an *energy conservation plan,* (a plan to prioritize your daily goals/activities and time use, simplifying tasks, and reducing the amount of energy you expend in accomplishing necessary tasks). Supportive discussions about the effects of fatigue/low energy on your life may result in new ways to

* The use/publication of figures/images in this book taken from the CDC website does not indicate endorsement or accuracy of content presented in this book by the CDC or US government. These images are considered in public domain and can be used for educational purposes in electronic and print media. Click the links below images which directs you to specific CDC webpages for more information.

adapt to the condition. Counseling may also help remove any faulty negative feelings about yourself (i.e. feeling lazy or selfish) and replace them with strategies to help you feel more energy, reduce stress, and improve your self-concept.

Other general suggestions for coping with chronic fatigue:

- Avoid or change the activities that cause more fatigue.
- Schedule activities for when you have the most energy / set priorities.
- Reduce stressful situations as much as you can.
- Get plenty of rest and sleep.
- Ask for help when you need it.
- Eat a diet that is low in caffeine and junk food.
- Engage in physical activity approved by your healthcare provider.
- Find activities to refresh your mind or distract yourself (massage, funny movie, nature walk).
- Practice mindfulness and relaxation exercises.

REFERENCES

American Cancer Society, Managing fatigue or weakness. https://www.cancer.org/cancer/managing-cancer/side-effects/fatigue/managing-cancer-related-fatigue.html

Children's Oncology Group. Long-Term Follow-Up Guidelines for Survivors of Childhood, Adolescent and Young Adult Cancers, (V6, 2023). Website: www.survivorshipguidelines.org

Ebede CC, Jang Y, Escalante CP. Cancer-Related Fatigue in Cancer Survivorship. (2017) Med Clin North Am. 2017 Nov;101(6):1085-1097. doi: 10.1016/j.mcna.2017.06.007. Epub 2017 Aug 25. PMID: 28992856.

Lin PJ, Kleckner IR, Loh KP, et al. (2019) Influence of Yoga on Cancer-Related Fatigue and on Mediational Relationships Between Changes in Sleep and Cancer-Related Fatigue: A Nationwide, Multicenter Randomized Controlled Trial of Yoga in Cancer Survivors. Integr Cancer Ther. 2019 Jan-Dec;18:1534735419855134. doi: 10.1177/1534735419855134.

Shin, H., Dudley, W. N., Bhakta, N., et al. (2023). Associations of symptom clusters and health outcomes in adult survivors of childhood cancer: A report from the St Jude lifetime cohort study. *Journal of Clinical Oncology, 41*(3), 497- 507. https://doi.org/10.1200/JCO.22.00361

Williamson LR, Effinger KE, Wasilewski-Masker K, et al. (2021). Self-reported late effect symptom clusters among young pediatric cancer survivors. *Supportive Care in Cancer, 29*(12), 8077-8087. https://doi.org/10.1007/s00520-021-06332-4

RESOURCES

Website: ccgresources.org
All resources and references mentioned in this book are available on
the website and will be routinely reviewed and updated.

American Cancer Society (ACS)
Website: www.cancer.org
Search, *cancer side effects, fatigue*

Children's Oncology Group (V6, 2023). *Long-Term Follow-Up
Guidelines for Survivors of Childhood, Adolescent, and Young
Adult Cancers*
Website: www.survivorshipguidelines.org
Search, *managing cancer side effects, fatigue*

**Passport for Care, Survivor Care Plans by Children's Oncology
Group (V6, Nov 2023)**
Website: https://cancersurvivor.passportforcare.org
Survivors and family can find online updated tailored long-term
care plans which should be reviewed with their oncologist or
health care provider.

Figure 8-2. Health Benefits of Physical Activity
https://www.cdc.gov/physical-activity/php/public-health

GLOSSARY

energy conservation plan, a plan to prioritize your daily goals/activ-
ities and time use, simplifying tasks, and reducing the amount of
energy you expend in accomplishing necessary tasks

symptom clusters, a symptom that usually occurs at the same time
as a group of other symptoms, i.e. the symptom of fatigue is often
seen in survivors who also experience symptoms of pain, nausea,
stress, and/or sleep problems

9
Brain and Nerves

JOANNE QUILLEN, MSN, APRN, PNP-BC

Although the world is full of suffering, it is full also of the overcoming of it.
— *Helen Keller*

THE NERVOUS SYSTEM in the body has two main parts: the central nervous system (CNS) and the peripheral nervous system. The central nervous system is composed of the brain and the spinal cord. The peripheral nervous system is a network of nerves throughout the body. The CNS and peripheral nervous system work together to monitor, coordinate, and control all activities of the body. Changes in the functioning of the brain or nerves can profoundly affect both health and quality of life.

As the number of survivors who have received treatment affecting the nervous system increases, more is being learned about long-term effects on the CNS. These effects can impact survivors' education, social lives, relationships, and job performance.

This chapter reviews the cancer treatments that can cause changes in the brain and nerves, the signs and symptoms of such changes, methods to screen for these effects, and the medical management of these effects.

THE BRAIN

The brain is the body's main information processing center. This complex organ weighs approximately 3 pounds and is protected by membranes called *meninges*, a cushion of fluid (*cerebrospinal fluid*), and the skull. The three main structural parts of the brain are the brain stem, the cerebellum, and the cerebrum. The brain stem connects the brain to the spinal cord. It coordinates most of the functions necessary for survival, such as breathing, heart rate, and sleep. The cerebellum controls muscles to allow smooth and coordinated movement. It also monitors posture and balance. The cerebrum controls all voluntary, or conscious, activities of the brain, including speech, language, hearing, memory, and learning.

Brain damage and side effects

The brain can be damaged by tumor growth or treatments such as radiation, surgery, and chemotherapy. The survivors most at risk for brain damage are children and adolescents treated for leukemia, brain tumors, and tumors of the head and neck such as rhabdomyosarcoma.

The tissues of the brain are very sensitive to radiation. The dose and location of radiation and the child's age, sex, and individual vulnerability all play a role in how much the radiation will affect brain function. Those at highest risk are children under the age of 2. Children under the age of 5 are at very high risk and children ages 5 to 8 are at high risk. Girls show a greater sensitivity to radiation than do boys. However, any child whose brain is irradiated may develop long-term changes in brain function (MacDonald, 2018).

Advances in software have led to more precise planning of radiation treatment and decrease exposure to healthy uninvolved brain tissue and nearby healthy organs. These types of radiation therapy are: Intensity-Modulated Radiation therapy (IMRT) and proton therapy or proton beam therapy. Because the damage to healthy cells depends in part on the total dose of radiation, this discussion will first deal with children who received less than 2500 centigray (cGy) of whole brain radiation.

My daughter had a brain tumor (medulloblastoma). She had 30 rounds of proton radiation and 4 rounds of intense chemotherapy. Treatment really impacted her brain. She has a slower processing speed compared to her peers and also struggles with executive functioning. She has sensorineural hearing loss which means that her ears function normally, but the way her brain processes sound has caused hearing loss. She wears hearing aids which help but she still struggles to hear in noisy areas. Her pituitary gland was also impacted by the treatment, so she needs daily growth hormone injections. Our daughter developed hydrocephalus so has a ventriculoperitoneal shunt in her brain to drain off the excess cerebrospinal fluid into her belly. The shunt needed to be replaced after 5 years.

Radiation doses below 2500 cGy

Children who have stem cell transplants may receive radiation to the brain. Depending on the year children received transplants, they most commonly received 1000 to 1200 cGy of *total body irradiation* (TBI).

Cognitive late effects/learning difficulties. Children who received 1200 to 1800 cGy often develop learning difficulties that may be subtle. The changes are more pronounced in those who received 2400 cGy. Greater doses of chemotherapy into the brain from intrathecal medications or high-dose systemic methotrexate may increase the effects from the radiation. Very young children (younger than 5 and particularly those younger than 2) whose brains are growing and developing are more at risk than are older children and adolescents (Smibert E,1996; Brown RT, 1996). Changes in the way children or adolescents think, remember, and learn are called *cognitive late effects*.

Our family has not returned to "normal"; we have a "new normal." My daughter had a brain tumor which has left her with many long-term side effects – she has been forever changed physically and mentally by cancer. When she was diagnosed, I was told that there could be long-term side effects, but I didn't anticipate how they would constantly continue to impact our lives. Learning to live with these challenges has been hard. We did not have an end-of-treatment celebration because even though she was done with chemo, she still had a lot of rehabilitation to do (physical therapy, occupational therapy, and speech therapy). It didn't feel like we had a specific end date. We do celebrate her diagnosis day. It's always hard, but we try to bring joy and gratitude to it.

Physical changes to the head/face/teeth. The growth of the skull (cranium) of young children who receive cranial radiation may slow, leaving the child with a smaller head than normal. The areas on either side of the eyes may develop a slightly pinched look. This late effect develops in approximately 3 out of 10 children. Children under the age of 5 when treated are most at risk. Children exposed to total brain radiation may also develop oral and dental problems. Children under the age of 2 are most at risk for dental late effects. This is discussed in more detail in *Chapter 12, Head and Neck*.

Effects on emotions and social interactions. Parents of children who had cranial radiation sometimes report that the child's *affect* (i.e., emotions shown on the face) has changed. Rather than a face that reflects what one is thinking and feeling, the face expresses no emotion and appears expressionless. This can have a negative effect on socializing and making and keeping friends because facial expressions and other body language play a big role in effective communication. Other parents may notice a lack of or reduced curiosity and interest in friends, social life or leisure events. Although not much research has been done on these late-effects, they are included here because they occur in some survivors and can affect the way those survivors deal with the world. See *Chapter 2, Emotions* for more explanation of research related to emotional, behavioral and overall mental health of childhood cancer survivors.

My daughter was in kindergarten when she was diagnosed, and she's now a middle schooler. I feel like she is socially immature but mature in other ways. Going through cancer treatment taught her to know what she needs and how to advocate for herself. She has a slower processing speed so it's difficult for her to keep up socially-- middle school girls talk fast!

Sometimes I think the world is uncomfortable with my daughter dreaming big. In 8th grade, she wanted to take French, instead of staying in the Study Skills class with other kids with IEPs. Her principal kept telling her it would be so hard. And my daughter looked at her and said: "Hard is cancer. French is just a language." She took French for 4 years. It was hard. She failed quizzes here and there, but that's okay. Failure is okay. Not being given the opportunity isn't okay.

She has also had to learn to advocate for herself. And since this has been her entire life—she's pretty good at it. She's taken the lead on researching services at college—and I hope she continues to be the fierce self-advocate she has been in high school.

I received chemotherapy for two years. I developed Attention Deficit Disorder (ADD) during treatment. I am constantly working on focusing and taking control of my ADD.

Slower mental processing. Slow processing speeds can impact overall decision making and ability to make good judgment calls. The amount of information a survivor has available to make decisions may be lessened, because the process of considering options might be slower. Again, this is not a universal late-effect for all survivors, but it does affect a significant percentage of survivors who received cranial radiation (Krull, 2018).

Hormone production, puberty, and general health. Children who received cranial radiation doses of 1800 or 2400 cGy are at risk for problems with hormone production, puberty, and growth. Children who were younger than age 8 when they received radiation are at highest risk. There is also a small risk that the thyroid might not produce enough thyroxin. This risk increases if spinal radiation was also received. It is important to remember that the risk continues throughout life, and in some children, the effects do not appear until a decade or two after treatment has ended. These issues are covered in depth in *Chapter 10, Hormone-Producing Glands.*

Children, especially girls, who received radiation to the brain at a young age are at risk for becoming overweight. The exact reason why some children become overweight after radiation is unclear. This is discussed in *Chapter 18, Muscles and Bones.*

A rare effect from radiation to the brain that occurs during treatment and may be progressive is *leukoencephalopathy*. Children who develop this disorder may have lasting problems with balance (ataxia), difficulty swallowing (dysphagia), or speech problems (dysarthria). Leukoencephalopathy usually occurs in children or teens who relapsed and received cranial radiation plus high total doses of intravenous and/or intrathecal methotrexate.

Radiation doses above 2500 cGy

In the past, many children or teens with brain tumors received 3500 cGy to the whole brain with a boost of up to 5540 cGy to the tumor bed (i.e., the place where the tumor originated). Others received high-dose radiation only to the tumor itself. Currently, lower doses of radiation to the whole brain are used with many times the boost remains at 5500 cGy. Specific disabilities may partly depend on which area of the brain received the highest dose of radiation. However, in general, the higher the dose and the younger the age, the more dramatic the effect on brain functioning.

Higher doses of radiation cause slower brain processing speeds and greater drops in IQ scores. The location of the tumor also influences the type and severity of learning disabilities that may develop. For example, children with temporal lobe tumors may have problems with memory. Learning may also be affected by medications used to treat seizures or by surgical complications, hydrocephalus, vision problems, and hearing loss.

Children or adolescents with brain tumors who get very high-dose radiation to the brain can have multiple and life-altering late effects.

Brain tumor survivors can develop seizure disorders, gait and balance problems, hand/eye coordination problems, personality changes, and learning disabilities. Radiation to the pituitary and hypothalamus can cause problems with growth, puberty, and fertility (see *Chapter 10, Hormone-Producing Glands*). Vision problems, cataracts, and diminished hearing can also develop after radiation (see *Chapter 11, Eyes and Ears*). All of the above late effects from high doses of radiation to the brain can range from mild to severe. With the use of proton beam radiation, there is hope that the risks to healthy brain tissue will be minimized.

Chemotherapy

Chemotherapy used to treat leukemia and some sarcomas can also cause learning disabilities that are sometimes subtle. Intrathecal methotrexate and high-dose methotrexate with leucovorin rescue can cause learning disabilities, although usually much milder than those caused by radiation (Schatz, 2000). Therapy for acute lymphoblastic leukemia sometimes includes triple intrathecals (methotrexate, hydrocortisone, and ARA-C) and has been associated with learning disabilities similar to those seen with lower doses of radiation (Montour-Proulx, 2005). Very young children (younger than age 5 and particularly younger than 2) whose brains are growing and developing are more at risk from chemotherapy to the brain than are older children and adolescents.

Surgery to the brain

Surgery to the brain can cause a host of late effects. The body system and amount of damage depend on the part of the brain where the surgery was performed, the amount of healthy tissue removed, and complications after surgery.

As with all the late effects described in this book, cognitive late effects are not an all-or-nothing phenomenon. You may have none, a few, or many. The lists of possible problems are not meant to fit you into a category, but rather to cover all possibilities so that if they develop, they are identified, and treated early to give the best possible outcomes.

Signs and symptoms of brain damage and cognitive difficulties

Brain damage from cranial radiation was first recognized in the late 1970s because survivors were having difficulty in school. Some young survivors were easily distracted and had trouble learning. This spawned many studies of neurocognitive changes from treatment.

Signs/symptoms of cognitive problems resulting from radiation and/or chemotherapy:

- Handwriting
- Spelling
- Reading or reading comprehension
- Understanding math concepts, remembering math facts, comprehending math symbols, sequencing, and working with columns and graphs
- Remembering and copying shapes
- Using calculators or computers
- Learning to ride a bike or tie shoes
- Auditory or visual language processing: trouble with vocabulary, blending sounds, and syntax
- Attention deficits: becoming either inattentive, hyperactive, or both
- Short-term memory and information retrieval
- Social maturity and social skills
- Understanding facial expressions or gestures
- Understanding deceit, cunning, or manipulation
- Planning and organizational skills
- Showing emotions on the face (*affect*)

Cognitive problems usually develop within a year or two of radiation and progress over time. So, if your child prior to treatment could color within the lines and draw proportional figures but is gradually losing those abilities, the radiation and/or chemotherapy are probably the culprits. The effect on individual children is quite variable. Some children have no late effects, some develop very subtle disabilities, and others develop life-altering problems.

Suspect learning difficulties if any of the following learning changes occur:

- Your child was an A student prior to cancer and is now working just as hard and getting Cs.
- Your child takes 3 hours to do homework that used to take 1 hour.
- Your child reads a story and then has trouble explaining the plot.
- Your child frequently comes home frustrated from school, saying: "I just don't understand things as well as the other kids."
- Your child's teacher complains that your child "just doesn't pay attention" or "just needs to work harder."
- Your child says (s)he doesn't like school.

If any of the above situations occur, take action to begin the evaluation process before your child's self-esteem plummets. It is often hard to take this first step because some children affected by radiation and/or chemotherapy can often reason well and think clearly and may be above average academically in several areas. However, they may begin to struggle and fall behind their classmates on tasks that require fast processing skills, short-term memory, sequential operations, and organizational ability (especially visual).

Once identified, these difficulties can be addressed in school through extra help with memory enhancement, eliminating timed tests, improving organizational skills, and providing extra help in mathematics, spelling, reading, writing, and speech. Early intervention is key to success and can make a huge difference.

It is also important to remember that higher cognitive functioning often remains intact; but the impairment occurs in the process of taking in and managing of information called, *information processing*. Children who are gifted usually remain so; children with average abilities retain them. Their performance may be slower, they may require extra instruction in memory enhancement and organizational skills, but they can still achieve to their potential. There are thousands of survivors in their late teens and 20s who are successfully attending high school or college or pursuing professional careers.

Addressing these issues with the schools can be tough because these disabilities are very different from those normally familiar to the school system. It requires a lot of time and special effort to get the best and most appropriate education for survivors with cognitive problems. Older survivors need to learn how to advocate for themselves as they go to college or enter the workforce. These issues are covered in detail in *Chapter 4, Navigating the System.*

Additional signs and symptoms associated with radiation to the brain (for brain tumors, relapsed leukemia, or bone marrow transplant following relapse):

- Problems with balance and coordination
- Impaired growth
- Altered fertility with higher doses of radiation
- Early or delayed puberty
- Problems making and keeping friends
- Second cancers.

Children who had radiation to the head may also experience permanent hair loss or thinning hair, dental problems, hearing loss, and cataracts. (For more information, see *Chapter 11, Eyes and Ears* and *Chapter 12, Head and Neck*)

Seizure disorders

Seizure disorders are another lasting effect that can develop in the brain after surgery, radiation, or chemotherapy. They occur most commonly during treatment, although sometimes begin many years after therapy. Seizures are caused by electrical disruptions in the brain. There are many types ranging from mild partial seizures during which the child does not lose consciousness to generalized seizures that involve convulsions and loss of consciousness. Signs and symptoms of seizures include the following:

- Staring into space
- Not hearing people talking

- Glassy eyes
- Auras (i.e., an abnormal smell, taste, abdominal sensation, or emotion that precedes a seizure)
- Stiff body
- Smacking lips and mumbled words
- Convulsions
- Jerking or twitching in parts of the body

Methods to screen for and treat all these late-effects are covered in the next part of this chapter.

Neuropsychological testing for cognitive problems

Any child at risk for cognitive problems should have neuropsychological testing performed as soon as possible after diagnosis. This should happen after treatment starts when the child starts feeling better or after treatment ends. The first test is called a *baseline screening*.

Neuropsychological testing is performed by PhD- prepared neuropsychologists who specialize in evaluating how children learn and think. Testing usually takes 4 to 6 hours, and can be scheduled over 2 days for younger children or those who are easily fatigued. All of that time is spent with the child, and the parents are interviewed separately. The psychologist gives a series of general tests appropriate for the child's age level and then another series of more specific subtests based on the results of the general ones. Pediatric psychologists usually adjust the testing format and make it enjoyable for children. Children should be informed before testing appointments that the testing will be fun, and not to fear or worry.

The *baseline testing* is used as a yardstick to measure future changes in brain functioning. Many institutions perform baseline tests and repeat them every two to three years until adulthood. Parents and older survivors use the information from these tests to advocate for the most appropriate education and any special education or disability accommodations that might be necessary in school or college. The process for scheduling neuropsychological tests, applying for insurance or funds to pay for them, and advocating for the survivor's best education environment are covered in more detail in *Chapter 5, Navigating the System.*

Yearly follow-ups

Survivors at risk for long-term effects from treatment to the brain need extensive, periodic evaluations throughout their lives. These should include:

- an educational analysis every year while in school
- yearly dental exams
- yearly evaluations of puberty and growth,
- yearly eye and hearing examinations
- education about second cancers
- a discussion about any new problems that have developed

Medical management of brain damage/dysfunction

Because treatment that affects the brain can cause a wide constellation of medical late effects, medical management includes a thorough evaluation and referral to appropriate specialists. An important component of medical management is a clear discussion of the risks for specific late effects to the brain and nerves. These should occur at each follow-up visit, as some of the late effects do not arise until years after treatment and are in some cases progressive.

My daughter was only 6 when she was diagnosed. She is now 12 and doesn't really remember much about what life was like for her before cancer. I wouldn't say she struggles with anger about having cancer per say, but one of the long-term effects of treatment is she has huge, angry outbursts over any variety of things. We never know what will set it off.

As a parent, I really struggle with anger. I am angry at what cancer has done to my child. I even experience bitterness and feelings of resentment towards friends and family who have *"normal"* healthy children.

Medical care should include referrals not only to medical specialists, but also to professionals who can help address any psychological, social, or educational issues that arise. Many medical institutions have educational liaisons/specialists who help parents and survivors understand the laws governing appropriate education for those with special needs. Sometimes these specialists travel to the school to attend *Individualized Education Program (IEP)* meetings. An IEP is a plan or program developed to ensure that a child with an identified disability who is attending an elementary or secondary educational institution receives specialized instruction and related services. Some institutions have transition specialists who work with survivors as they shift from pediatric medical care to adult care. These specialists can also help survivors with educational and vocational planning.

Recent research has examined the role of cognitive remediation in helping survivors overcome learning problems caused by treatment (Paltin, 2018). This therapy teaches methods to improve memory, attention, and math skills. Children learn strategies that help them keep on task and lessen attention drift. They also learn ways to organize both their thoughts and work habits and practice ways to retain information.

Although children and adolescents may develop attention problems after treatment, these are not the type usually diagnosed as *attention deficit hyperactivity disorder* (ADHD), a chronic condition including difficulty with attention, hyperactivity and impulsiveness. Some researchers, however, are using medications effective for that disorder to treat survivors with attention problems, and these children are showing improved attentional skills. Parents and medical professionals need to perform a careful risk/benefit analysis for each child to determine if using these medications is appropriate.

Medical management of seizure disorders starts with a thorough evaluation from a pediatric or adult neurologist. Many medications are available to treat seizure disorders, and sometimes the survivor needs trials with different drugs to discover which ones are best to control the seizures with the least number of side effects. Parents should ask the treating physician about added side effects of these medications on the child's already impaired thought processes.

If medications do not help and the seizures interfere with daily life, surgery may be recommended. An excellent resource for understanding seizures and treatment options is *Seizures and Epilepsy in Childhood: A Guide for Parents, Third Edition*, by John Freeman, MD; Eileen Vining, MD; and Diana Pillas (Freeman, 2003). See description and full reference at end of the chapter.

Some clinics have support groups for long-term survivors where they can share experiences with their peers. Some follow-up clinics link survivors going to college or into the workplace with mentors who are several years ahead of them in the process. Mentors can provide a lifeline of advice, support, and friendship. Medical management should address all aspects of the survivor's life: social, educational, vocational, and medical.

Because the research and treatments are constantly changing, survivors, families, and physicians must become lifelong learners and keep informed about the newest research, medications and treatments. This provides great hope that some late effects that cannot be treated today may be able to be treated in the future.

NERVES

Peripheral nerves gather information and send it to the spinal cord and brain. The central nervous system processes the information and sends instructions to the body to react. For example, when one touches a hot stove, a sensory receptor in the hand senses the heat/pain and carries that information through nerves to the CNS. The brain then sends instruction through the nerves to the muscles of your arm/hand to pull the hand away from the stove.

The CNS receives billions of signals about conditions inside and outside the body and sends responses that allow coordinated and smooth functioning of all body parts and organs. Damage to nerves from radiation or surgery can disrupt or block these signals.

Children are remarkably resilient. After treatment for cancer ends, many resume normal activities at age-appropriate levels. But some children, particularly those who received cranial radiation, have chronic problems with strength and coordination. Others who had chemotherapy or radiation have persistent problems with sensation or motion.

Nerve damage

Chemotherapy, particularly vincristine, often causes acute peripheral neuropathies. Usually these are characterized by foot drop (when the front of the foot does not lift while walking), problems with balance, winging out of lower legs when running, and poor coordination. For some survivors, these symptoms persist for months or years. Survivors have noted changes in both muscle strength and sensation.

Children who relapse and have higher total doses of chemotherapy are much more at risk for persistent nerve problems than children or teens who are treated once and cured.

Surgery anywhere in the body can damage nerves and thus affect function or sensation. For example, both spinal cord and urinary tract surgeries can leave the survivor *incontinent* (i.e., unable to control urination or bowel movements). Survivors of limb-salvage surgery sometimes are left with no sensation to touch in certain areas of the limb.

Pressure on nerves from a prosthesis, wheelchair, or crutches can also affect nerve functioning.

Survivors of Hodgkin lymphoma (formerly called Hodgkin's disease) treated on older protocols, including high-dose radiation, can experience neuropathies that affect sensation and function. The neuropathies can also result from vincristine and vinblastine in the combination drug therapy they receive. They occur during treatment and may subside with time or persist.

Another rarely reported late-effect is numbness, tingling, and electrical sensations in arms and/or legs that worsen when bending or twisting the head or neck. These sensations usually occur within months of high-dose radiation that involves the spinal cord but can appear years afterwards. These symptoms usually resolve on their own within months.

A very rare late effect after radiation to the brain and intrathecal chemotherapy is atrophy or destruction of the optic nerve which can cause blindness. Another very rare complication of radiation to the head and neck is vocal cord palsy (the nerves that tell the muscles to control movement of your voice do not work). Pressure from tumors directly on nerves can also affect motion and function.

Signs and symptoms of nerve damage

- Twitching face
- Decreased strength in hands and feet
- Tripping frequently
- Poor coordination
- Pain
- Dulled or absent sensation
- Paralysis
- Decreased vision
- Changes in the voice

Screening and detection of nerve damage

A thorough follow-up visit should include a full neurological examination and a discussion about physical activities. Any indication that there may be damage to the nerves should result in a referral to a neurologist for further testing. Vision changes should be evaluated by an ophthalmologist. (See *Chapter 11, Eyes and Ears*)

Medical management of nerve damage

Survivors with nerve damage from treatment may benefit from a referral to physical therapy for help with coordination and strength problems. Occupational therapy (OT) is often helpful if hand/eye coordination and visual-spatial problems persist after treatment.

REFERENCES

Brown RT, Sawyer MB, Antoniou G, et al. (1996) A 3-year follow-up of the intellectual and academic functioning of children receiving central nervous system prophylactic chemotherapy for leukemia. *J Dev Behav Pediatr.* 1996 Dec;17(6):392-8. doi: 10.1097/00004703-199612000-00004. PMID: 8960568.

Freeman JM, Vining EPG, and Pillas DJ. *Seizures and Epilepsy in Childhood: A Guide. 3rd edition*, Johns Hopkins University Press, Baltimore, 2003, 426 pp. Kevin Farrell MD, FRCPC; https://doi.org/10.1046/j.1528-1157.2003.36203.x This book is an extremely useful resource for parents of children with epilepsy. and provides a systematic review of the medical and social aspects that can affect families of children with seizures.

Krull KR, Hardy KK, Kahalley LS et al. (2018) Neurocognitive Outcomes and Interventions in Long-Term Survivors of Childhood Cancer, Clin Oncol 36:2181-2189.

MacDonald SM, Bindra RS, Sethi R, and Ladra M, Principles of Radiation Oncology. In Gajjar A, Reaman GH, Racadio JM, Smith FO. (eds.), (2018) *Brain Tumors in Children*, Springer Nature, 33-37.

Montour-Proulx I, Kuehn SM, Keene DL, et al. (2005) Cognitive changes in children treated for acute lymphoblastic leukemia with chemotherapy only according to the Pediatric Oncology Group 9605 protocol. *J Child Neurol.* 2005 Feb;20(2):129-33. doi: 10.1177/08830738050200020901. PMID: 15794179.

Paltin I, Schofield HL and Baran J. (2018) Rehabilitation and Pediatric Oncology: Supporting Patients and Families During and After Treatment. *Curr Phys Med Rehabil Rep* 6, 107–114 (2018). https://doi.org/10.1007/s40141-018-0181-1

Schatz J, Kramer JH, Ablin A, Matthay KK. (2000) Processing speed, working memory, and IQ: a developmental model of cognitive deficits following cranial radiation therapy. *Neuropsychology.* 2000 Apr;14(2):189-200. doi: 10.1037//0894-4105.14.2.189. PMID: 10791859.

Smibert E, Anderson V, GodberT, *et al.* Risk factors for intellectual and educational sequelae of cranial irradiation in childhood acute lymphoblastic leukemia. *Br J Cancer* **73**, 825–830 (1996). https://doi.org/10.1038/bjc.1996.145

RESOURCES

Website: ccgresources.org

All resources and references mentioned in this book are available on the website and will be routinely reviewed and updated.

Children's Oncology Group. *Long-Term Follow-Up* Guidelines for Survivors of Childhood, Adolescent, and *Young Adult Cancers, Version 6.0 (October 2023)* Website: http://www.survivorshipguidelines.org Click under **Health Links** for:

Neurological System: *chronic pain, peripheral neuropathy, Raynaud's phenomenon*

Passport for Care, Survivor Care Plans by Children's Oncology Group (V6, Nov 2023)

Website: https://cancersurvivor.passportforcare.org

Survivors and family can find online updated tailored long-term care plans which should be reviewed with their oncologist or health care provider.

GLOSSARY

affect, the expressions on the face such as smiling, frowning, blank stare that reveal emotions such as happiness, sadness, boredom, pain, fear

ataxia, poor muscle control which causes problems with balance, and can affect walking, hand coordination, speech, and swallowing, and eye movements

attention deficit hyperactivity disorder (ADHD), a chronic condition including difficulty with attention, hyperactivity, and impulsiveness

baseline screening, the initial conditions found by observation and measurement at the beginning of a treatment or clinical trial which is used for comparison with later data or findings to identify and measure changes

cerebrospinal fluid, a clear, colorless fluid found within the tissue that surrounds the brain and spinal cord

cognitive late effects, after cancer treatments, the changes in the way children or adolescents think, remember, and learn

dysarthria, a speech disorder caused by damage to nervous system causing muscles that produce speech to weaken resulting in slurred speech

dysphagia, difficulty or discomfort in swallowing

incontinent, unable to control urination or bowel movements

Individualized Education Program (IEP), a special educational plan or program developed to ensure that a child with an identified disability who is attending elementary or secondary educational institution receives specialized instruction and related services: the plan/program is agreed upon between parents and the school system to assure that the student will be taught the same things as other students: reading, writing, mathematics, science, history, and other preparation for college or vocational training.

leukoencephalopathy, structural change of the white matter (protein cover) of the brain. When this happens, the message signal gets interrupted along the brain nerve pathways.

meninges, three membranes that line the skull and vertebral canal and enclose the brain and spinal cord

processing or information processing, how the mind takes in information and the flow of information as it is passes from one stage to another within a person's mind.

proton therapy or proton beam therapy, a type of radiation treatment that uses a beam of protons to deliver radiation directly to the tumor

total body irradiation, radiation given in a way to cover the whole body

10
Hormone-Producing Glands

LISA BASHORE, PhD, APRN, CPNP-PC, CPON

*The future enters into us, in order to transform itself in us,
long before it happens.*

— *Rainer-Maria Rilke, Letters to a Young Poet*

SOME GLANDS IN OUR BODY produce substances called *hormones* and are part of the endocrine system. Hormones are released in tiny amounts, but travel throughout the body to direct complicated processes such as growth, puberty, reaction to stress, temperature regulation, and urine output. Damage in the balance of these chemical messengers can profoundly affect both health and quality of life. **See Figure 10-1** Male and female glands of the endocrine system.

HYPOTHALAMIC-PITUITARY AXIS (HPA)

The hypothalamus and the pituitary gland (*hypothalamic-pituitary axis*) are located deep in the brain and are connected by a stalk. The hypothalamus and pituitary work together to control all the other glands in the endocrine system. The hypothalamus—often called the master gland—produces substances that tell the pituitary to release or stop releasing hormones.

The *hypothalamus-pituitary axis (HPA)* works somewhat like a thermostat. It is programmed to secrete specific hormones under certain conditions and continues to do so until receiving a message to shut

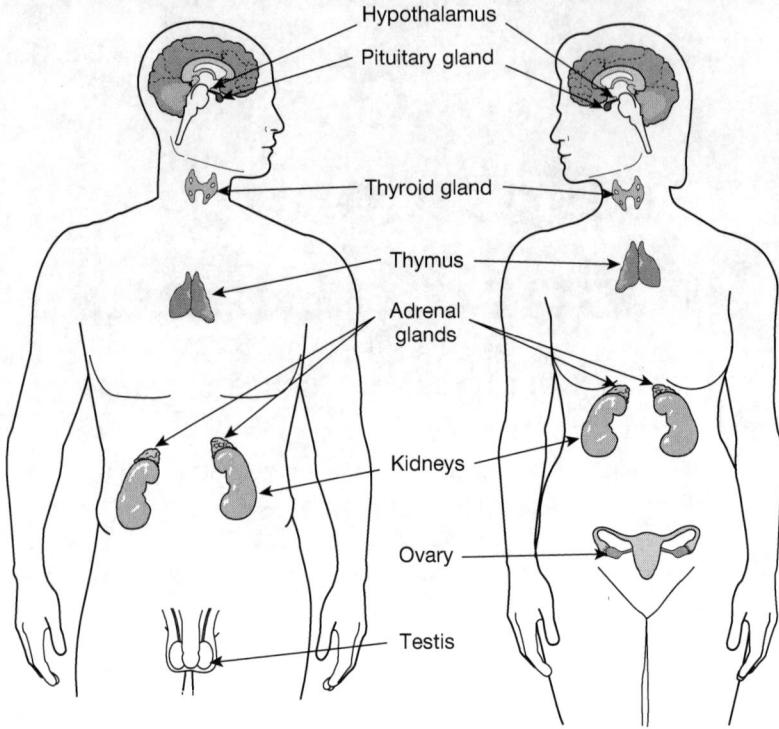

FIGURE 10-1. Male and female glands of endocrine system. (©*Alex's Lemonade Stand Foundation, 2025*)

off secretions (a feedback loop). For example, assume that the thermostat in your home is set at 70°. When the room temperature drops below 70°, the thermostat turns on the heater. The heater continues to run until the room reaches a preset temperature set in the thermostat (for example, 73°), and then the thermostat turns off the heater.

An example of this feedback loop system in the body is when puberty begins. When a girl reaches the age of puberty, the hypothalamus releases GnRH (gonadotropin-releasing hormone), which stimulates the pituitary to release FSH (follicle-stimulating hormone) and LH (luteinizing hormone). These hormones released start the development of the female ovaries. When the ovaries begin to mature and release hormones (*estrogen* and *progesterone*), the loop is complete, and puberty proceeds normally. If, however, the prepubescent girl received high-dose abdominal radiation, the LH and FSH are released, but the damaged ovaries do not respond. The HPA keeps pouring out LH and FSH to start puberty, but the loop is never connected, and the system never turns on. In this example, the girl would have high FSH and LH, but no estrogen and thus she would *not* begin puberty. **Table 10-1** shows hormones/substances each organ produces and their function in the body.

Damage to hypothalamus and pituitary gland

The hypothalamus and the pituitary gland are not normally damaged by chemotherapy. But abnormalities occur after radiation to the brain, face, or neck. The pituitary gland can tolerate higher doses of radiation. The hypothalamus is more delicate and can be affected by doses as low as 1800 to 2000 cGy, but each survivor is different. The amount of damage depends on total dose, method (proton; photon) used to deliver radiation, and age of the child when irradiated.

Growth hormone deficiency is the most common problem after radiation to the HPA. It is often not immediately obvious and tends to worsen over time. The survivors most affected by damage to the HPA are those who were treated for brain tumors. Almost all younger children treated with more than 3000 cGy to the brain experience growth disruptions.

Survivors whose growth is most likely to be affected are:

- Survivors of childhood brain tumors
- Surgery in the area near the HPA and high doses of radiation can both cause severe growth impairment
- Children exposed to radiation to the brain; the younger the age when irradiated, the more severe the effect on height
- Children who had spinal radiation (see *Chapter 18, Muscles and Bones*)
- Children who were treated with total body radiation prior to a *hematopoietic stem cell transplant* (this term includes bone marrow transplants). A single high dose of radiation causes more problems than radiation given in smaller doses. Children (especially girls) who enter puberty before age 8 (*precocious puberty)* are at the highest risk.

Table 10-1. Hormones in the hypothalamic-pituitary axis and functions

Hypothalamus Hormone	Pituitary Hormone	Function
Thyrotropin-releasing hormone (TRH)	Thyroid-stimulating hormone (TSH, also called thyrotropin)	Stimulates thyroid growth and secretion
Growth hormone-releasing hormone (GHRH)	Growth hormone (GH)	Increases body growth, muscle strength, energy, cognitive development
Gonadotropin-releasing hormone (GnRH)	Follicle-stimulating hormone (FSH)	Females: stimulates growth of ovarian follicles and female hormones Males: stimulates sperm production
Gonadotropin-releasing hormone (GnRH)	Luteinizing hormone (LH)	Females: stimulates ovulation and female hormones Males: stimulates testosterone production
Corticotropin-releasing hormone (CRH)	Adrenocorticotrophic hormone (ACTH)	Stimulates adrenal growth and secretions that help the body respond to emotions (especially stress)
None	Antidiuretic hormone (ADH or vasopressin)	Reduces the volume of urine
Prolactin-releasing factor Prolactin release-inhibiting factor	Prolactin	Regulates breast development and milk production in females

Short stature. An early linear growth spurt combined with sexual maturation can also result in short stature. Short stature occurs because the bones stop growing when sexual maturity is reached. When this happens at a young age, the child loses 2 or 3 years of additional growth.

Hormonal abnormalities. Children or adolescents who received high-dose radiation (more than 3000 cGy) to the area of the hypothalamus and pituitary often develop a variety of hormonal abnormalities. They are at risk for *growth hormone deficiencies,* early sexual development, deficiencies in production of LH, FSH, adrenocorticotrophic hormone (ACTH), and thyroid-stimulating hormone (TSH); and may produce too much prolactin. These problems may develop years after treatment, so these survivors need long-term endocrine follow-up.

Although this chapter describes each of these problems separately, survivors often have combinations of endocrine problems. There are numerous other problems from damage to the HPA that do not directly involve growth. These rare problems are listed below.

> Puberty was certainly stunted for me. I was baby-faced until my sophomore year of high school, and I didn't begin to hit puberty until I was 15. My younger brother, who was a year and a half younger, went through puberty at essentially the same time I did, the only difference being he was in middle school. It was difficult at times, having a higher voice than all my peers and not really filling out my body until I was well into high school, but my peers seemed very understanding. This was slightly difficult to deal with in sports because other boys my age were getting taller and stronger than I was. In the end, everything worked out. Just remember that although puberty can be more challenging as a survivor, you will get through it eventually!

Rare problems that can occur from damage to HPA:

- *Hyperprolactinemia* (higher levels of prolactin in the blood) can occur in children who receive more than 3000 cGy to the HPA. In females, prolactin is involved in breast development when there is adequate estrogen, progesterone, and growth hormone. Adolescents or women with too much prolactin stop having periods. Men who produce too much prolactin may have a lower sexual drive.

- *Panhypopituitary dysfunction* is when the pituitary gland does not make one or more hormones or does not make enough. It is a complication in children with brain tumors who get much higher doses of radiation to the HPA and replacement hormones may be needed.

Signs and symptoms of damage to the HPA

Signs and symptoms of damage to the HPA can take many forms. Common late effects are decreased growth, early or late puberty, and low levels of LH and FSH hormones.

Decreased growth. Decreased growth is a common problem for all children and adolescents on therapy for cancer. Many children experience catch-up linear growth after their cancer treatment ends. A few survivors continue to have slowed growth long after therapy ends. The symptoms may vary among children but may include:

- Significant changes in the growth percentiles (e.g., a child who used to be in the 90th percentile who is now in the 50th percentile)
- Below normal sitting height
- *Growth hormone deficiency (GHD)*, a rare condition in which the body does not make enough *growth hormone* (GH) that controls children's growth

Early (precocious) puberty. Precocious puberty can occur in children who were treated with cranial radiation.

Signs and symptoms of precocious puberty are:

- Physical signs of puberty in girls (e.g., breast development, underarm hair, body odor) before the age of 8
- Physical signs of puberty in boys (e.g., testicular enlargement, development of the penis, underarm hair, facial hair) before the age of 9 years
- Growth hormone deficiency

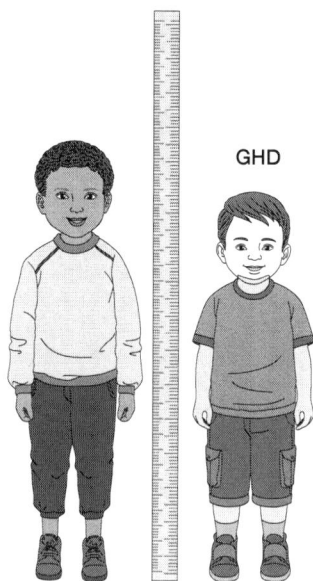

Children of the same age

FIGURE 10-2. Growth hormone deficiency (GHD) causes decreased or slow growth (©*Alex's Lemonade Stand Foundation, 2025*)

Late puberty. Puberty can also be delayed by treatment for childhood cancer. Normally, puberty begins by age 13 in girls and 14 in boys. However, if hormones produced by the pituitary (LH and FSH) are disrupted or decreased by treatment, girls and boys may not start puberty at the normal time.

Signs and symptoms of delayed puberty are:

- No signs of sexual maturation in girls (e.g., breast development, underarm hair, body odor) by age 13 years
- No signs of sexual maturation in boys, including underarm hair, deepening voice, and penial development by age 15 years
- Children who are shorter than their peers because they have not experienced a pubertal growth spurt.

Abnormal LH and FSH hormone levels. See **Table 10-2** for signs of abnormal LH/FSH levels in both females and males.

Table 10-2. Signs of abnormal LH/FSH hormone levels	
Outcomes of abnormal LH/FSH hormone levels during or after puberty	
Females	*Males*
Puberty stops	Puberty stops
Menstruation stops	Soft, small testicles
Changes in menstruation:	Low/absent sperm count
• duration/frequency	Changes in:
• other unusual changes	• libido
	• sexual performance
Signs of low estrogen:	
• hot flashes	
• vaginal dryness	
• low libido	
• sleep problems	
• painful intercourse	
• infertility	
LH, luteinizing hormone; FSH, follicle-stimulating hormone	

Screening and detection of damage to the HPA

Growth failure. Any child or adolescent who had radiation to the brain should be carefully screened for growth failure. A healthcare provider should measure standing height and plot it on a *growth chart* (graph that indicates if a child is growing normally for age) every 6 months. Sitting heights should also be obtained for any survivor who had radiation to the spine (i.e., total body radiation, mantle, spinal). The heights should be analyzed in light of the child's pre-cancer growth, current bone age (determined from a hand x-ray), stage of puberty, and height of parents.

> Healthcare providers (specifically endocrinologists) should discuss the signs and symptoms of HPA damage with survivors at risk and their parents (or older survivors) and complete a thorough yearly evaluation.

Any child who, after treatment, is growing slowly (i.e., less than 2 inches a year) or is in the fifth percentile or below for height should have additional tests:

- Bone age (measures the maturation of bones in the hand)
- Thyroid function tests
- Somatomedin-C (IGF1) and IGFBP3 (blood tests that measure the amount of hormone available to support normal growth)
- Bloodwork to check on the functioning of other major organs. All children with growth concerns should be referred to a pediatric endocrinologist.

Puberty status. All children should be evaluated for puberty status after radiation to the HPA, regardless of age. Any child who appears to be entering precocious puberty should have a bone age (x-ray of the hand) and GnRH testing done. Most facilities also test growth hormones in any child who appears to be entering precocious puberty because the two problems—slowed growth and early puberty tend to occur together. Children entering precocious puberty should be referred to a pediatric endocrinologist with experience treating survivors of childhood cancer. If your follow-up facility does not have such a specialist, you can find list of pediatric endocrinologists across the US at website: https://pedsendo.org and Search: *Patient resources, Find a pediatric endocrinologist.*

Some adolescents do not begin puberty at the normal age and need comprehensive evaluation by a pediatric endocrinologist that includes bone age, LH and FSH levels, *testosterone* or estradiol (*estrogen*) levels, and thyroid function tests for those who had high levels of radiation (of at least 3000 cGy) to the HPA. Consult an endocrinologist for further testing needs.

Medical management of damage to HPA

Healthcare providers (specifically endocrinologists) should discuss the signs and symptoms of HPA damage with survivors at risk and their parents (or older survivors) and complete a thorough yearly evaluation.

The following are the current methods used by most survivorship clinics to treat HPA problems:

- **GH deficiency.** Replacement GH is given in a daily injection (shot).
- **Low LH and FSH.** Females who produce no LH or FSH are usually treated with estrogen and synthetic progesterone (progestin). Adolescents and women with partial deficiencies may require only monthly progestin therapy to cause a period. Males with low LH are given sustained-release testosterone (through an injection into the muscle every 2 to 4 weeks, a daily patch on the skin, or in a cream).
- **Precocious puberty.** The drug Lupron® is given through a monthly or every three (3) month injection into the muscle to stop puberty until the time it should begin. Another medication, Supprelin is an implant placed just under the skin. Replacement GH and GHRH are given if the child also has low GH. Speak with your own health care provider about these options.
- **Hyperprolactinemia (too much prolactin).** This condition is treated with bromocriptine or a related medication.

Reevaluate after adult growth height reached to determine future treatment

Children who are growth hormone deficient should be evaluated again once they have achieved their adult height to determine if they require adult growth hormone replacement. Growth hormones affect many things other than growth, such as fat-to-muscle ratio, bone density, mood, cognitive function, and heart health. The criteria for receiving growth hormone in adulthood are stringent. Many children who are given growth hormone during childhood and adolescence do *not* need growth hormone into adulthood, but many do (although they need a smaller dose). There have been concerns about the long-term safety of growth hormones, and the safety of growth hormone replacement in children without any risk of malignancy has been established. However, the long-term use of growth hormone replacement in childhood cancers does not increase the risk of recurrence of cancer but may increase the risk of a subsequent primary cancer (Sripriya et al., 2013).

Doctors told me I wouldn't be able to have kids. I did egg retrieval before treatment even started when I was in college. My cousin would give me the daily shot in his frat house. I completed the rounds, but they told me that one side wasn't enlarged and I needed to try again. I said no. I decided that whatever was going to happen would happen. I was able to have children naturally and they are miracles!

Steroids are the biggest blessing yet also the biggest curse. During treatment I was on many different steroids that greatly affected my weight. Being a woman and a college student, this was something that took a serious toll on me. I gained weight all over, my face was often very swollen, and I couldn't do anything about any of it. Shortly after treatment, I was diagnosed with Type 2 diabetes. While now I am doing much better, it is something I struggled with after treatment because it was just another thing to add to the list of problems caused by treatment.

THYROID

The thyroid is a small, butterfly-shaped gland located in front of the trachea in the neck. The thyroid gland enlarges and becomes more active during puberty, pregnancy, or times of great stress.

The three hormones secreted by the thyroid are triiodothyronine (T3), thyroxine (T4), and calcitonin. T3 and T4, which contain iodine, have far- reaching effects on almost all tissues in the body and are intimately involved in physical growth, metabolism, and mental development. Calcitonin helps regulate the amount of calcium in the body. If T3 and T4 levels are low or nonexistent, growth hormone secretion is decreased and amount released is not effective.

The thyroid's functioning can be disrupted by radiation to the gland itself or to its regulator—the HPA. The pituitary gland produces TSH that prompts the thyroid to produce the exact amount of hormones needed by the body.

Thyroid damage

The thyroid is generally not affected by chemotherapy. If damage occurs, radiation is usually the culprit. Children or adolescents who had total body radiation, mantle radiation for Hodgkin lymphoma, or radiation to the head and/ or neck are at the highest risk for a malfunctioning thyroid. Several types of thyroid problems can develop after radiation.

> Survivors' healthcare providers should discuss the signs and symptoms of thyroid problems so they can be recognized and treated early.

Hyperthyroidism. Hyperthyroidism (low TSH and elevated T4) occurs when too much thyroxine is produced, causing the body to use energy faster than it should. It is not well understood but has been found in very small numbers of survivors who were treated with neck radiation.

Signs and symptoms of hyperthyroidism:

- Nervousness or anxiety
- Jittery
- Difficulty concentrating
- Feeling tired
- Muscle weakness or tremor
- Rapid or irregular heartbeat
- Increased sweating
- Diarrhea
- Weight loss
- Menstrual irregularities
- Bulging or protruding eyes
- Tenderness in the neck
- Poor exercise tolerance

Compensated hypothyroidism. High TSH and normal T4 may occur if the thyroid is working too hard. There are usually no symptoms. An irradiated and/or overstimulated gland is at increased risk for developing tumors, both benign and malignant. Most often, compensated thyroid dysfunction is found on routine screening of at-risk survivors. An elevation in the TSH is the first sign of thyroid gland dysfunction.

Primary hypothyroidism. Thyroid dysfunction can occur soon after radiation or 3 to 5 years after treatment. Survivors who received more than 1000 cGy of radiation to the neck (especially ≥ 3000 cGy or total body irradiation (TBI) are at risk for primary hypothyroidism (increased TSH and low T4). However, each survivor is different and close follow-up is necessary. Survivors of Hodgkin lymphoma, non-Hodgkin lymphoma, head and neck tumors, and those who had TBI prior to a *hematopoietic stem cell transplant* may develop this problem. Hypothyroidism sometimes occurs in patients treated with craniospinal radiation for leukemia.

Hypothyroidism is very common in Hodgkin lymphoma survivors who received mantle or radiation directed at the neck. Treatment at a young age may also increase the likelihood of developing a thyroid problem.

Signs and symptoms of hypothyroidism: (See Figure 10-3. Hypothyroidism, effects on the body)

Thyroid-stimulating hormone deficiency. This late effect, characterized by low TSH and T4 levels, is very uncommon but can occur after radiation to the head.

Thyroid cancer. Radiation to the neck can result in thyroid cancer later in life, so all survivors at risk need lifelong evaluation of thyroid function.

Screening and detection for thyroid problems

Free T4 and TSH levels should be checked every year after radiation to the head, chest, or neck, and when symptoms develop. Women who take oral contraceptive pills should also have their thyroid levels checked periodically.

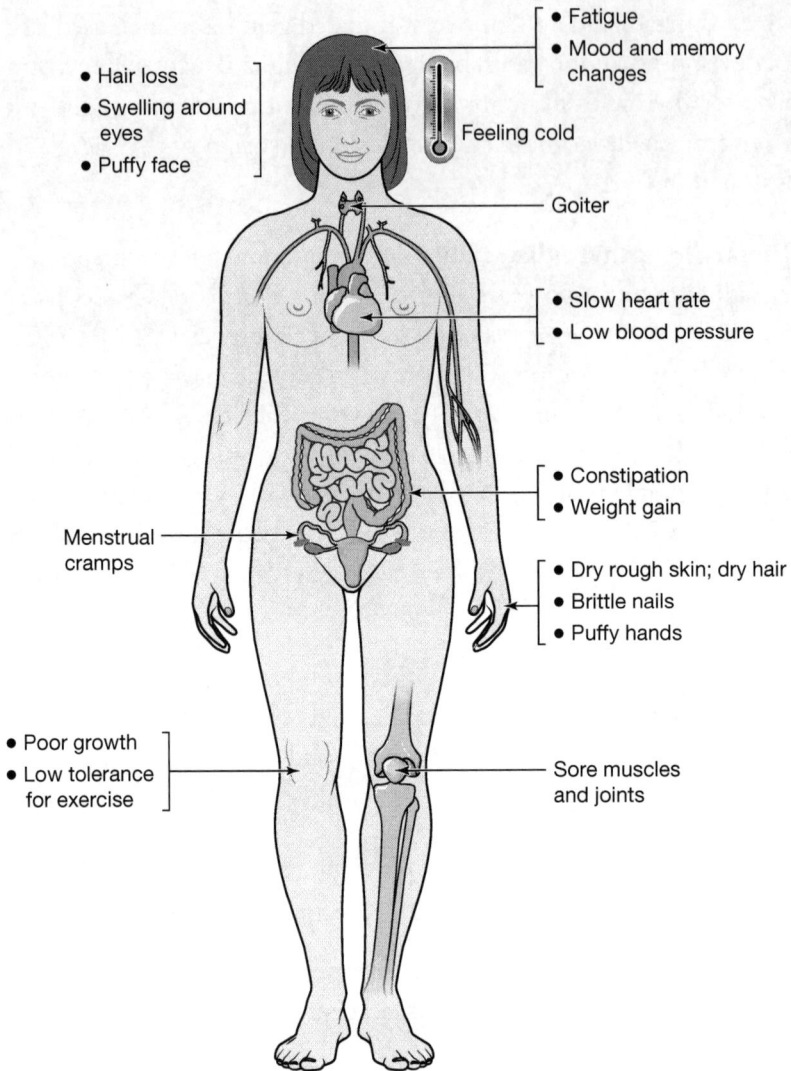

- Fatigue
- Mood and memory changes

- Hair loss
- Swelling around eyes
- Puffy face

Feeling cold

Goiter

- Slow heart rate
- Low blood pressure

- Constipation
- Weight gain

Menstrual cramps

- Dry rough skin; dry hair
- Brittle nails
- Puffy hands

- Poor growth
- Low tolerance for exercise

Sore muscles and joints

FIGURE 10-3. Hypothyroidism, effects on the body (©*Alex's Lemonade Stand Foundation, 2025*)

These are simple blood tests. At some facilities, radioactive iodine uptake by the thyroid is measured. At every yearly follow-up appointment, a survivor's thyroid should be palpated (felt by hand) and the linear growth of children and young adolescents should be assessed at each visit. If a healthcare provider can feel a thyroid nodule (bump), an ultrasound of the thyroid will be done to evaluate it. Some institutions now use ultrasound for screening.

Table 10-3 Laboratory tests, findings and treatments for thyroid diseases		
Condition	**Laboratory findings**	**Medical Management**
Compensated hypothyroidism	High TSH, normal T4	Daily thyroxine pill (suppress excessive gland activity
Primary hypothyroidism	High TSH, low T4	Replacement with thyroxine hormone pill
Low thyroid-stimulating hormone	Low TSH, low T4	Daily thyroxine pill
Hyperthyroidism	Low TSH, high T4	Radioactive iodine destroys thyroid gland, daily thyroxine pill

Thyroid problems can occur years or decades after treatment for cancer, so a yearly check is necessary for the rest of your life. If any abnormalities are detected during an examination, referral and follow-up by an endocrinologist or surgeon are necessary.

Medical management of thyroid problems

Survivors' healthcare providers should discuss the signs and symptoms of thyroid problems so they can be recognized and treated early. Although thyroid problems are common in survivors who had radiation to the head and neck, treatment is generally easy and effective. **Table 10-3** outlines laboratory tests, findings, and treatments for thyroid diseases.

Thyroid nodules. Patients with nodules detected by ultrasound should have a thyroid scan and evaluation by both an endocrinologist and a surgeon. See *Chapter 20, Subsequent Malignancies,* section on thyroid nodules. If the scan shows nodules, a biopsy should be performed.

> All survivors planning to become pregnant, should have a blood test to evaluate thyroid function because mothers with thyroid disease have higher risk of having children with neurological defects.

Pregnancy. Female survivors who are at risk for thyroid problems and are planning to become pregnant should have a blood test to evaluate thyroid function. Both the American Association of Clinical Endocrinologists and the American College of Endocrinology recommend that all women planning to become pregnant be screened before they conceive, because mothers with thyroid disease have a higher risk of having children with neurological defects.

TESTES

The testes are the male reproductive organs. These oval glands are each approximately 2 inches long when fully mature. They are enclosed in a sac called the *scrotum*. Each testicle contains hundreds of densely coiled tubes (called seminiferous tubules) that contain *spermatogonia*—cells that produce sperm. The creation of sperm depends on the presence of adequate FSH (follicle-stimulating hormone) and healthy germ cells.

Leydig cells, found throughout the testicles, produce the hormone *testosterone*. Leydig cell function is prompted by LH (luteinizing hormone). These two cell lines—spermatogonia and Leydig cells—react very differently to treatment for cancer.

Damage to the testes

The testes can be damaged by radiation, chemotherapy, or surgery. The following information is about *primary testicular failure*, when treatment affects the testes themselves.

Radiation: spermatogonia

Spermatogonia are very sensitive to radiation and any dose of radiation may cause abnormally low or permanent sterility.

When sperm production is permanently affected, reduced testicular size and softer testicles result. Survivors who have likely received these doses are:

- Boys treated for leukemia that is found in the testes
- Survivors of *hematopoietic stem cell transplant* whose conditioning included radiation
- Boys or adolescents with Hodgkin lymphoma treated with *inverted-Y* radiation.
- Boys or adolescents with soft tissue sarcomas in the thigh, groin, or abdomen

If damage to sperm-producing cells occurs before puberty, the first clue that there is a problem occurs when the testes do not grow to a normal size during puberty. These boys develop secondary sexual characteristics (e.g., facial hair, deepening voice), but the testes remain small and soft. If the teen is rendered infertile by treatment after puberty, his testicles may become softer and smaller over time.

Radiation: Leydig cells

Compared to spermatogonia, testosterone-producing Leydig cells are very resistant to radiation. Whereas male sperm production is affected quickly by small amounts of radiation, it takes approximately 2000 or more cGy to the testes before Leydig cells start to become damaged. However, each survivor is different and close follow-up is important.

Cranial or craniospinal radiation given to children with ALL or brain tumors (other than those near the pituitary) rarely causes damage to testosterone production.

Chemotherapy

Sperm production. Chemotherapy can be devastating to the production of sperm, although sperm production may resume months to years after chemotherapy ends. The drugs that most affect sperm are the alkylating agents most often used in current protocols including, cyclophosphamide, ifosfamide, and many stem cell transplant conditioning treatments. The higher the doses of these drugs, the more damage may occur to the sperm-producing cells.

Chemotherapy used to treat boys with leukemia does not usually affect sperm production unless high doses of cyclophosphamide were given. Vinblastine, bleomycin, and etoposide used to treat other cancers can temporarily affect sperm production, but the majority of survivors, over time, recover the ability to produce sperm. However, each survivor is different so close follow up is important. See the current Long-Term Follow-Up Guidelines for Survivors of Childhood, Adolescent, and Young Adult Cancers, Version 6.0 (October 2023) http://www.survivorshipguidelines.org/.

Abnormalities in puberty or sexual function. Patients treated during adolescence can have low testosterone and high LH. There can also be a lowering of libido despite a normal testosterone level. For a survivor experiencing any abnormalities in puberty or sexual functioning, a thorough evaluation may help determine the cause and identify solutions. Many adolescents and men with low-functioning Leydig cells feel much better when taking supplemental testosterone.

> It is vital to determine whether a survivor has *primary or secondary testicular failure* so he can get the best treatment. Each survivor is different, so close follow-up is important. If there is no damage to the testes but they have been shut down by the brain, they can be stimulated with hormones to produce sperm.

Secondary testicular failure. Spermatogonia and Leydig cell functioning can also be affected by damage to the HPA as well; this is called *secondary failure*. It's vital to determine whether a survivor has *primary or secondary testicular failure* so he can get the best treatment. High doses of radiation to the HPA in the brain can shut down both Leydig cells and sperm production. However, each survivor is different, so close follow up is important. If there is nothing wrong with the testes but they have been shut down by the brain, they can be stimulated with hormones to produce sperm.

Surgery
Surgery can also affect sexual functioning in males. If a survivor had an abdominal lymph node dissection, side effects can include impo-

Table 10-4. Symptoms of primary and secondary testicular failure	
Primary testicular failure*	**Secondary testicular failure**
• absence/change in libido (sex drive) • low or absent sperm count • increased breast tissue size	• lack of secondary sex characteristics • lack of facial and pubic hair • decreased testes size • decreased libido • impotence (lack of erection) • low testosterone levels
*If damage directly to the testes; **damage to the HPA	

tence or inability to ejaculate. For more information, see *Chapter 15, Kidneys, Bladder, and Genitals*. Surgery for a brain tumor involving the hypothalamus or pituitary also can disrupt the functioning of the testes.

Signs and symptoms of damage to the testes

Signs and symptoms of damage to the testes depend on age during treatment. If testosterone producing Leydig cells are damaged before puberty, boys usually do not go into puberty. If the Leydig cells are damaged after puberty, survivors may lose interest in sex and may become impotent.

If the sperm-producing cells are damaged before puberty, the testes won't grow as large as they normally would have. Survivors will have testosterone, so they will look like a normal male and can function sexually like a normal male, but the testes will be smaller and softer. If sperm-producing cells are damaged after puberty, sexual functioning will be unaffected, but the survivor may not produce sperm. Therefore, function is normal, but the survivor may be infertile.

Screening and detection for damage to testes

Survivors should receive a thorough annual evaluation if they received chemotherapy or radiation that might have damaged their testes. Evaluation by an endocrinologist is important and an examination may include the following:

- A complete history, including height, weight, and age when puberty occurred in all members of the family. The history should rule out other causes of precocious or delayed puberty. A careful physical evaluation, including evaluation of facial hair, underarm hair, pubic hair, length of penis, and size of testes.
- Analysis of a semen sample and a discussion about ejaculations, erections, and libido and about fertility
- Growth plotted on a chart to evaluate growth progression
- LH, FSH, and testosterone levels
- Prolactin level if radiation was given to the HPA

> Survivors should receive a thorough annual evaluation if they received chemotherapy or radiation that might have damaged their testes. Evaluation by an endocrinologist is important.

Recovery of sperm production sometimes occurs 10 or more years after treatment. These tests should be repeated yearly for men who have a low sperm count.

Medical management of deficient or lack of sperm-production

Male survivors who do not produce sperm as a result of direct damage to the testes must simply wait to see if sperm production recovers over time. They should have periodic sperm counts and evaluations of testosterone production, as testosterone replacement may improve a sense of well-being.

Even if adolescents have no sperm production after treatment ends, it can return. Healthcare providers should explain if new information in reproductive technology, such as intracytoplasmic sperm injection, and testicular tissue preservation is available for survivors who might want to father a child. Survivors should not assume that they are infertile; they should use birth control (including condoms) unless they are trying to become a parent. Survivors can find more information on fertility options at a local reproductive endocrinologist. (See *Chapter 3, Relationships* for more information about sexuality, birth control, marriage/life partnerships/fertility).

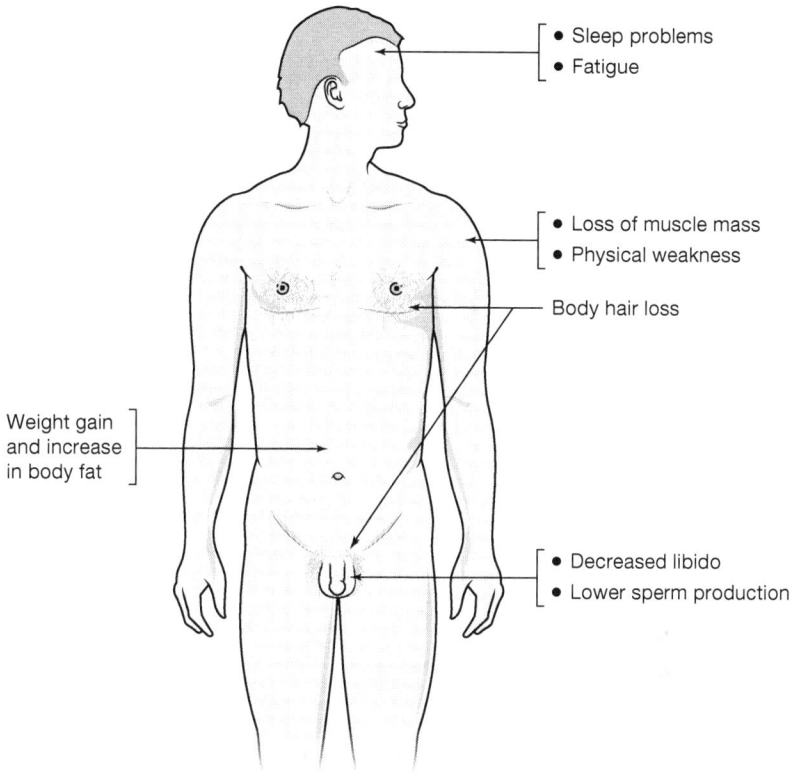

FIGURE 10-4. Common signs of low testosterone (©*Alex's Lemonade Stand Foundation, 2025*)

Adolescents or adults with primary Leydig cell damage need replacement testosterone. A testosterone patch or injection into the muscle every 2 to 4 weeks are the most common methods of supplementation for males with low testosterone. The treatment begins at the time of normal puberty. Boys with Leydig cell damage should be treated by a pediatric endocrinologist with experience treating survivors of childhood cancer. Common signs of low testosterone are important to consider.

> Medical management also includes counseling to help cope with the possibility of late effects on sexuality and fertility.

High-dose radiation to the HPA can cause *hyperprolactinemia*. Treatment with bromocriptine can sometimes resolve the symptoms, which include decreased libido, impotence, and low testosterone. Talk to your doctor about this medication and further information. Children or adolescents with tumors in the pelvis who receive high doses of abdominal radiation may have nerve damage that affects sexual functioning. Even with hormone replacement, these survivors sometimes continue to have sexual problems. Working closely with a pediatric endocrinologist and urologist will help survivors achieve the best possible outcome given their treatment.

Counseling. Medical management also includes counseling to help cope with the possibility of late effects on sexuality and fertility. For infertile males, counseling is helpful to explore other ways to become a parent (such as using donor sperm or adoption). Also, education about the difference between infertility (the inability to father a child biologically) and impotence (the inability to have or maintain erections) is tremendously important. The majority of male survivors of childhood cancer are able to have satisfying sexual relationships. (See *Chapter 3, Relationships* sections on sexuality, marriage and life partners, fertility.)

OVARIES

Ovaries are the main reproductive organs of the female. They are approximately 1½ inches in length when fully developed after puberty and are located in the abdomen on either side of the uterus. The major functions of the ovaries are development of eggs (ova) and production and release of sex hormones. Normal ovarian function is crucial for optimal growth, puberty, and fertility. Each ovary contains a finite number of eggs, so any damage to them is irreparable. The good news is that the ovaries are very treatment resistant, and it takes a considerable amount of radiation or chemotherapy to damage them.

I had a tumor in my pelvic region and had several rounds of radiation to eliminate it. Before I received radiation, a surgeon tried to move my ovaries out of the way so that they would not be affected by the treatment. The tumor was eradicated, but my ovaries were damaged. I essentially experienced full ovarian failure, and I had to see an endocrinologist during middle and high school to make sure I was receiving my hormones. I now take birth control and see an OB/GYN, but I do not menstruate like most women and will never be able to get pregnant or give birth.

Damage to the ovaries

The ovaries' functioning can be disrupted by radiation to the glands themselves or to their regulator—the HPA. Damage to the ovaries is called *primary ovarian failure* and damage to the HPA is called *secondary ovarian failure.*

Radiation to ovaries

Female children or adolescents who had radiation to the abdomen (which included the ovaries) or had TBI are at the highest risk for primary ovarian failure or insufficiency.

The effect of radiation on the ovaries is dependent on age and dosage. In older adolescents, the ovaries may be damaged at lower doses of radiation. During puberty, higher radiation doses can cause the ovaries to shut down. Once an ovary fails, it totally stops producing eggs and hormones. It is an "all-or-nothing" gland.

Older girls who stop having their periods after doses of up to about 1000 cGy may resume their normal cycles months to years after treatment ends. However, each survivor is different, so close follow up is important.

TBI prior to stem cell transplant can also cause ovarian failure.

Young girls may not start puberty, and adolescents past puberty may stop having periods. Some female transplant survivors never develop secondary sexual characteristics (e.g., breasts, pubic hair) or start menstruating.

The preceding information concerns primary ovarian failure—damage to the glands themselves. Female survivors who had high-dose radiation to the pituitary or hypothalamus (for treatment of brain tumors or rhabdomyosarcoma) are at risk for secondary ovarian failure—reduction in hormones regulating the ovaries. The hypothalamus secretes GnRH, which stimulates the pituitary gland to release FSH and LH. FSH regulates ovarian follicular growth and LH regulates ovulation. Young girls who received cranial radiation for leukemia have a slightly increased risk for precocious (early) puberty.

Chemotherapy

Primary failure of the ovaries has been associated with chemotherapy, but it usually takes very high doses to cause damage. High doses of busulfan combined with Cytoxan as a pre-transplant regime often causes ovarian damage. Sometimes older survivors of childhood cancer experience an *early menopause* (menopause that begins in the 20s or 30s instead of the 40s or 50s). As this risk can affect when and if survivors are able to have children, it is important to discuss this with your physician.

Girls treated for leukemia before or after puberty generally retain good ovarian function. The majority of girls treated for ovarian germ cell tumors remain fertile if they have one intact ovary and their uterus.

A great concern of many female survivors is their ability to have healthy children if they become pregnant. For more information, see *Chapter 3, Relationships* and Children's Oncology Group, Long-Term Follow-Up Guidelines for Survivors of Child, Adolescent, and Young Adult Cancers, Version 6 (October 2023) (www.survivorshipguidelines.org)

Signs and symptoms of ovarian problems

The signs and symptoms of ovarian problems depend on age. If ovaries fail before puberty, female survivors will *not* start puberty. They may grow pubic hair, prompted by the adrenal glands, but they do not develop breasts or begin menstruation.

Survivors who were treated after puberty may stop having periods, get hot flashes, and have decreased interest in sex.

Girls with precocious puberty begin to develop breasts and pubic hair before the age of 8. In addition to possible psychosocial problems, precocious puberty causes the growth of long bones to slow or stop. Girls whose precocious puberty is not stopped can be very short in height.

Screening and detection of endocrine problems

Survivors who received chemotherapy or radiation that might have damaged the ovaries should get a thorough annual evaluation. Also, any girl showing signs of puberty before age 8 or who has not begun puberty by age 14 needs an examination by a pediatric endocrinologist. A full evaluation of ovarian function includes the following:

- A thorough history, including information about puberty (or lack of it), menstruation (e.g., date of first period, date periods stopped), menstrual irregularities, pregnancies, difficulties becoming pregnant, libido, height of parents, age at which mother and sisters began menstruating, and symptoms of hypothyroidism (e.g., dry skin, constipation, sensitivity to cold)

- A complete physical, including height, weight, stage of puberty, and uterine size

- FSH, LH, and estradiol levels beginning at puberty

- If a survivor does not have a period by age 14 and has few or no secondary sexual characteristics (e.g., breast growth, pubic or underarm hair), referral to a pediatric endocrinologist is necessary.

- If a survivor once had periods, but periods have stopped for more than 6 months, or if she has hot flashes or breast discharge, referral to an endocrinologist is necessary.

Teenagers who have never had a period or whose periods have stopped should also have the following tests:

- Bone age (x-ray of hand)
- Ultrasound of ovaries
- Blood tests: Free T4, TSH, DHEAS, testosterone, prolactin, and *anti-mullerian hormone*. Anti-mullerian hormone is a measure of ovarian reserve and the risk of primary ovarian failure.

Medical management of ovarian failure

The medical management of girls whose ovaries have shut down is somewhat controversial. Consequently, it is extremely important that survivors be followed by a pediatric endocrinologist experienced in treating survivors of childhood cancer. An internist, family practice healthcare provider, or pediatrician may be able to provide care after a pediatric endocrinologist has thoroughly evaluated the situation and recommended treatment.

Some healthcare providers treat prepubertal girls experiencing ovarian failure with estrogen first, then add progesterone after a year.

Growth hormone is suggested if the girl is growth-hormone deficient. When the girl is fully mature (with complete breast development, pubic and underarm hair), she is maintained on birth control pills.

Girls experiencing precocious puberty are given medication to stop puberty so they will continue to grow normally. When the drug is discontinued, normal puberty begins. Survivors at risk for premature ovarian failure may want to consider *oocyte (egg) or embryo freezing* if they may want to have a child in the future. In addition, post-pubertal girls who need a stem cell transplant can also undergo a procedure to procure oocytes for future use.

For information about fertility and pregnancy, see *Chapter 3, Relationships*. For information on your fertility risk and ask your health care provider to assess your fertility risk based on your cancer treatment.

ADRENAL GLANDS

There are two adrenal glands, one on top of each kidney. Each gland is roughly triangular in shape and approximately 1 1/2 inches long and a 1/2 inch wide. The outer portion of the gland (cortex) secretes aldosterone, cortisol, and androgens (sex hormones). Aldosterone regulates the excretion of sodium (salt) and potassium in urine. Cortisol (hydrocortisone) has several important jobs, including guiding the body's reactions to stress and to inflammatory and allergic reactions. The adrenals are stimulated and controlled by adrenocorticotropin, produced by the pituitary gland.

Adrenal gland damage

Children or adolescents who had a kidney removed (e.g., treatment for Wilms tumor or kidney cancer) or an adrenal gland removed (e.g., for a neuroblastoma that started in an adrenal gland) usually function quite well with only one remaining gland. Abdominal radiation almost never damages the adrenal glands. Brain irradiation, however, can occasionally disrupt the functioning of the adrenal glands if the HPA was affected, which is rare and only in higher doses of radiation to the pituitary.

Signs and symptoms of adrenal insufficiency

The signs and symptoms of adrenal insufficiency are weight loss, lethargy, low stamina, low blood pressure, irritability, depression, craving for salty foods, darkening of areas of the skin, weakness, and vomiting. These symptoms can appear gradually or suddenly worsen during periods of stress—for example, during an illness or after an accident.

Symptoms of an adrenal crisis (acute onset of symptoms) include pain in the lower back, abdomen, or legs; severe vomiting and diarrhea; dehydration; low blood pressure; and loss of consciousness. *Left untreated, it can be fatal.* A temporary form of adrenal insufficiency may occur when a person who has been receiving a glucocorticoid hormone (such as prednisone) for a long time suddenly stops taking the medication.

Screening and detection for adrenal gland problems

Problems with the adrenal glands are rare after treatment for childhood cancer. However, cortisol levels should be checked in the following situations:

- If one adrenal gland was removed and the other gland received high doses of radiation
- If the pituitary received more than 5000 cGy of radiation

Healthcare providers should check cortisol levels in both the morning and evening. If cortisol is low, referral to an endocrinologist is necessary for further testing.

Medical management of cortisol deficiency

Treatment for cortisol deficiencies is replacement hydrocortisone given once in the morning or in two equal doses. Higher doses are needed if you are ill or undergoing anesthesia.

METABOLIC SYNDROME

There is evidence that survivors of childhood cancer are at increased risk for *metabolic syndrome*, which consists of a group of symptoms that, themselves are chronic conditions, and include obesity, insulin resistance, high cholesterol level, and high blood pressure. Though, each of these chronic conditions are independently potentially serious long-term effects of cancer treatment. This syndrome can lead to type 2 diabetes and cardiovascular disease. Some types of treatment predispose children to metabolic syndrome, and an endocrinologist is best able to diagnose this late effect. Treatment will vary based on which symptoms the child or young adult exhibits. Please speak with your own survivorship team for more information and refer to *Chapter 5, Staying Healthy*.

REFERENCES

Children's Oncology Group. Long-Term Follow-Up Guidelines for Survivors of Childhood, Adolescent, and Young Adult Cancers, Version 6.0 (October 2023) Available online: http://www.survivorshipguidelines.org Click under Health Links for: Endocrine System: Central Adrenal Insufficiency, Growth Hormone Deficiency, Hyperprolactinemia, Hypopituitarism, Precocious Puberty, Thyroid Cancer

Chemaitilly W, Li Z, Brinkman TM, et al. (2022). Primary hypothyroidism in childhood cancer survivors: Prevalence, risk factors, and long-term consequences. *Cancer, 128*(3), 606-614. https://doi.org/10.1002/cncr.33969

Chemaitilly W, Liu Q, Van Iersel L, *et al*. (2019). Leydig Cell Function in Male Survivors of Childhood Cancer: A Report from the St Jude Lifetime Cohort Study. *Journal of Clinical Oncology, 37* (32), 3018-3031. doi: 10.1200/JCO.19.00738.

Chemaitilly W, Li Z, Krasin MJ, et al: (2017) Premature ovarian insufficiency in childhood cancer survivors: a report from the St. Jude Lifetime Cohort. *J Clin Endocrinol Metab* 102(7):2242-50, 2017.

DeMayo FJ, Zhao B, Takamoto N, & Tsai SY. (2002). Mechanisms of action of estrogen and progesterone. *Annals of the New York Academy of Sciences, 955*, 48–406. https://doi.org/10.1111/j.1749-6632.2002.tb02765.x

Eugster EA. (2019) Treatment of Central Precocious Puberty. (2019) *J Endocr Soc.* 2019;3(5):965-972. Published 2019 Mar 28. doi:10.1210/js.2019-00036

Khaddour K, Hana CK, Mewawalla P. (2023) Hematopoietic Stem Cell Transplantation. [Updated 2023 May 6]. In: StatPearls [Internet]. Treasure Island (FL): StatPearls Publishing; 2023 Jan-. Available from: https://www.ncbi.nlm.nih.gov/books/NBK536951/

Kota AS, Ejaz S. Precocious Puberty. [Updated 2023 Jul 4]. In: StatPearls [Internet]. Treasure Island (FL): StatPearls Publishing; 2023 Jan-. Available from: https://www.ncbi.nlm.nih.gov/books/NBK544313/

Nyström A, Mörse H, Nordlöf H, et al. Anti-müllerian hormone compared with other ovarian markers after childhood cancer treatment. Acta Oncol 58(2):218-24, 2019

Raman S, Grimberg A, Waguespack SG, et al. (2015) Risk of Neoplasia in Pediatric Patients Receiving Growth Hormone Therapy—A Report from the Pediatric Endocrine Society Drug and Therapeutics Committee, *The Journal of Clinical Endocrinology & Metabolism*, Volume 100, Issue 6, 1 June 2015, Pages 2192–2203, https://doi.org/10.1210/jc.2015-1002

Sklar CA, Antal Z, Chemaitilly W, et al: Hypothalamic-pituitary and growth disorders in survivors of childhood cancer: an endocrine society clinical practice guideline. J Clin Endocrinol Metab 1;103(8):2761-2784, 2018

RESOURCES

Website: ccgresources.org
All resources and references mentioned in this book are available on the website and will be routinely reviewed and updated.

Children's Oncology Group. (V6, 2023). *Long-Term Follow-Up Guidelines for Survivors of Childhood, Adolescent, and Young Adult Cancers*
Website: www.survivorshipguidelines.org
Click under **Health Links** for: **Endocrine System**: *central adrenal insufficiency, growth hormone deficiency, hyperprolactinemia, hypopituitarism, precocious puberty, thyroid cancer*
Reproductive System: *female health issues, male health issues*

Oncofertility Consortium
Website: https://oncofertility.msu.edu
The Oncofertility Consortium is an international, interdisciplinary initiative originally designed to explore the urgent unmet need associated with the reproductive future of cancer survivors and continues to explore the relationships between health, disease, survivorship, treatment, gender, and reproductive longevity.

Passport for Care, Survivor Care Plans by Children's Oncology Group (V6, Nov 2023)
Website: https://cancersurvivor.passportforcare.org
Survivors and family can find online updated tailored long-term care plans which should be reviewed with their oncologist or health care provider.

Pediatric Endocrine Society
Website: https://pedsendo.org
Search for, *growth hormone deficiency, patient resources, Find a pediatric endocrinologist*
Email: info@pedsendo.org

GLOSSARY

anti-mullerian hormone, hormone produced by the granulosa cells in female ovarian follicles; levels of this hormone can indicate fertility

early menopause, menopause that begins in the 20s or 30s instead of the 40s or 50s

estrogen, sex hormones that have the primary role of human reproduction or sexual function. In females, they are primarily important to the health of the uterus.

FSH, follicle-stimulating hormone

GnRH (gonadotropin-releasing hormone), hormone that stimulates the pituitary gland to release FSH and LH

hormones, substances released in tiny amounts throughout the body to direct complicated and vital body processes such as growth, puberty, reaction to stress, temperature regulation, and urine output

hypothalamic-pituitary axis (HPA), the hypothalamus and pituitary glands that work together to control all other glands in the endocrine system

hematopoietic stem cell transplant (HPSCT) or stem cell transplant, formerly known as bone marrow transplant, involves administering healthy stem cells (e.g., bone marrow, cord blood, or peripheral blood) to patients after the bone marrow has been destroyed by disease, chemotherapy (chemo), or radiation.

hyperprolactinemia, higher levels of prolactin in the blood

hypothalamic-pituitary axis (HPA), the hypothalamus and pituitary work together to control all the other glands in the endocrine system

Leydig cells, found throughout the testicles produce the hormone, testosterone

luteinizing hormone (LH)

metabolic syndrome, a cluster of conditions that occur together including obesity, insulin resistance, high cholesterol level, and high blood pressure that increase risk of heart disease, stroke and type 2 diabetes. Survivors of childhood cancer are at increased risk for metabolic syndrome.

oocyte (egg) or embryo freezing, also called oocyte cryopreservation, a procedure to preserve a woman's eggs (oocytes) for future use. In the future, eggs can be thawed, fertilized, and transferred to the uterus as embryos.

primary ovarian failure, direct damage to the ovaries due to chemotherapy or radiation

primary testicular failure, failure of testes to function properly and produce sperm

testicular failure (secondary) failure of testes to produce sperm caused by a problem in the hypothalamus or the pituitary gland

progesterone, sex hormones that have the primary role of human reproduction or sexual function

secondary ovarian failure, direct damage to the HPA causing the ovaries not to function properly

spermatogonia, cells that produce sperm

stem cell transplant or hematopoietic stem cell transplant (HPSCT), involves administering healthy hematopoietic stem cells (e.g., bone marrow, cord blood, or peripheral blood) to patients after the bone marrow has been destroyed by disease, chemotherapy (chemo), or radiation

testosterone, a sex hormone produced in both males and females; it functions as the major sex hormone in males and is essential to the development of male growth and masculine development

11
Eyes and Ears

JOANNE QUILLEN, MSN, APRN, PNP-BC

The best and most beautiful things in the world cannot be seen, nor even touched. They must be felt in the heart.
— *Helen Keller*

EYES AND EARS can be damaged by treatment for some types of childhood cancers. Each eye is constructed of several layers of tissue that each react differently to cancer treatment. Some parts of the eye are resistant to damage, but other parts are extremely sensitive to cancer treatment. Hearing can be affected by chemotherapy (most notably the family of drugs that includes cisplatin) and radiation. Frequent ear infections and certain intravenous antibiotics can also damage hearing. This chapter covers the various late effects involving eyes and ears, the risk of developing them, and how to manage them if they occur.

Any of the late effects described in this section should be treated by an ophthalmologist skilled in treating survivors of childhood cancer.

EYES

The eye is the organ of sight. This nearly spherical body has numerous layers. At the front is the transparent cornea; through the cornea, the colored iris is visible. The space between the cornea and the iris is the anterior chamber, which is filled with a clear fluid called *aqueous humor*. In the center of the iris is a space called the *pupil* that contracts or expands to control the amount of light entering the eye. Directly behind the pupil is the lens of the eye. The cavity behind the lens is

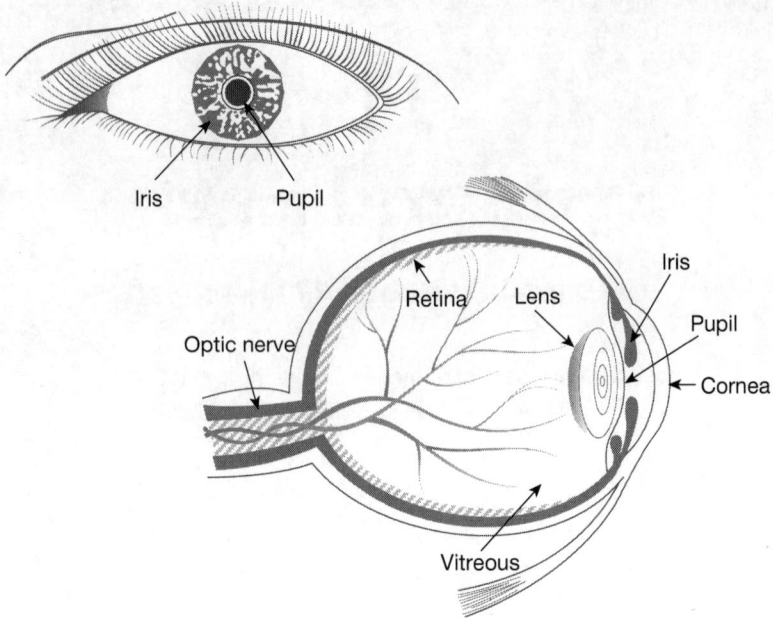

FIGURE 11-1. Anatomy of the eye. (©*Alex's Lemonade Stand Foundation, 2025*)

filled with a gel-like substance called the *vitreous humor*. The thin layer that lines this cavity is the *retina* which detects the light signals that enter the eye. The *optic nerve* transmits light information from the retina to the brain. **Figure 11-1** shows the anatomy of the eye.

> Both of our girls had 6 months of VEC chemotherapy and PRN laser/cryotherapy. They have both had chemotherapy injections into their eyes. Our oldest had 3 rounds of IAC at Jefferson. All of this to shrink and kill the tumors on their retinas and prevent them from spreading to the brain. One of our girls will only have peripheral vision in her left eye with close to normal vision in her right. The other will likely have normal vision in both eyes.

Eye damage

The eye can be damaged by radiation, treatment with steroids, or surgery. Vision can also be harmed if the optic nerve is damaged anywhere between the eye and the brain which can happen from radiation, a tumor pressing on the optic nerve, or a tumor in the brain causing high fluid pressure around the brain and optic nerves. In addition, tumors in the *brainstem* (where the brain meets the spinal cord) can cause problems with eye movement or double vision.

When a cancer is in the eye, as in retinoblastoma, the affected eye might have to be surgically removed (called *enucleation*); this occurs less often now than in the past because of newer radiation techniques and chemotherapy protocols. Small and medium-sized retinoblastomas are often treated with some combination of chemotherapy, cryotherapy (freezing treatment), and photocoagulation (laser treatment). Large or advanced tumors may require enucleation. See more information about retinoblastoma on website of American Academy of Ophthalmology: https://www.aao.org/eye-health/diseases/what-is-retinoblastoma

The eye is exposed to low-dose radiation during *total body irradiation* (TBI) prior to some types of stem cell transplants. High-dose radiation is used to treat retinoblastoma, rhabdomyosarcoma, and other tumors around the eye. The eye may also be exposed to radiation given to treat brain tumors or leukemia.

Common problems of the eye after treatment

- Hypoplasia (slowed growth of the bones around the eye)
- Dry eye
- Shrinkage of the lacrimal duct, which drains tears from the eye
- Loss of vision
- Cataracts

A common late effect is slowed growth (hypoplasia) of the orbits (eye sockets), which are the bony structures in the skull that protect the eyes. Each orbit is made up of seven bones, all of which can be damaged by radiation. This late effect is most noticeable in survivors who were treated at a very young age with more than 4000 cGy in the areas of the growing bones. Survivors with severe hypoplasia sometimes benefit from reconstructive surgery after the bones in the face are fully grown.

Cataracts (when the lens of the eye becomes opaque) are a frequent late effect of radiation treatment. Cataracts can cause vision loss, but they can often be treated with surgery. Higher doses of radiation cause more damage and shorten the time before cataracts appear. Cataracts appear earlier and become more severe if the child was treated at a young age. In addition, single, larger doses of radiation cause cataract formation more often than the same total dose given in several smaller fractions. Long-term steroid use (including prednisone and dexamethasone) or busulfan chemotherapy can also cause cataracts. See more information on cataracts on the American Academy of Ophthalmology website: https://www.aao.org Search: *what are cataracts*.

Graft-versus-host disease and/or radiation can cause mild to severely dry eyes. Symptoms include irritation, burning, pain, blurred vision, sensitivity to light, and the feeling that a foreign body is in the eye. Dry eyes can be eased by using artificial tears.

Loss of vision can involve *central vision* (the detailed vision used for reading) or the *peripheral visual fields* (side vision). Loss of peripheral vision can result from damage to the retina or optic nerve or damage to the visual areas of the brain from brain surgery.

Less common late effects to the eye or eye socket from radiation can include:

- Permanent loss of the eyelashes
- Hemorrhaging of small damaged blood vessels in the retina (telangiectasias) typically occurring 3 to 5 years after treatment
- Adhesions and scarring that limit the ability of the lids to fully close, making the eyes drier
- Inflammation of the cornea (called *keratitis*), with sensitivity to light and pain at the surface of the eye
- Ulcers, holes, or scarring of the cornea after treatment
- *Glaucoma* (increased pressure within the eye) which can also be caused by steroid use
- Secondary cancers

Surgery, stroke, and some medications can also cause problems with the eyes and vision. If there is damage to the part of the brain that controls the muscles that move the eyes, this can result in an eye that does not move normally, and the two eyes not being lined up with one another. If this happens at an early age, the brain may start to ignore one eye, and the eye can lose vision as a result (called amblyopia). Amblyopia may need to be treated with *patching therapy* (patching the good eye to improve vision in the eye that is not being used). Surgery may help improve the alignment of the eyes, but surgery cannot always restore a full range of movement.

Signs and symptoms of eye damage

When children are old enough to talk, and certainly by school age, visual disturbances are usually detected and treated. However, if changes are gradual, a child may get used to them, and identification of visual late effects can be delayed.

The following are signs and symptoms of late effects to the eye:

- Blurry vision
- Double vision
- Blind spots or a decrease in visual field (range of vision)
- Increased sensitivity to light
- Difficulty with night vision
- Floaters across the field of vision that change or light up
- Pain in the eye
- Decreased tearing or excessive tearing/watering of eyes
- Persistent dry, scratchy eyes or eyelids

Follow-up screening and detection for eye damage

You should be seen regularly by an ophthalmologist with experience treating survivors of childhood cancer if you:

- Had total body radiation
- Received high-dose radiation to one or both of the eyes or nearby structures
- Received radiation for a brain tumor or leukemia that included an eye in the radiation field
- Used steroids for a prolonged period

The ophthalmologist should perform a thorough evaluation that includes evaluation of vision, a test for glaucoma, checking for cataracts, and examination of the retina.

Survivors not at high risk for eye damage will usually have a brief eye examination as part of their yearly follow-up examination. This should include a visual examination of the eyes and a vision test using a Snellen letter chart, or a picture chart for children who cannot read letters. Even children as young as age 3 can identify simple pictures on charts specially designed for preschoolers. Any abnormalities should result in a referral to an ophthalmologist.

For additional information about vision tests you should have based on your specific treatment, you and your healthcare provider can refer to the Children's Oncology Group's survivorship guidelines at www. survivorshipguidelines.org.

Medical management of eye damage

If you have any visual changes, you should be followed by an ophthalmologist skilled in treating survivors of childhood cancer. If you have cataracts or glaucoma, you may need glasses, medications, and/or surgery. Survivors who had one or both eyes removed will need a series of well-fitted prostheses as they grow, and education about caring for the prostheses.

A survivor's healthcare team should also provide referrals to resources to assist with adjustments related to limited vision. Special arrangements should be made with schools to provide preferential seating, eyewear protection, and other necessary accommodations.

Childhood survivorship clinics or programs can provide detailed information about educational regulations and opportunities for young people with visual impairments. For more information about education, see *Chapter 4, Navigating the System.*

Artificial tears and ointments are used to protect the cornea and preserve vision in survivors with chronic dry eyes. A severe problem with dry eyes can sometimes be fixed by closing the tear draining ducts with either plugs or surgery (called *punctal ligation*). It also helps to avoid anything that contributes to dry eyes such as wind, fans, smoke, low humidity, or air conditioning.

Survivors who develop corneal ulcerations as complications of dry eyes may need to be treated with antibiotic eye drops.

Radiation-induced cataracts are progressive. Exposing these cataracts to extra sunlight may speed the progression. Sunlight can also aggravate glare symptoms from cataracts. Wearing sunglasses with UV protection when outside may help children and teens with cataracts.

EARS

The ear, the organ of hearing, is made up of three main parts: external, middle, and inner ear. The external ear includes the outer portion (auricle) and the external auditory canal. The middle ear is a cavity separated from the external ear by the eardrum and contains three small bones. The inner ear contains the cochlea (which is responsible for hearing), the vestibule (which senses position in space and motion), and the semicircular canals (which control equilibrium). **Figure 11-2** shows the anatomy of the ear.

Ear damage

Ears and hearing can be damaged by chemotherapy, high-dose radiation, and some antibiotics.

Chemotherapy

Some anticancer drugs, primarily cisplatin, can cause substantial hearing loss in the high- to ultra-high-frequency range—6,000 to 12,000 Hertz (Hz). The degree of hearing loss is greater in younger children and those who receive higher cumulative doses of cisplatin. If more damage occurs, the lower frequencies also can be affected. Carboplatin is also associated with hearing loss but to a much lesser degree. Radiation to the head can intensify the hearing loss from cisplatin.

The damage generally occurs in both ears and is irreversible. Sometimes ringing in the ears (*tinnitus*) or a sensation of drifting in space or having objects drift around you (*vertigo*) can also occur. Children most at risk for chemotherapy-caused hearing loss are those treated for brain tumors, germ cell tumors, osteosarcoma, and neuroblastoma.

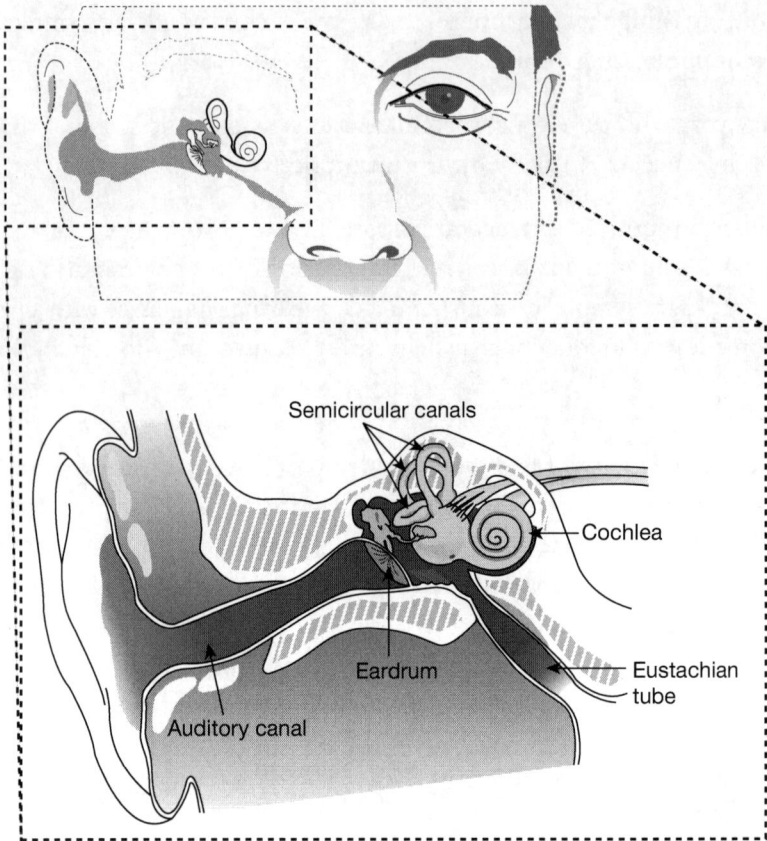

FIGURE 11-2. Anatomy of the ear. (©*Alex's Lemonade Stand Foundation, 2025*)

Radiation

Survivors who had head and neck tumors treated with higher doses of radiation often develop hearing loss.

The most common diseases treated with high-dose radiation that can affect the ears:

- Nasopharyngeal carcinomas
- Other soft tissues around the ear (rhabdomyosarcoma)
- Parameningeal sarcomas
- Brain stem gliomas
- Medulloblastomas
- Ependymomas

Children treated with less than 2400 cGy of cranial radiation (e.g., for leukemia or prior to stem cell transplantation) rarely develop any late effects in the ears.

Outer ear infections, which are common after high-dose radiation, can impair hearing by drying out and thickening the external ear canal and eardrum. Chronic middle ear infections (otitis media) can also be caused by radiation due to damage to the eustachian tube which is responsible for drainage of the middle ear. When the eustachian tube cannot drain properly, middle ear infections can become chronic.

The glands that produce earwax (*cerumen glands*) may produce less wax, and earwax that is produced sometimes becomes crusty and impacted. While the earwax is impacted, hearing is decreased and trapped moisture can increase the risk for ear infections. This late effect can also occur in survivors who developed graft-versus-host disease after stem cell transplantation. Impacted earwax can be removed by your healthcare provider. It is strongly discouraged to use cotton-tipped applicators or other objects in the ear canal because they can actually push impacted earwax further into the ear canal.

Risk factors for permanent hearing loss in children/teens treated for cancer:

- Treatment with cisplatin, and to a lesser extent, carboplatin
- High doses of radiation to the head and/or neck
- Younger age at time of treatment
- Surgery involving the ear, brain, or auditory nerve
- Treatment with certain antibiotics such as gentamicin (generally used for serious infections or fever when blood counts are low)
- Chronic ear infection
- Treatment with diuretics (drugs that help the body get rid of excess water)
- Poor kidney function

Signs and symptoms of hearing loss

Hearing loss should be suspected if your child has *any* of the following symptoms:

- Does not startle or respond to loud noises
- Does not respond to your voice consistently
- Has a hard time understanding or following directions after age 3
- Does not have clear speech
- Fails to develop sounds or words that are appropriate for their age
- Uses gestures instead of words

Lesser signs and symptoms of hearing loss which are typically associated with chemotherapy but should be suspected if your child:

- Confuses like-sounding words
- Drops sounds off words or reports not hearing sounds such as *th, f, sh, s, t, k, g, ch,* and *v*
- Reports (s)he can hear but not understand words and speech
- Has difficulty hearing in noisy situations or environments

Any parents who have a concern regarding their child's hearing and notice any of the above symptoms, should have the child's hearing evaluated by an audiologist.

School-aged children who have lost some hearing may withdraw socially or have trouble in school. They may also describe ringing in their ears or dizziness.

Follow-up screening and detection for ear damage

After treatment ends, appointments at the follow-up clinic should include an ear examination to look for infection, wax buildup, and eardrum perforation or scarring. Survivors should also have their hearing tested periodically following completion of treatment, because chemotherapy can have an impact on hearing up to 5 years after completion of the last round. Healthcare providers of survivors who had head or brain radiation may recommend periodic hearing tests because hearing problems can also sometimes develop several years after radiation. Anyone with abnormal test results should be referred to an *audiologist* or *otolaryngologist* (ear, nose, and throat doctor) for a thorough evaluation to determine whether assistive technology would be helpful.

The most widely used method to test the hearing of children with cancer is *pure tone audiometry*. These tests should be administered by an experienced pediatric audiologist. Extended high-frequency audiometry may be used to test for hearing loss in the high-frequency range (4,000 to 20,000 Hz). This is especially important for younger children with limited language because many consonants (*th, f, p, s*) are in this range. If a child cannot hear these consonants it may be very hard to acquire clear speech, so early intervention can make an important difference. Children at risk for hearing loss should also be tested for speech and language disorders.

For more information, see *American Speech and Hearing Association* website in Resources at the end of the chapter.

> My daughter suffered hearing loss as was expected. We did not have a lot of support for that during her school years. At the time, we were feeling relieved to survive a life-threatening situation, and the hearing loss seems like a minor challenge. Unfortunately, as school began, we realized the hearing loss *was* a huge problem and not just for learning but for her social development. It really caused her to feel isolated and left her feeling shy and excluded a lot of the time. I wish that I had known more, explored options and done more in terms of getting her support at that time, but I have learned I cannot go back and not to beat myself up about that.

Medical management of ear damage

Medical management includes treating middle or external ear infections, and in some cases, placing tubes in the ears. Survivors with *tinnitus* (ringing in the ears) may benefit from intervention and should be evaluated by an audiologist or otolaryngologist. State-of-the-art hearing aids are needed for those with permanent hearing impairment. Newer digital technology can minimize background noise and maximize speech sounds, unlike hearing aids of the past. Proper fitting and follow-up testing are crucial. It is also important to develop a routine for maintaining the aids, cleaning the ear molds and replacing the batteries. Ear molds will need to be replaced periodically. An alert that hearing aids need to be checked is if you hear *feedback* or high-pitched noise from the hearing aids. They should be taken to the audiologist to be checked.

For those with profound hearing loss, fostering language development with speech reading and signing is vital. Using the closed captioning while watching television can also be helpful. Coping with the emotional and psychological effects of hearing loss in children and teens is an essential component of care.

Educators sometimes need the support and direction of medical caregivers. For instance, an *FM system* (a special type of assistive listening device) can be used by hearing-impaired children in school to amplify the teacher's voice. The teacher wears a microphone that transmits the voice via radio waves to a receiver that can be attached to the child's hearing aids, in a speaker mounted in the classroom, or to a personal speaker on the child's desk. Your child's healthcare provider should give you detailed information about educational regulations for young people with hearing loss. For more information about education, see *Chapter 4, Navigating the System*.

The American Academy of Audiology offers information about hearing loss on the consumer website at *www.howsyourhearing.org*. In addition, the Children's Oncology Group's survivorship guidelines include an informational resource about hearing loss at *www.survivorshipguidelines.org*. See list of all Resources at the end of the chapter.

REFERENCES

Long-Term Follow-Up Guidelines for Survivors of Childhood, Adolescent, and Young Adult Cancers, Version 6.0 (October 2023). http://www.survivorshipguidelines.org/ Search *Sensory*, then subcategories: cataracts, eye health, hearing loss

Moke DJ, Luo C, Millstein J, et al. (2021) Prevalence and risk factors for cisplatin-induced hearing loss in children, adolescents, and young adults: A multi-institutional North American cohort study. *The Lancet Child & Adolescent Health, 5*(4), 274-283. https://doi.org/10.1016/S2352-4641(21)00020-1

RESOURCES

Website: ccgresources.org
All resources and references mentioned in this book are available on
  the website and will be routinely reviewed and updated.

American Academy of Audiology
  Website: www.howsyourhearing.org
  The website provides extensive resources for families, features
  *Find an audiologist, Managing hearing loss and balance con-
  ditions, anew over-the-counter hearing aids resources: questions
  and answers*
  11730 Plaza America Drive, Suite 300; Reston,VA 20190

American Academy of Ophthalmology
  Website: https://aao.org
  Search: *what are cataracts, eye health, diseases*

American Society for Deaf Children
  Website: https://www.hearingloss.org
  inquiries@hearingloss.org

American Speech-Language-Hearing Association
  Website: www.asha.org
  Search, *Pure-tone testing in children*

Hearing Loss Association of America
  Website: https://www.hearingloss.org
  inquiries@hearingloss.org
  Phone: (301) 657-2248

Hearing impairment - books
  Ogden, Paul W. (1996). *The Silent Garden: Raising Your Deaf
  Child.*
  Washington, DC: Gallaudet University Press.
  Schwartz, Sue. (2007). *Choices in Deafness: A Parent's Guide
  to Communication Options, 3rd ed.* Bethesda, MD: Woodbine
  House.

National Eye Institute
  Website: https://www.nei.nih.gov/

Passport for Care, Survivor Care Plans by Children's Oncology Group (V6, Nov 2023)

Website: https://cancersurvivor.passportforcare.org
Survivors and family can find online updated tailored long-term care plans which should be reviewed with their oncologist or health care provider.

GLOSSARY

amblyopia or lazy eye, type of poor vision usually in just one eye resulting from a weakness in one eye over the other. The brain does not recognize one eye over the other and causes poor vision in one of the eyes

audiologist, a professional who uses technology, creative problem solving, and social skills to help them identify and treat hearing, balance, tinnitus, and other audiology disorders

cataracts, when the lens of the eye becomes opaque

central vision, the detailed vision used for reading

cerumen glands, glands that produce earwax

cryotherapy, freezing treatment

diuretics, medications that help the body get rid of excess water

enucleation, surgical removal of the eye

FM system, a special type of assistive listening device that operates like a tiny radio station with its own frequency. One part is a microphone that the speaker wears (teacher in a class). As the teacher speaks, the microphone sends a signal to a receiver that you wear on your ears or in your hearing aids and the speaker's voice goes directly to you, making it easier to hear.

glaucoma, increased pressure within the eye

graft-versus-host disease (GvHD), a systemic disorder that occurs when the graft's immune cells recognize the host as foreign and attack the recipient's body cells. *Graft* refers to transplanted, or donated tissue, and *host* refers to the tissues of the recipient. It is a common complication after allogeneic hematopoietic stem cell transplant

keratitis, inflammation of the cornea

otolaryngologist, medical doctor who diagnosis and treats diseases of the ear, nose, and throat

patching therapy, patching the good eye to improve vision in the eye that is not being used

peripheral visual fields, side vision

photocoagulation, laser treatment

punctal ligation, surgery to treat severe dry eyes which closes the tear draining ducts

pure tone audiometry, the use of earphones placed on the child, who is then asked to raise a hand if they hear a beep

tinnitus, ringing in the ears

total body irradiation (TBI), a type of radiation therapy that delivers radiation to the entire body commonly used for the treatment of certain blood cancers before a bone marrow transplant

vertigo, dizziness or sensation of "drifting in space"

12
Head and Neck

LISA BASHORE, PhD, APRN, CPNP-PC, CPON

I never knew so young a body with so old a head.
— *Shakespeare, The Merchant of Venice*

THE HEAD AND NECK can be affected both by tumors that occur in the head and neck and the treatment used to destroy the tumors. Even treatment for cancers elsewhere in the body can affect the vital structures and functioning of the head and neck.

This chapter covers damage to bones, teeth, glands, and other tissues in the head and neck, including signs and symptoms, methods to detect late effects in the head and neck, and the medical management of late effects. Some survivors who were treated for tumors in the head and neck do *not* develop any late effects.

ORGAN DAMAGE

The parts of the head and neck that most often suffer long-term damage from treatment for childhood cancer are the bones, soft tissues, *esophagus*, mucous membranes, teeth, salivary glands, and taste buds. (See **Figure 12.1**, Possible damage to bone and soft tissues of the head and neck (excluding the brain). For information about parts of the head and neck not covered in this chapter, see *Chapter 9, Brain and Nerves, Chapter 10, Hormone-Producing Glands,* and *Chapter 11, Eyes and Ears*.

Bone growth

Bone growth in the skull, face, and jaw can be slowed or stopped by radiation. Craniofacial abnormalities, including soft tissue and bone

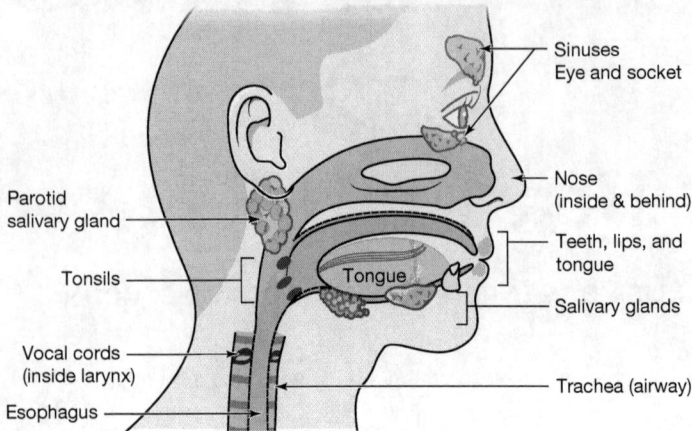

FIGURE 12-1. Possible damage to bone and soft tissues of the head and neck (excluding the brain) (©*Alex's Lemonade Stand Foundation, 2025*)

growth, are impacted. This growth disruption is less likely to be found in children given radiation for hematopoietic cell transplant with chronic graft versus host disease (GVHD) and those children who have received radiation to the head and neck region. Graft-versus-host disease is one of the long-term effects of cancer treatment elsewhere in the body that can affect the head and neck. In addition, children who have received radiation to the craniofacial region for rhabdomyosarcoma experience significant craniofacial abnormalities. However, each survivor is different, and long-term follow-up is important.

Young children who were given higher doses of radiation to the *bony orbit* (eye socket) of the eye to treat retinoblastoma or rhabdomyosarcoma close to the eye often have an altered appearance because the radiation causes the socket to grow less than the untreated socket. If the radiation is given to only one eye, the face appears more asymmetrical as the child grows.

Soft tissues

Children or adolescents treated with radiation for rhabdomyosarcoma, nasopharyngeal carcinoma, or sarcomas of the head and neck can have soft tissue (tendons, muscles, skin, fat, and connective tissue) damage as well as underlying bone damage in the irradiated areas.

Soft tissue damage can include scarring and blood vessel damage in the irradiated tissues. This damage can reduce blood supply to the affected area that slows healing and weakens bones.

Children or adolescents with Hodgkin lymphoma who received *mantle radiation* (radiation to lymph node areas in the neck, chest, under the arms. and sometimes the belly) are also at risk for underdevelopment of the structures in the areas irradiated, typically resulting in slender necks, narrow chins, and shortened distance between the shoulders. Mantle radiation was used to treat Hodgkin lymphoma from the 1970s to the 1990s, but its use was stopped because of its many serious side and late effects. Subsequent research showed that more selective use of radiation was as effective and led to changes in how it is used to treat Hodgkin lymphoma specifically. However, the risk for subsequent malignancies including breast cancer may occur even in lower doses of radiation.

Blood vessels

Carotid artery disease and an increased risk of stroke have been associated with radiation therapy to the neck in adults. Studies to determine whether survivors of childhood cancer who received radiation therapy to the neck are at risk for developing carotid artery disease are currently being conducted (see *Chapter 13, Heart and Blood Vessels*).

Sinuses

Most children and adolescents treated with chemotherapy and/or radiation suffer from serious damage to the mucous membranes in the nose and mouth. Many have severe *ulcerations* (mouth sores) that are painful and cause great difficulty with eating and drinking. For the majority of survivors, these sores heal, leaving no lingering difficulties. However, for a small group, mucous membrane changes persist. Scarring in the nasal passages can interfere with normal mucus production and drainage, resulting in chronic sinus infections. Survivors can develop a constant post-nasal drip or a thick, continuous drainage from the nose. Other late effects include pain in cheekbones or above eyebrows, headaches, and *halitosis* (bad breath).

These effects tend to be dose-related. The people most likely to suffer from painful sinus infections are those who received high-dose radiation to the mouth and sinuses. Children or adolescents who were given more than 4000 cGy to these areas are most likely to have these problems.

Teeth

The development and appearance of teeth can be affected by both radiation and chemotherapy. Radiation is more likely to cause problems when given in high doses to young children. Teeth that have not fully developed and have not yet erupted are also at risk. The damage to these tooth buds can be significant and result in the non-development of adult teeth.

Abnormalities of the teeth that can develop from radiation or chemotherapy include the following:

- Absent teeth
- Abnormally small teeth
- Short or thin roots
- Small crowns
- Poor bite (called *malocclusion*)
- Poor enamel
- *Incomplete calcification* (not enough minerals and calcium for healthy tooth enamel)
- Frequent cavities
- Enlarged *pulp chambers* (space in center of tooth containing nerves and blood supply)
- Baby teeth that don't fall out at the usual time during a child's development

Mouth

Saliva is a mix of secretions from the parotid gland (near the ear), sublingual gland (under the tongue), and submandibular gland (under the lower jaw) that lubricates the mouth and aids in taste and digestion. Decreased production of saliva (called *xerostomia*) affects overall well-being in many ways, including dry mouth. Dry mouth can result in food not tasting good, teeth riddled with cavities, bad breath, and bone decay.

The dose of radiation to the saliva-producing glands and the percentage of the glands that are radiated affect the amount of saliva produced. Children treated for head or neck soft tissue sarcomas are most at risk. Most glands regain the ability to secrete if the total dose of radiation to the area was less than 4000 cGy. Graft-versus-host disease of the salivary glands can also affect saliva production.

Survivors with persistent problems with dry mouth can find information and support from the Sjögren's Foundation at (800) 4-SJOGREN or www.sjogrens.org.

Taste

Changes in taste continue to bother some survivors long after treatment ends. Radiation can cause long-term taste problems because it can destroy the taste buds, as well as cause dry mouth by damaging the salivary glands. Lack of saliva affects the taste buds' ability to identify particular tastes.

Esophagus

The esophagus is the tube that carries food and liquids from the mouth to the stomach. In Hodgkin lymphoma survivors treated with mantle radiation and others treated with direct radiation to the chest, neck, and spine, stomach acid can flow up into the esophagus, causing a burning sensation and tissue irritation. Over time, the esophagus can swell, causing an inflammation called *esophagitis*. This condition can be painful and can reduce the desire to eat. *Barrett's esophagus* (which is changes in the cells of the esophagus) can occur in association with reflux in those whose gastrointestinal tracts were irradiated.

Severe esophagitis can lead to bleeding from the inflamed portion of the esophagus or the formation of scar tissue. This narrowing of the esophagus—called *esophageal stricture*—is often accompanied by choking and delayed stomach emptying causing discomfort.

In addition, some survivors have trouble swallowing because of damage from a tumor, prolonged vomiting from chemotherapy that damaged the esophagus, or complications from surgery or a tumor in the part of the brain that controls swallowing.

Vocal cords

Radiation to the neck can cause damage to the vocal cords and changes in the voice. The voice can become high and thin and hoarse as a result of doses of 3000 cGy or more of radiation to the neck. However, each survivor is different, and long-term follow-up is important.

Esophageal strictures

Esophageal stricture is a narrowing of the esophagus that can happen due to the effects of radiation to the head and cervical and thoracic regions. In addition, survivors of hematopoietic cell transplant who develop GVHD may develop gastroesophageal strictures.

Gastroesophageal reflux (GER)

Gastroesophageal reflux (GER) occurs when the end of the esophagus (food tube) does not close completely and allows acid and food in the stomach to back up into the esophagus. This can cause pain and discomfort (heartburn) and damage the lower esophagus. The damage can cause narrowing of the esophagus and over time, cancer. Other symptoms of GER include: non-cardiac pain, nausea, sore throat or feeling of a lump in your throat or difficulty swallowing, and asthma symptoms (coughing, wheezing, difficulty breathing). Occasional acid reflux can be manageable at home, but continuous (chronic) acid reflux can damage your esophagus tissue over time and might need treatment.

SCREENING AND DETECTION

Screening for problems in the head and neck starts with a careful physical examination of the sinuses, nostrils, and throat. The examination also includes close attention to how your teeth look, how your breath smells, and the condition of the skin and soft tissues in the head and neck. Your healthcare provider should ask questions about your eating habits and digestion, your dental health, and any pain or discomfort in the head and neck region.

Sinus infections. If the physical examination and discussion uncover possible sinus infections, a sinus x-ray should be ordered and a referral made to an ear, nose, and throat specialist, if necessary. Survivors with headaches or migraines should be referred to a neurologist for a thorough evaluation.

Difficulty swallowing and gastrointestinal discomfort. If you have a history of indigestion, difficulty swallowing, or stomachaches, your healthcare provider at the survivorship clinic may order tests to see how the stomach empties. These could include an upper gastrointestinal series, which is an x-ray examination of the upper gastrointestinal tract that includes the esophagus, stomach, and duodenum, or a *barium swallow*, which focuses on the esophagus. Esophageal strictures or esophagitis should be evaluated and treated by a gastroenterologist.

Oral health. You should get a complete dental examination and cleaning every 6 months if you are a survivor of childhood cancer. Your dentist should refer you to an *orthodontist* (a dentist with expertise in treating irregularities of the teeth or jaws) if you have problems with teeth crowding or improper bite.

MEDICAL MANAGEMENT

Medical management of late effects in the head and neck depends on your symptoms.

Oral health. Careful dental and orthodontal care is necessary if you have crooked teeth, crowded teeth, or an improper bite. Before beginning any orthodontal treatment, the orthodontist will need to carefully examine a full x-ray of the entire mouth to evaluate root length and general health of teeth.

Preventive antibiotics. If your spleen was removed during treatment, discuss with your doctor and dentist the need to take antibiotics prior to invasive medical procedures (for example, a colonoscopy). If you have an endoprosthesis (device used to replace cancerous bone), you may also need to take antibiotics prior to dental work to prevent an infection. Be sure to mention the endoprosthesis and ask about antibiotics when you schedule any dental work or invasive medical procedures.

Sinuses. Sinus medication is usually the first treatment for chronic sinus problems. In some cases, the ear, nose, and throat specialist may recommend watchful waiting to see if you stop having infections as you grow. In other cases, surgery may be necessary to clear out your sinuses and allow for proper drainage of mucus through your nasal passages.

Dry mouth. Frequent fluid intake, especially of water, and artificial saliva may be recommended if you have decreased salivary flow.

Gastroesophageal reflux (GER). Problems with reflux require an examination by a gastroenterologist who has experience treating survivors of childhood cancer. Your gastroenterologist or primary care provider may recommend antacids (to neutralize stomach acid), motility medications (to help move food through the digestive system), acid suppressers (to reduce heartburn), or acid blockers (to prevent production of stomach acid).

If you have gastroesophageal reflux (GER) (also known as esophageal reflux), you may be given instructions to do the following:

- Eat several small meals instead of three big ones.
- Avoid eating for three hours before going to bed.
- Raise the head of your bed four to six inches (not with pillows — the head of the bed needs to be raised).
- Avoid exercising, bending over, or lying down right after eating.
- Lose any excess weight
- Avoid foods that cause more reflux. Some of the most likely to cause problems are acidic foods, such as tomatoes or citrus fruits, and spicy or fatty foods.
- Avoid coffee, tea, chocolate, and alcohol, as they can also worsen reflux.
- Avoid smoking because smoke prevents the muscle at the bottom of the esophagus from closing properly. Tobacco also decreases saliva.

- Esophageal dilation (i.e., widening of the esophagus). This procedure may be necessary if you suffer from esophageal strictures.

REFERENCES

Asdahl PH, Oeffinger KC, Albieri V, et al. (2021). Esophageal disease among childhood cancer survivors - a report from the Childhood Cancer Survivors Study. *Pediatr Blood Cancer* 68(8):e29043. doi: 10.1002/pbc.29043. Epub 2021 Apr 12. PMID: 33844445; PMCID: PMC9124525.

Children's Oncology Group. (2023). *Long-Term Follow-Up Guidelines for Survivors of Childhood, Adolescent, and Young Adult Cancers*, v. 6. (www.survivorshipguidelines. org)

https://www.cancer.org/cancer/types/hodgkin-lymphoma/after-treatment.html

Mattos VD, Ferman S, Araújo Magalhães DM, et al. (2019). Dental and craniofacial alterations in long-term survivors of childhood head and neck rhabdomyosarcoma. *Oral Surg Oral Med Oral Pathol Oral Radiol.* 127(4),272-281. doi: 10.1016/j.oooo.2018.12.012. Epub 2018 Dec 21. PMID: 30685390.

Milgrom, SA, van Luijk, P, Pino, R, et al. (2021). Salivary and dental complications in childhood cancer survivors treated with radiation therapy to the head and neck: A pediatric normal tissue effects in the clinic (PENTEC) comprehensive review. *Int J Radiat Oncol Biol Phys.* S0360-3016(21)00443-0. doi: 10.1016/j.ijrobp.2021.04.023. Epub ahead of print.

RESOURCES

Website: ccgresources.org
All resources and references mentioned in this book are available on the website and will be routinely reviewed and updated.

Children's Oncology Group. *Long-Term Follow-Up Guidelines for Survivors of Childhood, Adolescent, and Young Adult Cancers, Version 6.0 (October 2023)*
Website: http://www.survivorshipguidelines.org
Click under **Health Links** for: *dental health, osteoradionecrosis*

FACES—The National Craniofacial Association
Website: https://www.faces-cranio.org

Let's Face It
Website: https://media.dent.umich.edu/faceit

Locks of Love
Website: https://locksoflove.org/
A nonprofit organization that provides hairpieces to financially disadvantaged children under the age of 21 suffering from long-

term medical hair loss. (It does not provide hairpieces for temporary hair loss due to chemotherapy and radiation.)

234 Southern Blvd, West Palm Beach, FL 33405-2701

Phone: (888) 896-1588 or (561) 833-7962

Passport for Care, Survivor Care Plans by Children's Oncology Group (V6, Nov 2023)

Website: https://cancersurvivor.passportforcare.org

Survivors and family can find online updated tailored long-term care plans which should be reviewed with their oncologist or health care provider.

Sjögren's Syndrome Foundation,

Website: https://sjogrens.org

GLOSSARY

barium swallow, an imaging test to check on the health of the esophagus using barium to coat the walls of the esophagus so that it can be examined by x-ray

Barrett's esophagus, a disorder in which stomach acid damages the lining of the esophagus

bony orbit, eye socket

carotid artery disease, narrowing or blockage of the blood vessels in the neck that supply blood to your brain and head and which increases the risk of stroke

cranial, relating to the skull

esophageal stricture, a narrowing of the esophagus (food tube) that carries food and liquid from your mouth to your stomach

esophagitis, a condition in which the lining of the esophagus or "food tube" becomes swollen and irritated by stomach acid that flows back into it

esophagus, the "food tube" that carries food and liquid from your mouth to your stomach

gastroesophageal reflux (GER), when the end of the esophagus (*food tube*) does not close completely and allows acid and food in the stomach to back up into the esophagus causing pain and discomfort

halitosis, bad breath

incomplete calcification, not enough minerals and calcium for healthy tooth enamel

malocclusion, when the teeth are not aligned properly resulting in poor bite

mandible, jawbone

mantle radiation, a radiation treatment in which the neck, chest, and armpit area are exposed to radiation, this method is rarely used today

orthodontist, a dentist who specializes in correcting irregularities in the teeth or jaw

pulp chamber, space in the center of a tooth that contains nerves and blood supply

ulceration, an open sore that develops on the skin, mucous membranes, or the lining of the stomach

upper gastrointestinal series, an x-ray examination of the upper intestinal tract that includes the esophagus, stomach, and the first part of the small intestine

xerostomia, a condition in which there is not enough saliva to keep the mouth wet; also known as "dry mouth"

13

Heart and Blood Vessels

JOANNE QUILLEN, MSN, APRN, PNP-BC

The human heart has hidden treasures, in secret kept, in silence sealed.
— Charlotte Brontë, Evening Solace

CERTAIN TYPES OF RADIATION and chemotherapy can affect the cardiovascular system (i.e., heart, blood vessels, heart valves, and pericardium). Problems can occur during treatment, or months to years after treatment ends. Because children, teens, and adult survivors can appear well and be active despite heart damage, it is important to know if you are at risk and to obtain careful follow-up screening and testing to identify and treat problems early. It is also reassuring to find out if your particular treatments did not increase your risk of any of these problems.

THE HEART

The heart is a four-chambered, muscular organ that pumps blood throughout the body. It is approximately the size of a clenched fist and is located beneath the breastbone (sternum) in the center of the chest cavity. It is a hollow organ with thick walls of cardiac muscle. A double-walled sac, the *pericardium,* surrounds the heart and helps anchor it in place with connections to the diaphragm and sternum.

The heart has two sides, separated by a thick, muscular wall called the *septum.* The two upper chambers of the heart are called the *right atrium* and *left atrium.* The lower chambers are the left and right ventricles. The atria (plural for *atrium*) receive blood coming in from

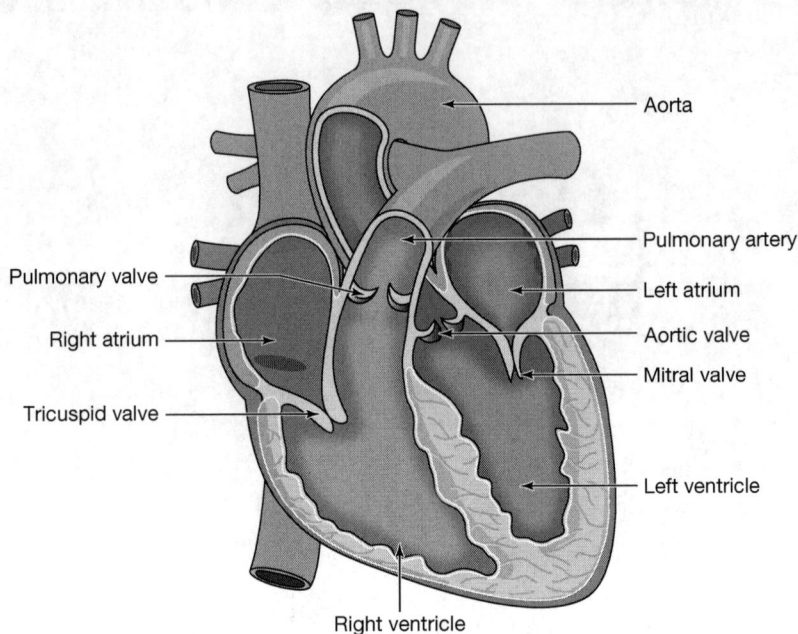

FIGURE 13-1. Anatomy of the heart and valves. (©*Alex's Lemonade Stand Foundation, 2025*)

the lungs and the body. They squeeze blood into the ventricles, which then pump it out to the lungs and body.

Valves in the heart prevent blood from flowing backward. The valve between the left atrium and the left ventricle is called the *mitral valve*, and the valve between the right atrium and right ventricle is called the *tricuspid valve*. Two other valves are located between the ventricles and the major blood vessels; one leads to the lungs (called the *pulmonary valve*) and the other to the rest of the body (called the *aortic valve*). **Figure 13-1** shows the anatomy of the heart and valves.

Heart muscle damage from treatment

The muscles in the heart are made up of cells called myocytes. By 6 months of age, an infant heart contains the adult number of myocytes. Further growth of the heart occurs from growth of these existing cells. Chemotherapy drugs called anthracyclines—daunorubicin (Cerubidine®), doxorubicin (Adriamycin®), epirubicin, and idarubicin—sometimes damage or destroy myocytes. The remaining cells enlarge and stretch to try to compensate for the damage. This can cause thin and stiff ventricular walls, which reduce the heart's ability to contract effectively.

If the muscle of the heart is weakened, the heart may not pump as well as usual. This is called *cardiomyopathy*. Some survivors with early-stage cardiomyopathy don't have any symptoms, while others have problems if the heart can no longer keep up with the demands brought on by growth, pregnancy, isometric exercise (e.g., weight lifting, pull-ups, push-ups), or activities of daily life.

Chemotherapy

The number of cells destroyed or damaged is related to several factors: dose of anthracyclines, whether the heart was also irradiated, and other risk factors, such as being female and age (children younger than age 2 are at highest risk). In addition, there are other risk factors that are not yet known or understood especially now that we are learning more about genetic risks for heart dysfunction.

Anthracyclines can also interfere with the rhythm of the heart and how signals are carried through the heart to make it beat regularly. Children treated with anthracyclines may be at risk for rhythm and conduction problems of the heart that can result in irregular heartbeats, called *arrhythmias*.

Some patient treatment plans incorporate drugs such as dexrazoxane (Zinecard®) to see if they will minimize damage from anthracyclines. This drug is typically given with every anthracycline dose in cancer treatment trials. During the last three decades, researchers have learned more about the long-term cardiac effects of anthracyclines, and lower cumulative doses are now being used whenever possible.

All survivors who were given anthracyclines should be periodically checked for cardiac damage for the rest of their lives. You and your healthcare provider should refer to the guidelines and recommended screening schedules online at: Children's Oncology Group, *Long-Term Follow-Up Guidelines for Survivors of Child, Adolescent, and Young Adult Cancers*, V6 (Oct 2023). See Resources for website and link for the current recommendations for appropriate life-long screening based on treatment exposure. Also, many survivors with changes in the pumping ability of the heart have no symptoms and the changes may not at all interfere with life activities. Consequently, it is important for survivors to know about possible cardiac effects, be checked for them on a regular basis, and discuss any abnormal test results with their healthcare providers.

Anthracyclines are not the only drugs that can damage the heart. Very high doses of cyclophosphamide (Cytoxan®) given in preparation for a stem cell transplant may also cause heart damage. The walls of the left ventricle may thicken, leading to heart problems years or decades later. This rare complication may worsen if the child or teen also had radiation to the chest and/ or received anthracyclines.

The risk of developing heart problems may be greatest for survivors who had changes in their cardiac function noted on an electrocardiogram (EKG) or echocardiogram during or shortly after the end of therapy. Very long-term research studies are needed to determine who is most at risk.

Radiation

Radiation can cause several late effects to the heart. Children or teens at possible risk for late effects are those who received spinal radiation (for central nervous system–brain/spine tumors), chest radiation (for Hodgkin lymphoma or non-Hodgkin lymphoma), left flank radiation (for Wilms), or radiation directly to the heart. Modern radiation techniques using lower total doses, *hyperfractionation* (smaller doses more often), and cardiac shielding (protecting the heart from radiation) are much less likely to cause damage. It is hoped that the use of proton therapy (radiation therapy that uses protons instead of x-rays) will reduce damage to healthy organs.

Whether the heart sustains injury after radiation treatment depends on several factors, including the following:

- *Total radiation dose* (amount of radiation delivered at each visit x the number of visits)

- Dose of *radiation fractions* (amount of radiation delivered at any individual visit)
- Extent and areas of the heart treated
- Presence of tumor in or next to the heart
- Chemotherapy drugs used

Age, weight, blood pressure, family history, smoking, and cholesterol levels do not change the likelihood of developing heart damage, but can magnify its effect later in life in those who have damage.

Damage to the heart muscle from high-dose radiation can lead to restrictive cardiomyopathy and arrythmias. *Restrictive cardiomyopathy* is when the heart muscle becomes stiff and the heart cannot adequately fill with blood. This may lead to problems in the pumping action of the heart. Valves in the heart can also be damaged by radiation (see later section in this chapter about valve damage).

Signs and symptoms of heart damage

The signs and symptoms for radiation-induced heart damage vary widely. Most damage is caused by higher doses of chemotherapy/radiation and older radiation techniques. Children and adolescents treated for Hodgkin lymphoma with mantle radiation using modern doses and heart shielding may still develop heart problems, and need to be followed over time to see if any long-term late effects develop. Some of the coronary arteries cannot be protected by shielding because of their location.

Restrictive cardiomyopathy. Restrictive cardiomyopathy can develop months, years, or decades after treatment for childhood cancer ends.

Early signs and symptoms of restrictive cardiomyopathy include:
- Increasing fatigue
- Decreased ability to exercise
- Shortness of breath, especially with exercise
- Feeling full after only a few bites of food
- Increased difficulties with regular activities of daily life

If you have any of the risk factors for heart damage, these signs and symptoms should prompt you to get a thorough evaluation of your heart. Fatigue alone can be caused by a multitude of things, but if it is getting worse or is accompanied by other symptoms, get it checked out.

Later signs and symptoms of restrictive cardiomyopathy include:

- Swollen lower legs and feet (called edema)
- Rapid or irregular heartbeat
- Rapid breathing
- Difficulty exercising
- Dizziness
- Chest pain

Arrhythmia. The electrical pathways that control the heart's rhythm can be damaged by treatment, which can result in arrhythmia (i.e., abnormally fast, slow, or irregular heartbeat). You may be asymptomatic or may have some of the following symptoms:

- Palpitations (a feeling that the heart is beating strongly)
- Rapid heartbeats
- Skipped beats
- Dizziness or lightheadedness
- Fainting

Some healthcare providers (doctors and nurse practitioners) are not aware of the risks for heart problems from your treatment for childhood cancer. If you find this to be the case, get a second opinion from a healthcare provider who is well versed in cardiac late effects associated with cancer treatment.

Screening and detection for cardiac damage

Survivors at risk for late cardiac damage are those who received anthracyclines and/or radiation to the heart (which can occur during radiation to the chest, whole lung, left kidney, and possibly the spine). Even if there are no symptoms, any survivor who received these therapies should have an annual examination to identify risk for cardiac deterioration, to help decide the best medical management, and to guide lifestyle choices. You need to share your cancer treatment summary with your healthcare provider as they need to be aware of radiation/chemotherapy/medications you were exposed to and the possible risks to the heart.

The minimum testing should include:

- Thorough medical history
- Fasting blood levels of cholesterol (lipid panel)
- Physical examination
- Chest x-ray
- Echocardiogram
- 12-lead EKG
- Baseline cardiac stress test to get a clear picture of oxygenation of heart muscle

The type of routine cardiac screening for survivors of childhood cancer depends on the treatment received. For *cardiomyopathy*, an echocardiogram is done (how often is based on a variety of factors). Cardiac magnetic resonance imaging (MRI) provides additional information for survivors diagnosed with cardiomyopathy. Routine screening for survivors who received treatment that could affect the heart must be performed for the rest of their lives.

Any changes in the ECHO/EKG or other cardiac tests require a consultation with a cardiologist experienced in treating survivors of childhood cancer.

Intervals between screenings may be longer for those at lesser risk. Ongoing research is helping to define the types of evaluations necessary and determine how often they need to be done. You and your healthcare provider should refer to the guidelines and recommended screening schedules online at: Children's Oncology Group, *Long-Term Follow-Up Guidelines for Survivors of Child, Adolescent, and Young Adult Cancers*, V6 (Oct 2023). See Resources for website and link.

When special circumstances/changes arise when the heart undergoes increased stress, survivors at risk for cardiac problems should get baseline evaluation and systematic follow-up testing.

Examples of activities that stress the heart include:

- Starting an exercise program
- Being pregnant
- Getting general anesthesia
- Taking growth hormone
- Doing isometric weight lifting (e.g., bench presses or squats)

Some survivors report that they have to insist on referrals to a cardiologist because they are often young and healthy looking and may see healthcare providers who are not familiar with cardiac late effects from cancer treatment.

Many survivors with heart damage have no symptoms, so it is especially important to get thorough follow-up from a healthcare provider with experience treating survivors of childhood cancer.

Medical management for heart damage

Routine screening for damage to the heart is usually done by pediatric oncologists or internists. If abnormalities are identified (e.g., pericardial thickening, ventricular wall stiffness), a referral to a cardiologist with experience treating survivors of childhood cancer should be made.

Treatment of cardiomyopathy from anthracyclines or radiation may include ACE inhibitors (such as enalapril) and beta blockers (such as propranolol). Cardiac glycosides (such as digoxin) and diuretics, such as furosemide (Lasix®), are also used for survivors with congestive heart failure. In some rare cases of severely progressive disease, heart transplantation is considered.

Lifestyle counseling is necessary for survivors with heart damage. The discussion should emphasize eating a healthy diet, maintaining a normal weight, developing an exercise program, reducing stress, and not smoking cigarettes, vaping, or using street drugs. Many healthcare providers caution survivors at significant risk for heart problems to limit *isometric exercise* as it can stress the heart, but they encourage *aerobic exercise*. Examples of isometric exercises are weight lifting, wrestling, and rock climbing.

Cardiac rehabilitation may also improve heart function and quality of life for survivors with heart damage.

Medications and illegal drugs

Some prescription drugs can be toxic to the heart. If you have cardiac problems, get a list from your cardiologist of medications to avoid. Some over-the-counter medications include ingredients that can stress the heart; it's important to read labels and avoid taking medicines that contain pseudoephedrine. Pregnant survivors at risk for heart damage from anthracyclines should see an obstetrician who specializes in high-risk pregnancy, as well as a cardiologist.

Many illegal drugs (such as cocaine and various forms of amphetamines, including ecstasy and crystal methamphetamine) stress the heart and should not be taken. A rapid rise in blood alcohol levels can cause an irregular heartbeat, so excessive or binge drinking should be avoided.

Preventing heart problems

You cannot prevent the damage already done to the heart from chemotherapy or radiation. However, you *can* control some things that can lessen your risk of heart damage worsening as you age.

To keep your heart as healthy as possible, you can:
- Not smoke or vape (or quit if you smoke now)
- Not use drugs that stress the heart, such as cocaine, ephedra, pseudoephedrine, diet pills, or sport performance-enhancing drugs
- Eat only healthy fats (e.g. lean protein – chicken, fish – especially salmon and tuna, turkey, tofu and low-fat or fermented dairy products such as yogurt and kefir) and make sure fats are only 30 percent of your calories
- Maintain a healthy body weight
- Exercise at least 30 minutes every day (but if you have heart problems now, check with your cardiologist before starting an exercise program and minimize *isometric exercises*)

- See *Chapter 5, Staying Healthy* for more information
- See a cardiologist if you are female, plan to get pregnant, and had anthracyclines and/or radiation to your heart

BLOOD VESSELS

The human body has three types of blood vessels: arteries, veins, and capillaries. Arteries are large vessels that carry blood away from the heart. They branch into smaller arteries and then into arterioles. Arterioles eventually split into capillaries, which are vessels so small that blood cells have to flow through single file. The thin walls of the capillaries allow exchange of gases (i.e., oxygen and carbon dioxide), nutrients, and waste products. Capillaries merge into venules, which in turn merge into veins. Veins return blood to the heart. Arteries that carry oxygen to the heart muscle itself are called *coronary arteries*.

Blood vessel damage from treatment

Coronary artery disease and atherosclerosis. The interiors of healthy blood vessels are usually smooth, but radiation can roughen them inside. These rough spots provide sites for fatty deposits (plaques) to develop in coronary arteries and other arteries and veins. Calcium deposits can harden the plaques, resulting in *atherosclerosis* (hardening of the arteries). When this happens in the coronary arteries in the heart, it is called *coronary artery disease*.

Survivors of Hodgkin lymphoma have been studied extensively due to the risk of vascular injury in the field of radiation (e.g., carotid arteries in the neck). An inflammatory process that damages the endothelial lining of the blood vessels is suspected. In these studies, survivors of Hodgkin lymphoma who did not have neck irradiation also had increased premature carotid artery disease, and the reason is not yet understood.

Atherosclerosis can cause three problems:

1) The fatty deposits narrow the blood vessels, reducing flow of blood.

2) Layers of plaque decrease the strength and elasticity of the arteries.

3) Plaques roughen the lining of the vessel, allowing platelets to form clots at the rough spots.

If a clot breaks free, it can block blood flow in narrow arteries, reducing or stopping the supply of oxygen to that area. When oxygen is slowed to areas of the heart, *angina* (chest pain) results. If the clot blocks a coronary artery completely, it causes a heart attack.

Healthy lifestyle can make a difference

The tendency to develop atherosclerosis is related not only to treatment for childhood cancer, but also to family history, weight, and lifestyle choices such as diet, exercise, and smoking.

- Smoking vastly increases the risk of heart disease. The nicotine in cigarettes increases the heart rate and accelerates plaque formation that narrows arteries. It also damages the lungs, reducing their efficiency. Consequently, the heart must pump faster to deliver adequate oxygen to the cells of the body. Vaping is more intense than smoking.

- A diet high in saturated fat can lead to high levels of cholesterol. This can increase the chance of developing fatty deposits in the arteries, making a heart attack or stroke more likely. Health experts now suggest eating as little dietary cholesterol as you can, under 300 milligrams (mg) a day (see below for foods recommended for a heart healthy diet).

- Exercise helps maintain a healthy weight, increases lung capacity, and strengthens body muscles, including the heart. A note of caution is that if you received anthracyclines or radiation to the heart, you should consult your follow-up healthcare provider prior to starting an exercise program.

- High blood pressure based on your age (any blood pressure greater than 140/90) is a risk factor for heart disease and promotes atherosclerosis. High blood pressure is the initial sign of heart changes. Your physician may prescribe medications to lower your blood pressure.

A healthcare provider who specializes in treating survivors of childhood cancer cautions:

A significant problem that we are just beginning to understand is the effect of cranial radiation and chemotherapy in promoting premature coronary artery disease. Leukemia (ALL) survivors, especially those treated with cranial radiation, have an increased inci-

dence of obesity and are more likely to be physically inactive. Obesity and physical inactivity at a young age are significant risk factors for the development of high blood pressure, diabetes, and dyslipidemia (high LDL cholesterol, low HDL cholesterol, high triglycerides) and these aid in the development of premature coronary artery disease. Because of this, it is essential that survivors exercise, eat a prudent diet, and get regular follow-up.

Activities *you can do* to help slow the atherosclerotic process and keep blood pressure low include:

- Eat a diet low in saturated fats, cholesterol, salt, and processed foods with reduced amount of meat, poultry, dairy products (except for low-fat yogurt and kefir), limit whole eggs (use egg-whites or egg substitutes).
- Eat more whole grain breads, oats, bran, fruits, and vegetables.
- Eat foods high in fiber, such as potatoes, turnips, sweet potatoes, peas, beans (especially black beans), lentils, and nuts (almonds, walnuts, pistachios).
- Exercise regularly (30 minutes every day).
- Keep body fat low and monitor your *body mass index (BMI)* with your health care provider. BMI is a screening tool based on height and weight that helps health care providers evaluate weight categories that may lead to health problems.
- Limit alcohol intake (including beer).

Medical problems such as hypothyroidism, high blood pressure, high cholesterol, and diabetes can increase your risk of developing atherosclerosis.

Raynaud's phenomenon can also develop in long-term survivors with vascular disease. This is when the fingers and toes become white or bluish due to spasms of the arteries leading to the hands. It is usually precipitated by cold or emotion, and affected individuals often have a genetic predisposition for developing Raynaud's. This may also occur in survivors treated with vincristine/bleomycin. The condition is usually chronic, but it may improve slowly over several years in some survivors.

Signs and symptoms of coronary artery disease/heart attack

Coronary artery disease. Risk of coronary artery disease and heart attack is lower for patients who had lower doses of radiation using modern techniques, and higher for patients treated with high doses of radiation and no heart shielding.

Signs and symptoms of coronary artery disease are as follows:
- Chest pain (or pressure-like sensation)
- Chest, neck, or jaw pain upon exertion
- Indigestion upon exertion
- Shortness of breath upon exertion

Heart attack and decreased oxygen. Symptoms of inadequate oxygen to the heart and heart attack are as follows:
- Crushing chest pain
- Pain or numbness down the left arm
- Shortness of breath
- Sweating
- Nausea
- Feelings of impending doom

Many of these signs and symptoms can be caused by other illnesses or conditions; however, it is prudent to get an evaluation if any of these symptoms are present. **Do not ignore any of these symptoms; seek medical attention right away**.

Screening and detection for coronary artery disease

Screening and detection for coronary artery disease includes some of the tests described above for the heart. A stress test is also needed. Routine cholesterol screening for those at risk for coronary artery disease is also essential.

Medical and surgical management

Medical management should involve frequent surveillance for symptoms in at-risk survivors. You and your healthcare provider should refer to the guidelines and recommended screening schedules online at: Children's Oncology Group, *Long-Term Follow-Up Guidelines for Survivors of Child, Adolescent, and Young Adult Cancers*, V6 (Oct 2023). See Resources for website and link.

A variety of medications and lifestyle modifications are used to treat coronary artery disease. Advanced coronary artery disease is sometimes treated with a coronary artery bypass graft (open heart surgery) or balloon dilation angioplasty.

HEART VALVES

The valves that control the flow of blood in the heart can become stiff or leaky after high-dose radiation to the chest (e.g., mantle radiation to treat Hodgkin lymphoma).

Signs and symptoms of valvular disease

Valvular disease may be asymptomatic or it may cause symptoms such as the following:

- Shortness of breath
- Fatigue
- Palpitations
- Rapid heartbeat
- Swelling of ankles
- Prominence of veins in the neck
- Cough
- Difficulty with exertion

Screening and detection for valve problems

Regular and lifelong screening using an echocardiogram is done to check for possible valve problems caused by radiation to the heart. You and your healthcare provider should check the current guidelines and recommended screening schedules online at: Children's Oncology Group, *Long-Term Follow-Up Guidelines for Survivors of Child, Adolescent, and Young Adult Cancers*, V6 (Oct 2023). See Resources for website and link.

Medical and surgical management of heart valve damage

Medical management should involve frequent surveillance for symptoms in at-risk survivors. A variety of medications and lifestyle modifications may be used to treat heart valve damage. Severe damage to valves in the heart may require surgery to replace the valves. This care should be directed by a cardiologist.

If you have valve damage or have had a valve replaced, you should take an antibiotic before dental work or any other invasive procedure (such as a colonoscopy). The antibiotic can help prevent *endocarditis*, a serious heart infection caused by bacteria entering the bloodstream during the procedure. The healthcare provider who will do the procedure (dentist or doctor) should write the prescription for you.

PERICARDIUM

Pericarditis is an inflammation of the sac surrounding the heart. Acute pericarditis usually occurs during treatment or within the first year after treatment. Delayed acute pericarditis, a rare occurrence, usually resolves within a few months but may persist for years.

Constrictive pericarditis occurs when the sac surrounding the heart becomes tough and inelastic. This can result in an accumulation of fluid that can interfere with the heart's ability to pump efficiently. Constrictive pericarditis can occur years after treatment.

Signs and symptoms of pericarditis

The signs and symptoms of **delayed acute pericarditis** include the following:

- Fever
- Shortness of breath
- ST wave changes (elevation) on the EKG

The signs and symptoms of **constrictive pericarditis** include the following:

- Chest pain
- Wheezing
- Shortness of breath
- Decreased ability to exercise

Screening and detection for pericarditis

Screening for pericarditis is the same as for other cardiac problems. However, if you develop any of the symptoms listed above, you should see your healthcare provider immediately to get an examination. Pericarditis can develop quickly and can be life-threatening.

Medical and surgical management of pericarditis

Radiation-induced pericarditis is treated with medications and sometimes with surgery.

Recommended schedule of life-long follow-up tests

Although recommendations evolve as more research is done, the current recommendations for heart evaluations after taking anthracyclines and/or having radiation to the heart can be found online by accessing Section 77 (p. 87) of: *Children's Oncology Group, Long-Term Follow-Up Guidelines for Survivors of Child, Adolescent, and Young Adult Cancers*, V6 (Oct 2023). See Resources for website and link.

REFERENCES

Armenian SH, Armstrong GT, Aune G, et al. (2018) Cardiovascular disease in survivors of childhood cancer: insights into epidemiology, pathophysiology, and prevention. *J Clin Oncol*. 2018 Jul 20;36(21):2135-2144. doi: 10.1200/JCO.2017.76.3920.

Cheng SW, Wu LL, Ting AC, et al. (1999) Irradiation-induced extracranial carotid stenosis in patients with head and neck malignancies. *Am J Surg*. 1999 Oct;178(4):323-8. doi: 10.1016/s0002-9610(99)00184-1.

Childrens Oncology Group. Long-Term Follow-Up Guidelines for Survivors of Childhood, Adolescent, and Young Adult Cancers, Version 6.0 (October 2023) http://www.survivorshipguidelines.org/

Chow EJ, Leger KJ, Bhatt NS, et al. (2019, April 15). Paediatric cardio-oncology: Epidemiology, screening, prevention, and treatment. *Cardiovascular Research, 115(5),* 922-934. https://doi.org/10.1093/cvr/cvz031

Lipshultz SE, Diamond MB, Franco VI, et al. (2014, August 19). Managing chemotherapy-related cardiotoxicity in survivors of childhood cancers. *Pediatric Drugs, 16(5),* 373-389. https://doi.org/10.1007/s40272-014-0085-1

Meeske KA, Nelson MD, Lavey RS, et al. (2007) Premature carotid artery disease in long-term survivors of childhood cancer treated with neck irradiation: a series of 5 cases. *J Pediatr Hematol Oncol*. 2007 Jul;29(7):480-4. doi: 10.1097/MPH.0b013e3180601029.

RESOURCES

Website: ccgresources.org
All resources and references mentioned in this book are available on the website and will be routinely reviewed and updated.

Children's Oncology Group. (V6, 2023). *Long-Term Follow-Up Guidelines for Survivors of Childhood, Adolescent, and Young Adult Cancers*
Website: www.survivorshipguidelines.org
on home page, see **Health Links,** and click, *cardiac system, heart health, cardiovascular risk factors*

Passport for Care, Survivor Care Plans by Children's Oncology Group (V6, Nov 2023)
Website: https://cancersurvivor.passportforcare.org
Survivors and family can find online updated tailored long-term care plans which should be reviewed with their oncologist or health care provider.

GLOSSARY

aerobic exercise, physical activity that uses your body's large muscle groups, is rhythmic and repetitive. It increases your heart rate and how much oxygen your body uses. Examples of aerobic exercises include walking, cycling, and swimming. It reduces your risk of heart disease, diabetes, high blood pressure, and high cholesterol.

angina, chest pain

aortic valve, valve that controls flow from the ventricles into your aorta, the major blood vessel that takes oxygen-rich blood to the rest of the body

arrhythmia, irregular heartbeat

atherosclerosis, hardening of the arteries

body mass index (BMI), a screening tool based on normal height/weight charts that helps health care providers evaluate whether a patient's weight may lead to health problems

cardiac shielding, protecting the heart with a protective covering while radiation is administered

cardiomyopathy, chronic disease of the heart muscle which makes it harder for the heart to pump blood; depending on the type, heart muscle could become thicker, stiffer or larger than normal

constrictive pericarditis, when the sac surrounding the heart becomes tough and inelastic and can interfere with the heart's ability to pump efficiently

coronary arteries, arteries that carry oxygen to the heart muscle

coronary artery disease, when plaque builds up in the coronary arteries and hardens, blocking the blood flow and forming clots

edema, swelling caused by fluid trapped in your body's tissues.

endocarditis, a serious heart infection caused by bacteria entering the bloodstream

hyperfractionation, newer treatment protocols giving smaller doses of radiation more often

isometric exercise, exercises in which your muscles are engaged, but they are not changing length; examples are weight lifting, wrestling, and rock climbing

mitral valve, the valve between the left atrium and left ventricle that prevents the blood from flowing backward

pericarditis, inflammation of the sac surrounding the heart

pulmonary valve, valve that controls flow of oxygen-poor blood to the lungs where blood gets rid of carbon dioxide and gains new oxygen-rich blood

radiation fractions, amount of radiation delivered at any individual visit

Raynaud's phenomenon, fingers and toes become white or bluish due to spasms of the arteries leading to the hands, usually triggered by cold or emotion

restrictive cardiomyopathy, when the heart muscle becomes stiff and the heart cannot adequately fill with blood

total radiation dose, amount of radiation delivered at each visit times the number of visits

tricuspid valve, the valve between the right atrium and right ventricle that prevents the blood from flowing backward

14

Lungs

LISA BASHORE, PhD, APRN, CPNP-PC, CPON

The living body is a machine which winds its own springs:
the living image of perpetual motion.
— *Julien Offroy de la Mettrie*

LUNG FUNCTION IS AFFECTED by cancer treatment in children, which can involve your breathing, ability to exercise, and overall quality of life.

THE RESPIRATORY SYSTEM

Most air enters the body through the nose. As it passes through the nose and nasal cavity, it is warmed, moistened, and filtered.

The *pharynx* (throat) is the area where the passages from the nose and mouth come together. This area leads to the *esophagus* (a tube to the stomach) and the *larynx* (which contains the vocal cords). When you swallow, a flap of tissue called the *epiglottis* covers the larynx to prevent food from getting into the lungs. (see **Figure 14-1**, The respiratory system).

The larynx leads to the trachea—the main passageway to the lungs. The lungs are two organs that surround the heart and fill up most of the space in the ribcage. The lungs are divided into sections called lobes. The left lung is slightly smaller and has fewer lobes than the right lung.

The trachea branches into two tubes called *bronchi*, which divide into smaller and smaller tubes called bronchioles. These tiny tubes end in air sacs called alveoli. The air you breathe carries oxygen that

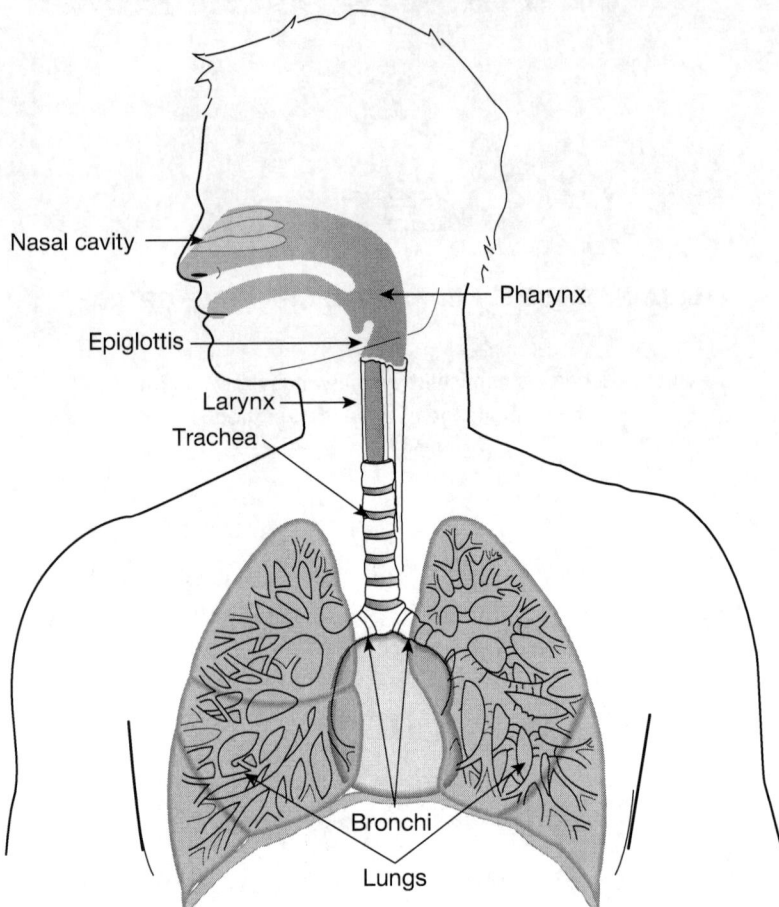

FIGURE 14-1. The respiratory system (©*Alex's Lemonade Stand Foundation, 2025*)

moves across the air sac walls into blood in capillaries in exchange for carbon dioxide. This carbon dioxide exits the body when you exhale (**Figure 14-1**).

Damage to the lungs

Lung damage from treatment can reduce your lungs' ability to expand and thus the amount of air they can hold (called *restrictive lung disease*). Lung growth and chest size can be affected in some survivors who were treated at a very young age and those children who develop scoliosis, which may impact pulmonary function. Treatment can also cause scarring in the lungs (called *pulmonary fibrosis*) which reduces the exchange of oxygen for carbon dioxide in the air sacs. *Obstructive lung disease* (narrowing of the airways) can also occur. A combination of these problems can develop after treatment for childhood cancer.

I only have one lung. They removed the other because my cancer was on the pleural lining of my lung, so they couldn't just take out a portion. Thankfully my other lung has moved and expanded more, which makes up for some of it. This made my heart move over more to the center/right side.

I only have one lung due to my removal. I follow-up with my oncologist for this but not that frequently. The only time I notice a problem is when the weather changes. If it is really cold, I feel like the air is taken from me. If it's humid, I feel myself trying to gasp for air.

Lungs can be damaged by both radiation and chemotherapy. Certain types of chemotherapy drugs can intensify the damaging effects of radiation. Lung damage is common in survivors of hematopoietic stem cell transplants who develop chronic graft-versus-host disease.

Radiation

The lungs are located in the chest cavity. If the chest is irradiated during childhood or adolescence, the growth of bones in the area (spine, ribs, and sternum) as well as muscles in the chest wall can be slowed or stopped. Survivors treated for cancer and who had *mantle radiation* (used before 1990) or radiation to the lungs (chest radiation) may have smaller chests than do those treated only with chemotherapy. This reduces the area in which the lungs can expand and contract. Survivors who received radiation to one side of the body (e.g., those treated for Wilms tumor) can develop curvature of the spine (*scoliosis*) that can also affect the space occupied by the lungs.

A small number of children and adolescents who received high-dose radiation to the lung area develop *radiation pneumonitis* during treatment. They may recover from the pneumonitis on their own or may require treatment with corticosteroids for a period of time. If the pneumonitis worsens, it can result in *pulmonary fibrosis*. Pulmonary fibrosis occurs when lung tissue becomes scarred and loses its elasticity. The amount of air the lungs can hold (lung volume) is then reduced, and the amount of gases exchanged (oxygen and carbon dioxide) is lowered.

Pulmonary fibrosis can develop months to years after treatment and can either stabilize or continue to get worse. Symptoms depend on the amount of lung involved. Fibrosis usually occurs in those who had tumors in the chest or lungs or lung metastases from cancers in other locations and were treated with radiation. It can also occur in survivors who received total body radiation (TBI) as part of their preparation for stem cell transplantation.

The risk of developing pulmonary fibrosis or other pulmonary late effects is highest in survivors who received higher doses of radiation to the lungs/chest including TBI, certain chemotherapy drugs, or combinations of chemotherapy and radiation.

Children or adolescents who get relatively low doses of radiation––less than 1500 centigray (cGy) given in *fractions*––may develop mild or moderate restrictive pulmonary disease, but it usually does not affect daily life activities. Survivors should be evaluated yearly, and most can participate in sports and lead active lives. Survivors who receive doses of radiation >15 Gy (1500 cGy) are at risk for developing repeated lung infections.

Chemotherapy
Pulmonary fibrosis can also be caused by some chemotherapy drugs, such as bleomycin, busulfan, carmustine (BCNU), and lomustine (CCNU). Any combination of these chemotherapy drugs, including asparaginase combined with radiation to the chest (doses >10 Gy), increase the risk for pulmonary fibrosis. Survivors treated with these drugs can develop problems during treatment or many years after treatment ends. Survivors most at risk for pulmonary fibrosis are those who had doses of bleomycin, busulfan, BCNU, or CCNU.

Risk Factors for developing lung problems after bleomycin treatment:
- High total doses of bleomycin (400 units/m2 or more in all doses combined), or in combination with radiation and BCNU (>600 mg/m2) and busulfan (>500 mg/m2)

- Radiation to the chest or lungs especially in higher doses, or total body irradiation (TBI)
- Treatment with other chemotherapy drugs that can also damage the lungs
- Exposure to high oxygen levels (such as during general anesthesia or scuba diving)
- Smoking
- Inhaled drugs, such as smoking marijuana, vaping, or cocaine
- Young age when receiving bleomycin treatment

General anesthesia/sedation precaution. Oxygen and fluids should be monitored closely by an anesthesiologist if you need to be sedated for any reason. You should not be given high concentrations of supplemental oxygen. Too much oxygen to someone who was previously treated with bleomycin can cause edema (fluid buildup) in the lungs. This complication can be avoided with planning and communication ahead of time.

Follow-up screening and detection for lung damage

Part of comprehensive follow-up care should be a discussion about any risks to your lungs from treatment. If you are at risk, you should tell your healthcare provider how you breathe at rest and while exercising. Be aware of the signs and symptoms of common pulmonary late effects (see **Table 14-1**) and contact your healthcare provider if you experience any of these symptoms. Your PCP or pulmonologist can prescribe *bronchodilating medications* that relax the muscles around your airways and help clear mucus from your lungs and relieve symptoms of some lung conditIons such as asthma and COPD.

If you received treatment with bleomycin, BCNU, CCNU, or busulfan; chest, spine, or flank irradiation; or have any symptoms of fibrosis, you should have the following tests performed:
- Pulmonary function tests (PFTs) (see **Figure 14-2**)
- Chest x-ray
- Evaluation of chest wall growth
- Evaluation for *scoliosis* (curvature of the spine)
- Evaluation of trunk length and size of chest cavity

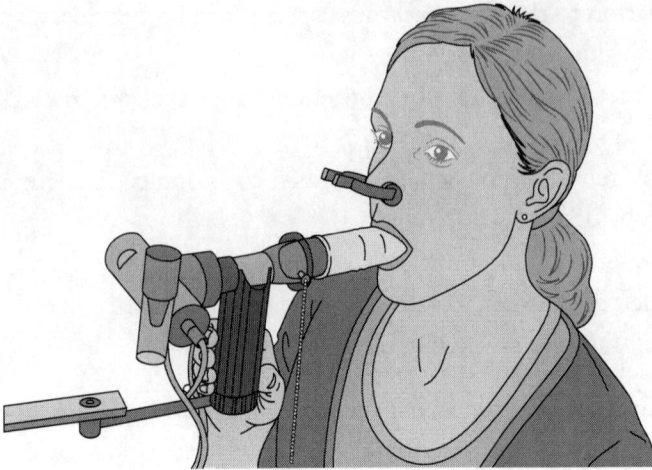

FIGURE 14-2. Pulmonary function testing (spirometry) (©*Alex's Lemonade Stand Foundation, 2025*)

TABLE 14-1 Signs and symptoms of common pulmonary late effects	
Pneumonitis	**Lung Fibrosis**
• cough • fever • shortness of breath • rapid heartbeat	• chronic cough (with or without fever) • shortness of breath • painful breathing • tiring easily during exercise • increasing difficulty with daily activities

Current guidelines recommend monitoring as needed during therapy or at two years after completion of therapy. If you have symptoms, or if the tests are abnormal, you will be monitored periodically. Most follow-up clinics perform PFTs. If a chest x-ray or PFTs suggest fibrosis, a referral to a pulmonologist is usually made for further evaluation.

Prior to receiving general anesthesia. If you received bleomycin, you should have PFTs before having general anesthesia. Make sure you tell the anesthesiologist about your cancer history, bleomycin treatment, and results of your PFTs.

Prior to scuba diving, survivors who had chemotherapy and/or radiation that can affect the lungs should have PFTs and possibly see a pulmonary specialist.

Medical management for lung problems

Yearly influenza vaccine and pneumococcal vaccine

All survivors who had pulmonary radiation or potentially lung-toxic chemotherapy should get a yearly influenza vaccine. They should also receive the *pneumococcal vaccine* once they have completed therapy and their immune system is functional—about 6 months to 1 year from most conventional therapy, and later for those who had a *hematopoietic stem cell transplant*. This vaccine will not prevent all types of pneumonia, because many types are due to organisms not covered by these vaccines.

Also, it is wise to protect oneself and take precautions to avoid close contact with anyone who has a respiratory infection: *an ounce of prevention is worth a pound of cure.*

Pulmonary fibrosis

If you have pulmonary fibrosis, you should maintain as active a lifestyle as possible to maximize lung function. You should also be seen periodically by a pulmonologist.

Careful management of upper respiratory infections is necessary if you have pulmonary fibrosis. If there are increasing signs of pulmonary distress, such as breathing difficulties, increased sputum production, or increased shortness of breath, call your healthcare provider.

No smoking, vaping or exposure to toxic fumes

If you are a cancer survivor, you should not smoke cigarettes or marijuana or vape/inhale any substance other than prescribed medications prescribed by your doctor. This is especially important if you had any treatment that is potentially toxic to your lungs. Your medical management should include a frank discussion about the dangers of smoking, vaping or inhalation of any foreign substance.

E-cigarettes and similar devices. E-cigarettes and other electronic nicotine delivery systems (ENDS) have become very popular in recent years, especially among younger people. They are sometimes used as substitutes for cigarettes or other tobacco products, but for many people, they are the first tobacco product used.

Makers of e-cigarettes and other ENDS often claim the ingredients are safe. But the aerosols (mixtures of very small particles) that these products produce can contain addictive nicotine, flavorings, and a variety of other chemicals, some known to be toxic or to cause cancer. The levels of many of these substances appear to be lower than in traditional cigarettes, but the amounts of nicotine and other substances in these products can vary widely because they are not standardized. The long-term health effects of these devices aren't yet known. (quote from: https://www.cancer .org Search: *risk-prevention, tobacco*).

Avoid toxic fumes. To protect your lungs, avoid fumes from chemicals, solvents, and paints and observe respiratory safety precautions in the workplace. For more information about keeping your lungs healthy after treatment for childhood cancer, visit www.survivorshipguidelines.org; toward the bottom of the home page, look for the heading "Pulmonary System" and click on the link below it to download the "Bleomycin Alert" pdf.

REFERENCES

American Cancer Society website: (https://www.cancer.org/cancer/risk-prevention/tobacco/health-risks-of-tobacco.html) *Health Risks of Using Tobacco Products.*

Armenian, Saro, Landier, Wendy, Francisco, Liton, Herrera, Claudia, Mills, George, Siyahian, Aida, et al. (2015). Long-Term Pulmonary Function in Survivors of Childhood Cancer. *Journal of Clinical Oncology*, 33, 1592-1600. https://doi.org/10.1200/JCO.2014.59.8318

Dietz AC, Chen Y, Yasui Y, et al. (2016). Risk and impact of pulmonary complications in survivors of childhood cancer: A report from the childhood cancer survivor study. *Cancer,* 122(23), 3687-3696. https://doi.org/10.1002/cncr.30200

Huang TT, Hudson MM, Stokes DC, et al. (2011) Pulmonary outcomes in survivors of childhood cancer: a systematic review. *Chest.* 2011 Oct;140(4):881-901. doi: 10.1378/chest.10-2133. Epub 2011 Mar 17. PMID: 21415131; PMCID: PMC3904488

Interiano RB, Kaste SC, Li C, et al. (2017). Associations between treatment, scoliosis, pulmonary function, and physical performance in long-term survivors of sarcoma. *Journal of Cancer Survivorship, 11*(5), 553-561. https://doi.org/10.1007/s11764-017-0624-1

Children's Oncology Group (V6, Oct 2023). *Long-Term Follow-Up Guidelines for Survivors of Childhood, Adolescent, and Young Adult Cancers,* (www.survivorshipguidelines.org) See: *Pulmonary System: bleomycin alert; pulmonary health*

RESOURCES

Website: ccgresources.org
All resources and references mentioned in this book are available on
the website and will be routinely reviewed and updated.

American Cancer Society - *Stay Away from Tobacco*
Website: www.cancer.org/cancer/risk-prevention/tobacco

Website: www.smokefree.gov
Created by the National Cancer Institute, the site includes tips
on how to quit and live chats with trained counselors.

Centers for Disease Control and Prevention (CDC)
U.S. Department of Health
Website: www.cdc.gov/quit
to quit smoking, practical guidance and resources
Website: www.cdc.gov/tobacco/site.html
Website: https://bit.ly/quitSTARTapp

Children's Oncology Group (V6, Oct 2023). *Long-Term Follow-
Up Guidelines for Survivors of Childhood, Adolescent, and
Young Adult Cancers*
Website: www.survivorshipguidelines.org
Click below to download individual Health Links:
Pulmonary System: bleomycin alert; pulmonary health

Passport for Care, Survivor Care Plans by Children's
Oncology Group (V6, Nov 2023)
Website: https://cancersurvivor.passportforcare.org
Survivors and family can find online updated tailored long-term
care plans which should be reviewed with their oncologist or
health care provider.

Physical activity basics and your health
Website: www.cdc.gov/physical-activity-basics/benefits/
Strategies for making regular physical activity a part of your life

GLOSSARY

***acute respiratory distress syndrome (ARDS)**,* a serious condition
that occurs when alveoli in the lungs are damaged and can no longer provide oxygen to the body

bronchodilating medication, medication that relieves the symptoms of lung conditions such as asthma, and chronic obstructive pulmonary disease (COPD) by quickly relaxing the muscle bands that tighten around the airways (bronchi) and allowing more air to come in and out of the lungs so that breathing requires less effort.

fibrosis, build-up of scar tissue

fractions, delivery of radiation in small amounts over the course of a week

hematopoietic stem cell transplantation (also known as stem cell transplant) formerly known as bone marrow transplant, a procedure that involves administering healthy stem cells (e.g., bone marrow, cord blood, or peripheral blood) to patients after the bone marrow has been destroyed by disease, chemotherapy, or radiation

mantle radiation, a radiation technique used from the 1970s to the 1990s which treated a large area of the neck, chest, armpits and mediastinum (area between the lungs) in order to cover all areas with cancer involvement. This technique is **rarely used** today in current treatment.

obstructive lung disease, lung disease that occurs due to blockages or obstructions in the airways that narrow the airways and make it hard to exhale all the air in your lungs. The main symptom is shortness of breath.

pneumococcal vaccine, vaccine given to help prevent or reduce effects of pneumonia bacteria

pneumonitis, inflammation of the tissue of the lungs. This inflammation can worsen if a person develops lung infections, such as pneumonia.

pulmonary fibrosis, formation of scar tissue in the lungs which makes the lungs stiffer and less elastic and reduces lung capacity, making it more difficult to breathe

pulmonary function tests (PFTs), a group of tests that measure how well your lungs work; how well you breathe; and effectiveness of your lungs in bringing oxygen to the rest of your body

radiation pneumonitis, pneumonitis (inflammation of the lungs) resulting from receiving high-dose radiation to the lung area *restrictive lung disease,* lung disease that reduces lungs' ability to expand and reduces amount of air the lungs can hold; shortness of breath is a major symptom

scoliosis, curvature of the spine

vaping, use of a battery-operated device to inhale an aerosol that may contain nicotine, flavors, or other chemicals

15

Kidneys, Bladder, and Genitals

JOANNE QUILLEN, MSN, APRN, PNP-BC

Prosperity is not without many fears and distastes;
and adversity is not without comforts and hopes.
— *Francis Bacon*

THE KIDNEYS AND BLADDER are part of the body's system for clearing waste (the excretory system). In earlier years, damage to these organs from treatment for childhood cancer was far more common than it is today. Chemotherapy drugs that can be toxic to these organs are now given in lower doses or with protective agents and intravenous (IV) fluids that flush them through the excretory system quickly, minimizing damage. Newer treatments of *hematopoietic stem cell transplants (HSCTs)* which is a procedure that inserts healthy stem cells into your body to replace damaged stem cells and *chimeric antigen receptor T-cell (CAR-T) therapy* which uses genetically altered immune cells (T cells) to recognize and attack the cancer, may cause some toxicity to kidney and bladder function. Organ shielding and use of lower doses of radiation have also decreased late effects, but some long-term survivors live with damage to the kidneys and bladder, and a small number of children on newer protocols still develop problems.

Late effects to the vagina, uterus, prostate, and nerves that control sexual function are covered in this chapter. Signs and symptoms, detection, and medical management of late effects to the kidneys, bladder, and genitals are presented. The genitals are organs in the body's reproductive system. Hormones that affect this system are covered in *Chapter 10, Hormone-Producing Glands*.

KIDNEYS

The kidneys, the main organs of the excretory system, are located at the bottom of the ribcage near the back of the body. These two bean-shaped organs are each about the size of a fist. Blood enters the kidneys from branches off the aorta (the main blood vessel that carries oxygen-rich blood from the heart). The kidneys regulate blood pressure, filter waste products from the blood, and control the amount of water, minerals, and vitamins in the blood that returns to the body. Inside each kidney are millions of microscopic structures that filter out large particles, such as white and red blood cells and most proteins, allowing them to return to the bloodstream. What remains in the kidney after this process is the yellow liquid called urine. Urine flows from the kidneys through long tubes (ureters) into the bladder, where it is stored until it is eliminated from the body by urination. **Figure 15-1** shows the anatomy of kidneys and bladder and location within the body.

Kidney damage

The kidneys can be impacted by surgery, chemotherapy, and radiation. The majority of children with Wilms tumor have one kidney removed. If they only receive a short cycle of chemotherapy and no radiation, the remaining kidney usually functions with no major problems. The remaining kidney enlarges and does the work of two kidneys. Protecting the remaining kidney is discussed later in this chapter, under "Medical management."

The vast majority of survivors of childhood cancer have good kidney function. Several long-term effects that may develop are: *nephritis* (inflammation of the kidneys), high blood pressure, kidney artery damage, and *tubular necrosis* (damage to kidney tubules, that filter out waste and fluid).

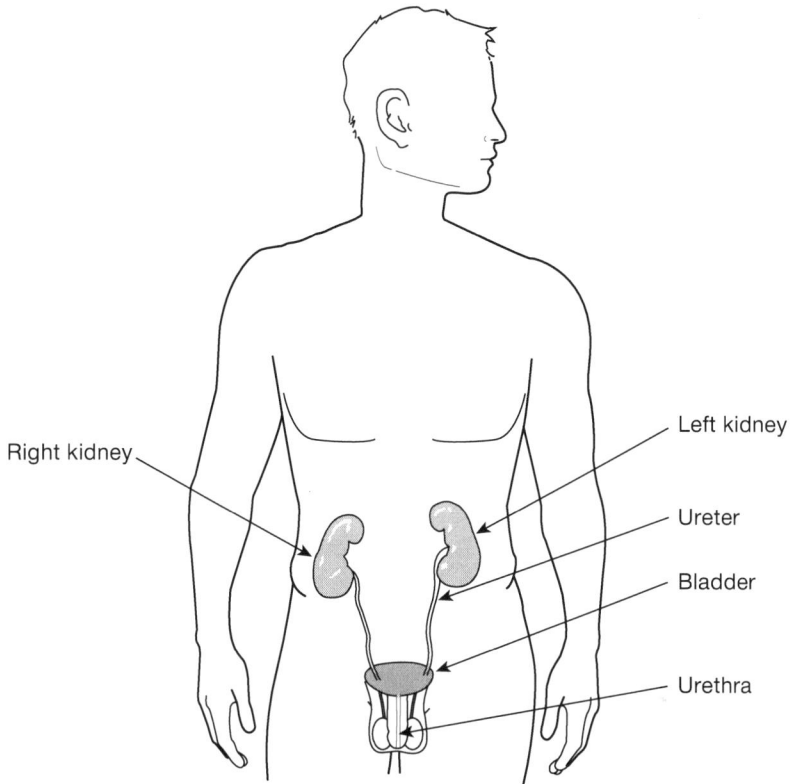

FIGURE 15-1. Anatomy of the kidneys and bladder (©*Alex's Lemonade Stand Foundation,* *2025*)

> My daughter had several months of chemo to shrink the tumor, then surgery to remove it and the kidney was removed as well. They could never definitively say if the tumor grew from the inside or grew into her kidney; it was removed as a precaution. Her remaining kidney has suffered some damage, but it appears to be stable and we continue with all of our follow-ups.

Radiation

Radiation delivered directly to the kidneys can cause dysfunction. Survivors who are at highest risk include those who received:

- Radiation to the whole abdomen for soft tissue sarcomas of the pelvis or abdomen; tumors of the kidney, abdomen, or pelvis; or abdominal lymphomas

- Total body radiation (TBI) before undergoing stem cell transplantation (e.g., bone marrow transplant, peripheral stem cell transplant, or cord blood transplant).

Chronic nephritis. *Chronic nephritis* (inflammation of the kidneys that lasts a long time) can develop after higher doses of at least 2000 centigray (cGy) to an entire kidney. If chemotherapy is given as well, lower doses of radiation (1000 to 1500 cGy) can cause injury. However, each survivor is different, so long- term follow-up is important. Chronic nephritis is also seen in stem cell transplant survivors who had TBI as part of their conditioning regimen. The likelihood of nephritis developing appears to depend on which chemotherapy drugs the survivor had prior to the transplant.

Chronic nephritis can develop during treatment or years after treatment is completed. It can lead to kidney failure or heart damage and thus requires close medical surveillance. Improved radiation techniques and kidney shielding have decreased the number of cancer survivors who develop nephritis.

Hypertension. The kidneys also help regulate blood pressure. High blood pressure (*hypertension*) means the heart is working overtime to push blood through arteries. High blood pressure can lead to heart disease, hardening of the arteries (*atherosclerosis*), or stroke.

Renal artery damage. Another rare late effect in long-term survivors who were treated with radiation to a field (area of the body) that included one or both kidneys (this includes Hodgkin lymphoma survivors who had their spleens irradiated) is renal artery damage or blockage. The main symptom is very high blood pressure that occurs years after treatment.

Chemotherapy

Acute renal toxicity. High doses of cisplatin can affect the kidneys. Some children or teens who received cumulative doses of at least 450 mg/m2 of cisplatin can develop *acute renal toxicity* during treatment. Also known as acute kidney injury, it develops quickly when kidneys lose their filtering ability and dangerous amounts of waste accumulate in the blood. Over time, a kidney can sometimes repair itself. In other cases, survivors need to take replacement magnesium. Cisplatin damage usually becomes apparent during or within a year after treatment. Carboplatin is less toxic to the kidneys; however, in combination with other therapies, it can also impact renal function.

Tubular necrosis. High doses of cyclophosphamide and/or ifosfamide can cause *necrosis* (death) of tubules in the kidneys. *Kidney tubules* filter out waste products and fluid and return substances to the blood that your body needs. If these drugs are given with radiation to the pelvis or abdomen, or if combined with other drugs that can damage the kidneys, the risk of kidney problems increases. These changes usually occur only in survivors who have had multiple relapses and received extremely high doses of these drugs.

Late effects. Some chemotherapy drugs, when combined with radiation, can increase the risk of late effects to the kidneys. These drugs include the following:

- Ifosfamide
- Cytoxan
- Cisplatin
- Carboplatin
- Dactinomycin

Persistent problems usually only develop in survivors who had severe kidney problems during treatment.

Signs and symptoms of kidney damage

Signs and symptoms of kidney damage include the following:

- Fatigue
- *Anemia* (not having enough red blood cells)
- Excessive urination during the night (*nocturia*)
- Weakness
- Retaining fluid (*edema*)
- High blood pressure
- Poor growth (this can be a sign of very poor kidney function)

Screening and detection

Survivors who received chemotherapy that can cause kidney problems need an evaluation of kidney function after the end of treatment. Survivors who were treated with chemotherapy and radiation to the abdomen or a kidney need an evaluation of kidney function either annually or every other year. Your evaluation should include the following:

- Physical exam
- Health history, including questions about frequency of urination, painful urination, and bedwetting
- Blood pressure
- Urinalysis, or urine test, to check for protein in the urine, a sign of kidney damage
- Blood tests for blood urea nitrogen (BUN) and creatinine (waste product of the body) levels, to measure how well the kidneys are working

For a complete list of the tests you should have based on your treatment, you and your healthcare provider can refer to the Children's Oncology Group's survivorship guidelines at www.survivorshipguidelines.org.

Medical management

If you have long-term kidney toxicities from treatment, you should be seen by a pediatric or adult *nephrologist* (kidney specialist). Because damage to the kidneys can resolve over time, expert medical care is needed while waiting to see if recovery occurs. In the very rare cases in which progressive kidney failure occurs, dialysis and/or kidney transplant may be necessary.

If you had radiation to one or both kidneys, regular checks of your blood pressure should be part of your medical care. You should visit your healthcare provider's office or your school clinic several times a year to have your blood pressure checked. Steps you can take to help keep your blood pressure in the healthy range are maintaining a normal weight, exercising daily, and eating less salt.

The primary concern of survivors with only one kidney (after treatment for Wilms and occasionally neuroblastoma) is protection of the remaining kidney. The kidney is naturally very well protected within the body. However, you should talk with your healthcare provider about the sports you play. Your healthcare provider may recommend that you avoid contact sports or use a kidney guard if you do participate. Each family needs to balance quality of life issues with protection when making decisions about sports activities.

Survivors with one kidney should also know the signs of urinary tract and kidney infections and seek treatment quickly to protect their single kidney. If you have burning upon urination, blood in the urine, painful urination, an urgent need to urinate frequently, or flank pain on the side of the remaining kidney, go to your healthcare provider as soon as symptoms develop. The key preventive step for urinary tract and kidney infections is to drink half your body weight in water, for example, if you weigh 120 pounds, drink 60 ounces of water daily.

There are certain categories of drugs, including some types of antibiotics, that can affect renal function. If you only have one kidney, don't use over-the-counter, herbal, or other medications without first discussing them with your nephrologist. Many of these are toxic to the kidneys, including *nonsteroidal anti-inflammatory drugs* (e.g., aspirin, ibuprofen, and naproxen) for pain, fever, or inflammation. **Remind your healthcare provider anytime you receive a prescription that you have** *only one kidney*.

> Survivors with only one kidney need to make sure their healthcare providers know of their special circumstances. Putting a card in with your driver's license that says you have only one kidney and/or wearing a medical alert bracelet will assist you in the unlikely event that you need medical care and are unable to tell emergency responders that you have a single kidney.

BLADDER

The bladder is a muscular bag located in the lower pelvis. The ureters from the kidneys carry urine to the bladder. Urine collects in the bladder until it is full. When the muscle of the bladder signals the brain that it is full, the brain orders muscle contractions that squeeze the urine out of the bladder. The urine flows through a tube called the urethra to the outside of the body.

Organ damage

The vast majority of survivors of childhood cancer have good bladder function. However, bladder damage, including *hemorrhagic cystitis* (blood leaking into the bladder from irritated blood vessels inside the bladder wall), *fibrosis* (scarring or hardening of the tissue in the bladder), or a bladder that doesn't grow to a normal size, can occur after treatment with cyclophosphamide or ifosfamide and/or radiation.

> My advice to other survivors and parents is to listen to the doctors but trust your instincts. If the doctors tell you something, and it doesn't feel right to you, ask follow-up questions. Our daughter was born with a rare bladder birth defect which we knew while I was pregnant, but that *defect* turned out to be a blessing in disguise. After her first surgery at one month to correct the bladder condition, they found the cancer, neuroblastoma. If she had not had that bladder surgery, they wouldn't have discovered the neuroblastoma as early. It was a rapidly developing cancer that went from non-existent to stage 4 in a month and a half, so it was a blessing that they found it early-on.

Radiation

Scarring and strictures. Survivors who had tumors in the bladder or pelvic area may have received high doses of radiation that can scar their bladders. A scarred (fibrotic) bladder does not stretch to hold urine or contract well to empty. A bladder that does not grow (or shrinks due to fibrosis) may meet the needs of a preschooler, but will be too small for an older child. Thus, intervention may be necessary years after treatment even though the injury to the organ has not progressed. Radiation can also cause narrowing (strictures) in the urethra, which causes difficult, painful urination.

Chemotherapy

Hemorrhagic cystitis. This condition is caused by cyclophosphamide (Cytoxan®) and ifosfamide. Children who were given *mesna* (a drug given with some types of chemotherapy to help protect the bladder from inflammation and serious bleeding), or who received cyclophosphamide by IV with lots of fluids to flush it through the bladder, rarely get cystitis. Survivors most at risk for hemorrhagic cystitis are those who:

- Received cyclophosphamide and/or ifosfamide for long periods of time with minimal flushing through the system.
- Had hemorrhagic cystitis during treatment and the problem persists. It does not tend to spontaneously occur years later.

Signs and symptoms of bladder damage

Hemorrhagic cystitis. Signs and symptoms of hemorrhagic cystitis are blood in the urine, lower abdominal pain, frequent and painful urination, an urgent need to urinate, and difficulties with urination.

Bladder scarring and bleeding ulcers. Radiation damage to the bladder can cause bleeding ulcers and scarring in the bladder. Survivors with this condition may have little or no bladder control (wetting or leakage) or may have to urinate very frequently.

Screening and detection

All survivors who had therapies that can harm the bladder should have a baseline and then yearly *urinalysis.* An assessment of the function of the urinary system also includes asking questions about the following:

- Incontinence
- Urine dripping
- Difficulty starting urination
- Painful urination
- Inability to completely empty the bladder

Survivors with hemorrhagic cystitis are at risk for bladder cancers and thus need education about signs and symptoms, as well as yearly evaluations.

Medical, surgical, and psychological care

Hemorrhagic cystitis. If you had treatment that could damage your bladder, and your urine test shows blood, it should be repeated in a week. If it is still positive, you should request a referral to a *urologist* (a medical doctor who specializes in diagnosis and treatment of the urinary system in men and women and also the reproductive system of men) with experience treating survivors of childhood cancer.

Chronic bladder infections. Survivors with chronic bladder infections need to drink lots of fluids. This can be challenging for parents of younger children. The following are suggested ways to encourage young children to drink more.

- Fill water bottles halfway, add a drop of food coloring, then freeze. Then add cold water to fill and add a different color.
- Use different kinds of cups with crazy-shaped straws.
- Flavor crushed ice with juice.
- Freeze juice in ice trays and add to drinks.
- Make juice popsicles.

Some survivors are at risk for cavities and obesity, so drink juice and energy drinks in moderation. Consider using flavor options lower in sugar and calories. It is important to brush your teeth often.

Scarred bladders. Bladder-stretching surgery for survivors with scarred bladders has not been very successful. At some large, university-affiliated children's hospitals, new surgical techniques are being developed to increase bladder size (called bladder augmentation) by stitching in pieces of tissue from other parts of the body. If you have a fibrotic bladder, occasional visits to specialists in the field at large pediatric hospitals can alert you to the newest developments in treatment.

Complete or partial bladder removal. Treatment for tumors in the bladder or pelvic area once included total removal of the bladder and placement of a *urinary diversion* (surgery that allows urine to flow out of the body through a tube in the abdominal wall). Children who had a urinary diversion need physical and psychological support as they grow. Such services can be found at childhood cancer survivors' clinic.

Newer treatments combine chemotherapy with removal of part of the bladder. In the majority of cases, survivors retain functional bladders.

GENITALS

Genitals are human reproductive organs.

Genitals of females. The female organs are the ovaries, uterus, and vagina. Ovaries, the organs that release eggs and produce sex hormones, are discussed in *Chapter 10, Hormone-Producing Glands*. The uterus is an organ with strong, muscular walls. The structure at the bottom of the uterus that connects it to the vagina is the cervix. The vagina is a muscular, tube-shaped organ. It is sometimes called the birth canal because it is the opening through which a baby is born. **Figure 15-2** shows the location of female genitals.

Genitals of males. This chapter focuses on the overall function of genitals in males. For information about the relationship between genitals in males and hormones, please see *Chapter 10, Hormone-Producing Glands*.

The testes are the male organs that produce sperm cells and the hormone testosterone. The testes are in a sac called the scrotum, located behind the penis. Each testis is made of coiled tubules called seminiferous tubules. Cells in the tubules produce sperm, which is stored in a structure called the epididymis. The prostate is a walnut-sized gland located just below the bladder. It makes fluid that is mixed with sperm cells to produce semen. The penis is the male organ through which sperm cells leave the body during sexual intercourse. **Figure 15-3** shows the male genitals.

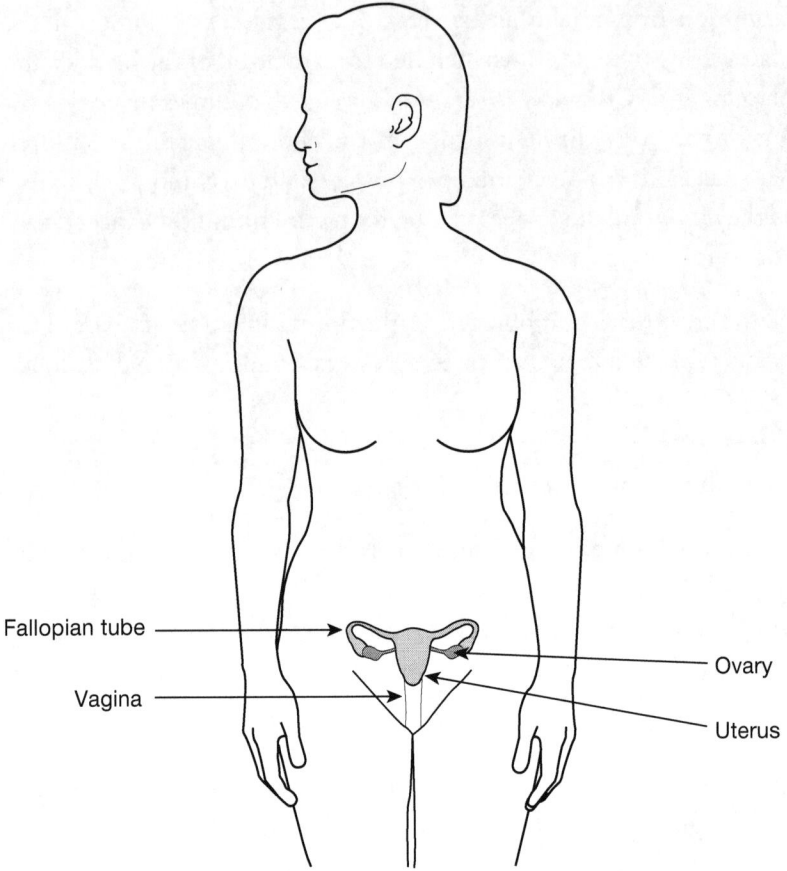

FIGURE 15-2. Anatomy of the female genitals (©*Alex's Lemonade Stand Foundation, 2025*)

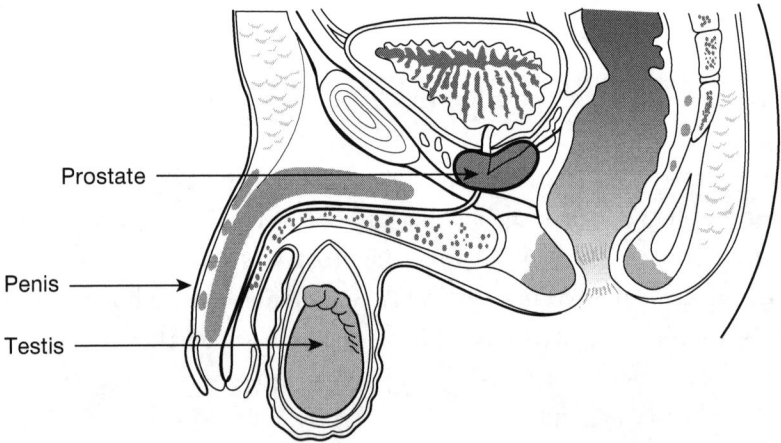

FIGURE 15-3. Anatomy of the male genitals (©*Alex's Lemonade Stand Foundation, 2025*)

Organ damage in females

Very few girls get tumors in the vagina or uterus. However, some female children or teens with tumors in the pelvic area (i.e., rhabdomyosarcoma, Ewing sarcoma, osteosarcoma) get high-dose radiation that can affect the growth and development of the vagina and/or uterus. Lower doses of radiation, when used with some types of chemotherapy that enhance radiation (e.g., dactinomycin and doxorubicin), can cause the same long-term effects as high-dose radiation alone.

Some female survivors who had abdominal tumors treated with radiation have permanent changes in the size and function of the uterus. These late effects are more likely in girls treated before puberty with more than 2000 cGy of radiation. The uterus of a girl treated after puberty usually is not damaged unless more than 4000 cGy of radiation is used. Radiation can stunt the growth of the uterus and can also cause it to become scarred (fibrotic) and less elastic. This type of damage to the uterus can cause miscarriages of pregnancies or low birthweight children. It occurs most often in survivors of Wilms tumor who had more than 2000 cGy of abdominal radiation and in Hodgkin lymphoma survivors who had radiation to the abdomen and chemotherapy (but not either alone).

Girls or teens who had more than 4000 cGy of radiation to a field that included the vagina can develop *fibrosis* (tissue gets scarred and tough and doesn't stretch well) and diminished vaginal development. This problem can also occur after lower doses of radiation if radiation-enhancing chemotherapy drugs (e.g., dactinomycin) are also given. Fibrosis can affect the size and flexibility of the vagina, which can alter sexual function and the ability to deliver babies vaginally.

Signs and symptoms in females

Uterine damage. Signs and symptoms of uterine damage include the following:

- Small uterus (your gynecologist will tell you this)
- Inability to get pregnant
- Difficulties with menstruation such as irregular periods or heavier than normal flow

- Miscarriage
- Low birthweight babies

Vaginal damage. Signs and symptoms of vaginal damage include the following:
- Abnormal vaginal bleeding
- Vaginal dryness
- Inability to have intercourse due to a small vaginal opening
- Painful intercourse

Organ damage in males

Male children or teens who had high-dose radiation to the abdomen for rhabdomyosarcoma, Ewing sarcoma, or osteosarcoma are at risk for damage to the prostate gland and the nerves that control sexual functioning. Boys or teens with testicular cancer or relapsed leukemia (in the testes) usually have a testicle removed and the area irradiated.

Low doses of radiation to the prostate can slow or stop the development of this organ. High doses (more than 5000 cGy) can cause the organ to atrophy (shrink). Because the prostate produces part of the fluid that makes semen, damage to it can reduce or eliminate ejaculation. Nerve damage from surgery or radiation can affect the ability to have an erection and can also affect ejaculation.

Survivors who had *radical lymph node dissections* (removal of many lymph nodes in an area of the body) sometimes accumulate excessive fluid in the testicles (called *hydrocele*). This late effect has been seen in long-term survivors of Hodgkin lymphoma, Wilms tumor, and paratesticular rhabdomyosarcoma.

Signs and symptoms in males

Prostate damage. Signs and symptoms of prostate damage include the following:
- Decreased volume of ejaculate (seminal fluid released upon *ejaculation*)
- Small or atrophied prostate (your healthcare provider will tell you this)

Nerve damage. Signs and symptoms of damage to nerves that control sexual function include the following:

- Inability to have an erection
- Inability to maintain an erection
- Inability to have an orgasm
- Having orgasms without ejaculation

Screening and detection for males and females

Frank discussions with your healthcare provider about changes in your sexual organs or sexual function are essential to identify and treat these late effects. Many people (including some healthcare providers) feel uncomfortable talking about sex and sexuality. However, sexuality is a vital part of your life that influences your sense of self and quality of life. Find a healthcare provider you trust who is comfortable discussing these issues so you can explore all of your options to address late effects involving your genitals.

Male survivors. Healthcare providers for males should take an age-appropriate history that focuses on any problems with *libido* (sex drive), sexual function, or fertility. For males, the prostate gland is felt manually, and sometimes an ultrasound of the organ is done to evaluate size. Late effects involving the testicles are covered in *Chapter 10, Hormone-Producing Glands*.

Female survivors. Healthcare providers for female survivors should take an age-appropriate history that focuses on any problems with libido, sexual function, or fertility. Female children and teens need regular evaluation of their sexual development to ensure that puberty is proceeding normally. Women and sexually active teens should have a yearly pelvic examination. This exam may need to be done under anesthesia or sedation for women or teens who have small vaginas or vaginal fibrosis. The uterus can be evaluated using ultrasound, computed tomography (CT) scan, or magnetic resonance imaging (MRI). Abdominal radiation that included the ovaries requires extensive evaluation, outlined in *Chapter 10, Hormone-Producing Glands*.

Medical, surgical, and psychological care

Females. Female teens and women with late effects that alter sexual functioning or fertility need to be referred to a *gynecologist* (a medical doctor specializing in the female reproductive system) and/or *endocrinologist* (a medical doctor specializing in the body's hormone-producing glands) for further evaluation, testing, and treatment. Women or female teens with vaginal late effects may need *vaginal dilations* (expansion of the vagina using tube-shaped devices) or reconstructive surgery. Survivors should consult a gynecologist with extensive experience doing these procedures. A woman with a small uterus or who has *uterine fibrosis* (scarring of the uterus) needs counseling about pregnancy. Pregnant women who had pelvic radiation should get their prenatal care from an obstetrician who specializes in high-risk pregnancies.

Males. Male teens or men with late effects that alter sexual functioning or fertility need to be referred to a *urologist* (doctor specializing in the reproductive tract of men) and/or *endocrinologist* (doctor specializing in the body's hormone-producing glands) for further evaluation, testing, and treatment. Males who had a testicle removed may want to discuss having a prosthesis (artificial body part) implanted. Those who develop a hydrocele usually have the fluid surgically drained.

Any survivor with sexual problems that result from treatment for childhood cancer needs both medical and psychological follow-up. A team approach that provides psychological help to address concerns about body image, fertility, or sexuality is crucial.

Centers with childhood cancer survivors' programs have multidisciplinary teams that include psychologists and social workers who are familiar with survivors' sexual issues and concerns. They can provide information, support, and one-on-one assistance with how to address these issues in relationships.

REFERENCES

Children's Oncology Group. (2023). *Long-Term Follow-Up Guidelines for Survivors of Childhood, Adolescent, and Young Adult Cancers*, v. 6. (www.survivorshipguidelines. org) under Health Links, Click, Appendix II (Entire set of Health Links) and click on topics: *urinary tract, bladder health, cystectomy, kidney health, neurogenic bladder, single kidney health*

Ginsberg, JP, Hobbie, WL, et al. (2004). Prevalence of and risk factors for hydrocele in survivors of Wilms Tumor. *Pediatr Blood and Cancer, 42*: 361–363.

Kapoor M et al. Malignancy and renal disease. (2001). *Crit Care Clin*, 17: 571–598.

Nada A, Jetton JG. (2021). Pediatric onco-nephrology: time to spread the word: Part I: early kidney involvement in children with malignancy. *Pediatr Nephrol.* 36(8):2227-2255. doi: 10.1007/s00467-020-04800-3. Epub 2020 Nov 27. PMID: 33245421.

RESOURCES

Website: ccgresources.org

All resources and references mentioned in this book are available on the website and will be routinely reviewed and updated.

Children's Oncology Group (2023). *Long-Term Follow-Up Guidelines for Survivors of Childhood, Adolescent, and Young Adult Cancers*, (V 6)
Website: www.survivorshipguidelines.org
Individual **Health Links**, search **Urinary Tract** topics: *bladder health, cystectomy, kidney health, neurogenic bladder, single kidney health*
Reproductive System: *ovarian or testicular reproductive health*

Passport for Care, Survivor Care Plans by Children's Oncology Group (V6, Nov 2023)
Website: https://cancersurvivor.passportforcare.org
Survivors and family can find online updated tailored long-term care plans which should be reviewed with their oncologist or health care provider.

GLOSSARY

acute renal toxicity (or acute kidney injury), when kidneys lose their filtering ability and dangerous amounts of waste accumulate in the blood

anemia, not having enough red blood cells

chimeric antigen receptor T-cell (CAR-T) therapy, a type of cancer treatment that uses genetically altered immune cells called T cells to recognize and attack cancer

chronic nephritis, inflammation of the nephrons of the kidneys that lasts a long time. It can affect kidney function leading to changes in urine and urination

edema, swelling caused by tiny blood vessels leaking fluid into nearby tissues; most often occurs in feet, ankles, legs but can occur in other parts of the body

ejaculation, sudden release of semen from the penis from sexual stimulation

endocrinologist, a medical doctor who specializes in diseases and disorders of the body's hormone-producing glands

fibrosis, scarring or hardening of the tissue in the bladder which makes it more difficult for the tissue to stretch

gynecologist, a medical doctor who specializes in the female reproductive system

hematopoietic stem cell transplant (HPSCT), formerly known as bone marrow transplant, involves administering healthy stem cells (e.g., bone marrow, cord blood, or peripheral blood) after the bone marrow has been destroyed by disease, chemotherapy (chemo), or radiation.

hemorrhagic cystitis, blood leaking into the bladder from irritated blood vessels inside the bladder wall

hydrocele, excessive fluid in the testicles

libido, sex drive

mesna, a medication used in those taking cyclophosphamide or ifosfamide to decrease the risk of bleeding from the bladder

nephrologist, a medical doctor who specializes in treating diseases of the kidneys

nephritis, inflammation of the kidneys that can affect kidney function leading to changes in urine and urination

nocturia, excessive urination during the night

nonsteroidal anti-inflammatory drugs, over-the-counter medications used for pain, fever or inflammation (e.g., aspirin, ibuprofen, and naproxen)

radical lymph node dissections, removal of many lymph nodes in an area of the body

tubular necrosis, damage that occurs to tube-shaped structures in the kidneys (tubules) that filter out waste products and fluid

urologist, a medical doctor who specializes in diagnosis and treatment of the urinary system in men and women and also the reproductive system of men

urinary diversion, a surgical procedure that allows urine to flow out of the body through a tube in the abdominal wall

vaginal dilations, expansion of the vagina using tube-shaped devices

16

Liver, Stomach, and Intestines

LISA BASHORE, PhD, APRN, CPNP-PC, CPON

Food is an important part of a balanced diet.
— Fran Lebowitz

THE LIVER, STOMACH, AND INTESTINES are part of the body's gastrointestinal (GI) system. This system gets useful nutrients from food to help the body grow and function well and perform different jobs. Some areas mix and store food, some help in chemical breakdown, and others absorb nutrients and store waste materials.

LIVER

The liver is the body's largest internal organ and one of the most complex. This wedge-shaped organ is located beneath the rib cage in the upper-right part of the abdomen. The liver performs thousands of functions that are essential to life. It transforms food into energy, removes toxins (e.g., alcohol and drugs) from the body, keeps blood clotting normally, and makes proteins. It regulates the supply of essential minerals and vitamins and also produces bile, a fluid needed for proper digestion. In addition, the liver helps filter many chemical substances and waste products from the blood.

Risk factors for damage to the liver

Hepatitis
For survivors who received treatments after 1990s, the risk for significant hepatic toxicity is low (Bardi et al, 2021). Inflammation of the liver is called hepatitis. There are many possible causes of liver inflam-

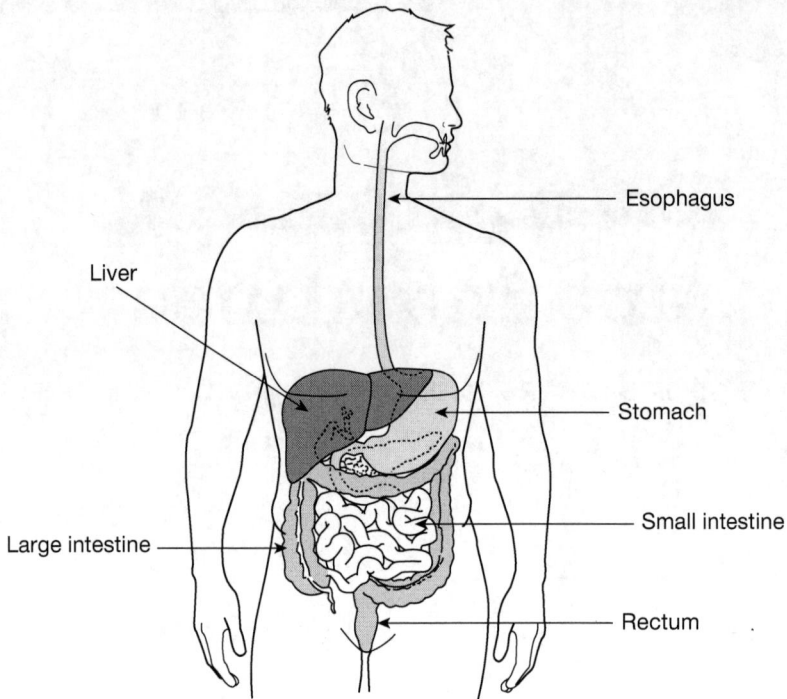

FIGURE 16-1. Location of the liver, stomach, intestines and rectum (©*Alex's Lemonade Stand Foundation, 2025*)

mation in childhood cancer survivors, including infection by viruses and damage from radiation and/or chemotherapy drugs. However, inflammation of the liver is relatively rare in survivors, especially in those treated for cancer in recent years.

Viral hepatitis

Hepatitis A. Hepatitis A is an infection caused by the hepatitis A virus (HAV), which is usually spread by contamination of food by human waste. Although in 2020, there were 15,000 new cases of HAV, in 2022 less than 4,500 new cases were reported, and as of 2023 the number was almost zero (http://www.cdc.gov/hepatitis). It is most common in international travelers, sexually active homosexual men, intravenous drug users, and daycare workers. Most healthy people who get hepatitis A have no long-term consequences from the infection. There is an effective vaccine that prevents hepatitis A infections. This type of hepatitis is not a late effect of childhood cancer.

Hepatitis B. Hepatitis B is an inflammation of the liver caused by the hepatitis B virus (HBV). Approximately 1 million Americans have chronic hepatitis B infections, including survivors who received blood transfusions prior to 1972 (blood products were not screened for this virus before 1972). In 2022 in the United States, 2,126 acute hepatitis B cases were reported but there was an estimated total of 13,800 acute hepatitis B virus (HBV) cases rates (http://www.cdc.gov/hepatitis). There is now an effective vaccine that prevents hepatitis B infections. The blood supply for transfusions is now well screened, and health-care workers are routinely vaccinated.

Hepatitis C. Hepatitis C is an inflammation of the liver caused by the hepatitis C virus (HCV). HCV was spread by blood transfusions that were received prior to effective testing of blood products and is currently spread by sharing needles for illicit intravenous drug use, and, less commonly, through sexual intercourse. Since 2020, the number of individuals diagnosed with Hepatitis C has decreased substantially, and may be due to under-reporting due to COVID, less risky health behaviors, and vaccination rates (http://www.cdc.gov/hepatitis). There is no vaccine for HCV.

If you are infected with HCV, there are five possible outcomes:

- Your body's immune system may eliminate the virus and you will have no further problems (this happens in 15 to 25 percent of persons infected).
- You may have a lifelong infection, but your liver will sustain no damage.
- You may develop liver inflammation, with or without symptoms.
- You may develop progressive inflammation and scarring of the liver. When this scarring (*fibrosis*) spreads throughout the liver and causes lumps, it is called *cirrhosis*. This process occurs over many years and usually results in symptoms. It can eventually lead to liver failure.
- In rare cases, liver cancer develops, but only after years of inflammation from chronic hepatitis C and cirrhosis.

Liver fibrosis

Liver fibrosis (excessive formation of scar tissue in the liver) develops from liver inflammation, which has a variety of causes. Liver toxicity can be measured by liver function tests during or after cancer treatment ends.

The risks for liver fibrosis in cancer survivors are:
- Chronic viral hepatitis
- Liver irradiation (abdominal radiation on the right side)
- High doses of drugs that can cause liver toxicity (e.g., methotrexate, 6-MP, 6-TG, dactinomycin)
- Hematopoietic cell transplantation

Risk factors for development of liver fibrosis due to radiation:
- amount of the liver that was irradiated
- radiation dose
- younger age at treatment
- at highest risk are those who had higher doses of radiation to the entire liver

Chemotherapy can also cause liver fibrosis. Very few children who received lower doses of methotrexate develop fibrosis. Even less frequently, mercaptopurine (6-MP), thioguanine (6-TG), and dactinomycin can affect the function of the liver.

Survivors of hematopoietic stem cell transplantation (e.g., bone marrow, peripheral stem cell, or cord blood transplants) may have several risk factors for chronic liver disease, including HCV infection, *iron overload* (*hemochromatosis*), and *chronic* (ongoing) *graft-versus-host disease* (GVHD) (when the graft, marrow or stem cells from the donor reacts against the *host* who is the person receiving the transplant). Liver damage can develop rapidly in transplant survivors.

Signs and symptoms of damage to the liver
Hepatitis C and liver fibrosis
Because HCV can silently damage the liver, you may not be aware of the infection until late, when it has already caused fibrosis and corresponding symptoms of nausea/vomiting, fluid in abdomen, and enlarged liver.

Symptoms of hepatitis C include the following:

- Abdominal pain
- Darkening of the urine
- Fatigue
- Fever
- Jaundice (yellowing of eyes and skin)
- Nausea
- Lack of appetite
- Vomiting

Screening and detection for liver damage

Most institutions recommend three blood tests (ALT, AST, and bilirubin – see definitions in glossary) to assess the health of the liver on entry to a long-term follow-up clinic and on an ongoing basis, if necessary. All survivors of childhood cancer regardless of treatment should also have a *serum ferritin test,* a blood test that measures the amount of ferritin (blood protein that contains iron) in the blood and is a check for iron-deficiency anemia. During your annual physical examination, your healthcare provider should *palpate* (feel) your abdomen to check for an enlarged liver. Any abnormal findings should result in further evaluation including an MRI of the liver to assess for excessive iron deposits in the liver. A referral to a *gastroenterologist* (a medical doctor specializing in digestive diseases and disorders) may be necessary for further evaluation and treatment.

Medical, surgical, and psychological management

Although currently the risk for developing hepatitis C is low, the following may be helpful for those survivors experiencing this chronic illness. There is no specific treatment for *acute HCV* (HCV that develops suddenly and goes away after the body successfully fights it off). As noted above, in 15-25 percent of people infected, their immune system eliminates the virus, and they have no further problems.

See a specialist. Survivors who experience chronic (long-lasting) HCV should see a specialist who treats liver problems/diseases. There are a number of medications to treat chronic HCV, including interferon alpha, which stimulates the immune system to fight the infection, and ribavirin, an antiviral antibiotic, which are usually given together. This combination treatment is effective in up to half of patients. Treatments for HCV may change or evolve over time, so keep in touch with a specialist if you have HCV to learn of the newest options.

Treatments for iron overload. Survivors who have excessive liver deposits based on ferritin levels and MRI findings may benefit from routine phlebotomy or chelation for *iron overload* (*hemochromatosis*).

Surgery. Some people who have had HCV infections for many years need a liver transplant, because the liver becomes so damaged that it can no longer perform its crucial functions.

Take precautions. If you have HCV or chronic liver fibrosis, the following can help to protect your liver:

- Don't drink alcohol—it greatly increases damage to the liver.
- Don't take over-the-counter medications, such as Tylenol˙ (acetaminophen) or Advil˙ (ibuprofen), herbal or dietary aids, or prescription medications, without first discussing them with your healthcare provider.
- Get vaccinated against hepatitis A and B
- See your healthcare provider regularly.

Transmission through sexual intercourse. HCV can be spread to a partner by sexual intercourse, so it is important to use barrier protection, such as condoms. Because there is no vaccine against HCV, a sexual partner of a survivor with HCV can also get the infection. Therefore, your sexual partner should be periodically screened for HCV. Rarely, HCV can be transmitted to an infant during pregnancy. It is important that female survivors with HCV tell their obstetrician and family physician about the infection.

Counseling and support. Counseling with a healthcare provider should be provided if you test positive for HBV or HCV to help you learn about and cope with these chronic diseases. Many people with HCV infections find comfort participating in support groups, which are available in many communities because HCV is so widespread.

For more information about HCV, visit the U.S. Centers for Disease Control and Prevention website at https://www.cdc.gov/hepatitis/, or call 1- 800-CDC-INFO (1-800-232-4636).

The American Liver Foundation has an informative website at www. Liverfoundation.org

STOMACH AND INTESTINES

The stomach is a muscular sac that contracts to mix food with digestive secretions. Glands in the stomach secrete acids and enzymes to help break down food and mucus to lubricate the digestive tract and coat the stomach wall.

Approximately three hours after arriving in the stomach, food moves into and through the small intestine (also known as the small bowel), where digestion of proteins, carbohydrates, and fats is completed and nutrients are absorbed into the bloodstream. Undigested material passes into the large intestine, also called the colon, where water and vitamins are reabsorbed, leaving behind undigested material called feces. The feces move into the rectum, then out of the body through the anus.

Damage to the gastrointestinal system

Survivors of childhood cancer sometimes develop fibrosis (excessive formation of scar tissue) or *chronic enterocolitis* (inflammation of the intestines).

Fibrosis can occur anywhere in the GI system, from the esophagus to the rectum, causing thickening of the inner walls that can lead to *strictures* (narrowing) or obstructions (blockages). Fibrosis can also occur outside of the GI tract in the form of *adhesions* (bands of scar tissue that cause surfaces of structures that are usually separate to stick together).

Fibrosis, strictures, and chronic enterocolitis can be caused by the following:
- Radiation (3,000 cGy or higher) and if the colon received > 45Gy
- Abdominal surgery

- Chemotherapy (with radiation)
- Chronic GVHD
- Infection

Fibrosis and chronic enterocolitis can cause adhesions, obstructions, ulcers, diarrhea, constipation, lactose intolerance, and malabsorption problems. Intestinal damage can appear months to decades after treatment ends. The colon and rectum are more often damaged by radiation than the stomach and small intestine.

Survivors who received low doses of radiation have a very low incidence of GI damage, while those who had multiple abdominal surgeries and higher radiation doses are at higher risk.

Another problem that can develop is slow emptying of the stomach and *reflux* (backflow) of food into the esophagus. These effects can occur after radiation or in survivors who had long-term problems with severe vomiting while in treatment. Reflux is a chronic problem. Barrett's esophagus (changes in the cells of the esophagus) can occur in association with reflux in those whose GI tracts were irradiated. For more information about late effects to the esophagus, see *Chapter 12, Head and Neck.*

The role of chemotherapy drugs in the development of GI late effects is not well understood. Certain drugs (i.e., dactinomycin, Adriamycin', daunorubicin) are known to increase the effects of radiation and thus may increase the likelihood of GI problems.

Signs and symptoms of damage to the stomach and intestines:

Signs and symptoms of damage to the stomach and intestines:
- Chronic diarrhea
- Chronic constipation
- Nausea and vomiting
- Persistent or severe abdominal pain or cramping or bloating
- Blood in the stool
- Anemia

- Loss of appetite
- Problems gaining weight or loss of weight
- Failure to grow or thrive

Failure to grow and thrive is the primary symptom of *malabsorption* or difficulty in the digestion or absorption of nutrients from food. It often is accompanied by persistent diarrhea. This problem usually begins during treatment and persists. Malabsorption does not suddenly occur years after treatment.

Small bowel obstructions (obstructions of the small intestine) generally begin abruptly. The signs and symptoms include abdominal pain, nausea, vomiting, and loss of appetite. The pain is sometimes described as "crampy." It may be in one specific area but is more commonly generalized. If the obstruction is complete, you cannot pass gas or have a bowel movement. Vomiting is caused by the increased pressure from the obstruction. The abdomen will become distended (enlarged) and if tapped will sound like a drum. **If this happens, it is a medical emergency and you need to get medical attention right away because it can be life-threatening.**

Screening and detection for damage to stomach and intestines

Your annual follow-up appointment should include a thorough physical examination and health history. You are at risk if you had one or more abdominal surgeries, abdominal radiation, or chronic GVHD after a stem cell transplant.

If you haven't reached your full adult growth, your height and weight should be plotted on a growth chart. Your healthcare provider should ask about your diet, any stomach or abdominal pains, and whether you have chronic diarrhea or constipation. If you have persistent symptoms, you should be referred to a gastroenterologist for further evaluation.

Certain abnormalities can be detected only with laboratory tests. A complete blood count (CBC) will show if you have anemia. Some clinics for cancer survivors test serum total protein and albumin levels every couple of years to check for liver and kidney disease and nutritional deficiencies.

Medical, surgical, and nutritional management of GI problems

Diet and nutrition. Many GI problems require low-fat, gluten-free, lactose-free, or low-residue diets. These are best undertaken under the guidance of a gastroenterologist and nutritionist.

GALLSTONES

An uncommon late effect after treatment for childhood cancer is *gallstones*, which are solid lumps of cholesterol or bilirubin that form in the gall bladder. Survivors who are most likely to develop gallstones are those who had abdominal radiation, stem cell transplants, and have cirrhosis of the liver.

Some people with gallstones are *asymptomatic* (having no symptoms), and the gallstones are discovered in routine x-rays. Asymptomatic gallstones are usually not treated. However, if a gallstone blocks a bile duct, then pain develops in the mid-right abdomen or upper right abdomen.

Other symptoms include fever, nausea, vomiting, and clay-colored stools.

If you have these symptoms, you should see your healthcare provider immediately. Gallstones are usually diagnosed with an abdominal ultrasound or CT scan. In the past, open surgery was done to remove the gall bladder. Now, the gall bladder is removed using laparoscopic surgery, which uses smaller incisions and usually results in a much shorter hospital stay.

REFERENCES

Bardi E, Mulder RL, van Dalen EC, et al. (2021). Late hepatic toxicity surveillance for survivors of childhood, adolescent and young adult cancer: Recommendations from the international late effects of childhood cancer guideline harmonization group. *Cancer Treatment Reviews*, 100, 102296. https://doi.org/10.1016/j.ctrv.2021.102296

Castellino S, Muir A, Shah A, et al. (2010). Hepato-biliary late effects in survivors of child-hood and adolescent cancer: a report from the Children's Oncology Group. Pediatr Blood Cancer. 2010 May;54(5):663-9. doi: 10.1002/pbc.22265.

Children's Oncology Group. (2023). Long-Term Follow-Up Guidelines for Survivors of Childhood, Adolescent, and Young Adult Cancers, v. 6. (www.survivorshipguidelines.org)

Strasser SI, Sullivan KM, Myerson D, et al. (1999) Cirrhosis of the liver in long-term mar-row transplant survivors. Blood. 1999 May 15;93(10):3259-66. PMID: 10233877

U.S. Centers for Disease Control (CDC)
www.cdc.gov/hepatitis/php/npr-2024/overview
www.cdc.gov/hepatitis-surveillance-2022

RESOURCES

Website: ccgresources.org
All resources and references mentioned in this book are available on the website and will be routinely reviewed and updated.

Children's Oncology Group. (V6, 2023). *Long-Term Follow-Up Guidelines for Survivors of Childhood, Adolescent, and Young Adult Cancers*
Website: www.survivorshipguidelines.org
Individual **Health Links**, search **Gastrointestinal System** topics: *gastrointestinal health, hepatitis, and liver health*

American Liver Foundation
Website: www.liverfoundation.org
Phone: 1-800-465-4837

Centers for Disease Control and Prevention, Viral Hepatitis
Website: https://www.cdc.gov/hepatitis
Phone: 1-800-CDC-INFO (1-800-232-4636)

GLOSSARY

ALT, a blood test to check the impact of cancer treatment or poten-tial damage to the liver

AST, a blood test to check the impact of cancer treatment or poten-tial damage to the liver

bilirubin test, a blood test to check the impact of cancer treatment or potential damage to the liver

acute HCV, hepatitis C that develops suddenly then goes away after the body successfully fights it off

adhesions, bands of scar tissue that cause surfaces of structures that are usually separate to stick together *asymptomatic,* not showing any symptoms

chronic enterocolitis, long-lasting inflammation of the intestines

chronic graft versus-host disease (GVHD), after stem cell transplant when the bone marrow or stem cells provided by the donor (*graft*) attack the tissues and organ of the child receiving the transplant (*host*). GVHD may be acute or chronic. Acute GVHD occurs within the first 100 days after the transplant, while chronic GVHD occurs or persists after day 100.

cirrhosis, severe scarring of the liver, a serious condition caused by many forms of liver diseases and conditions, such as hepatitis or chronic alcoholism

fibrosis, excessive formation of scar tissue in the liver

gallstones, solid lumps of cholesterol or bilirubin that form in the gall bladder

gastroenterologist, medical doctor specializing in digestive diseases and disorders

iron chelation therapy, medication taken by mouth or injected by healthcare provider which removes extra iron from your body

iron overload (hemochromatosis), when the body stores too much iron which can cause damage to your liver, heart and pancreas and needs to be treated as soon as possible

liver fibrosis, excessive formation of scar tissue in the liver

malabsorption, difficulty in the digestion or absorption of nutrients from food

palpate, to examine by feeling with the hand

reflux, backward flow of food and stomach acid into the esophagus ("food tube")

serum ferritin test, a blood test that measures the amount of ferritin (blood protein that contains iron) in the blood and is a check for iron-deficiency anemia

small bowel obstruction, blockage of the small intestine

stricture, narrowing

therapeutic phlebotomy, when blood is removed from your body (by healthcare provider by needle and tube) to rid blood of excess iron; this is repeated frequently and you need regular blood tests to monitor the amount of iron in your blood

17

Immune System

JOANNE QUILLEN, MSN, APRN, PNP-BC

The courage of life is often a less dramatic spectacle than the courage of the final moment; but it is no less a magnificent mixture of triumph and tragedy.
— *John Fitzgerald Kennedy, Profiles in Courage*

THE IMMUNE SYSTEM is the body's defense against harmful organisms and substances. It is made up of a variety of cells, organs, and systems, ranging from individual white cells to the entire lymphatic system. One of its primary functions is to fight infectious diseases such as influenza and the common cold. The immune system identifies foreign substances and neutralizes, eliminates, or breaks them down into harmless components.

Radiation, chemotherapy, stem cell transplantation, and removal of the spleen can result in decreased immune function (called *immunosuppression*) and decreased production of blood cells (called *myelosuppression*).

SPLEEN AND LYMPHATIC SYSTEM

The spleen is part of the *lymphatic system*—a body-wide network of vessels and organs. The tonsils, thymus, and spleen are organs composed of lymphoid tissue. The tonsils, located in the back of the throat, filter and destroy bacteria. The thymus, a small organ beneath the breastbone, plays a role in helping white blood cells mature. The spleen is an organ in the upper abdomen that has several important functions which include filtering old red blood cells, white blood cells, and platelets from the blood. It also stores red blood cells and performs other important functions of the immune system. **Figure 17-1** shows the various parts of the lymphatic system.

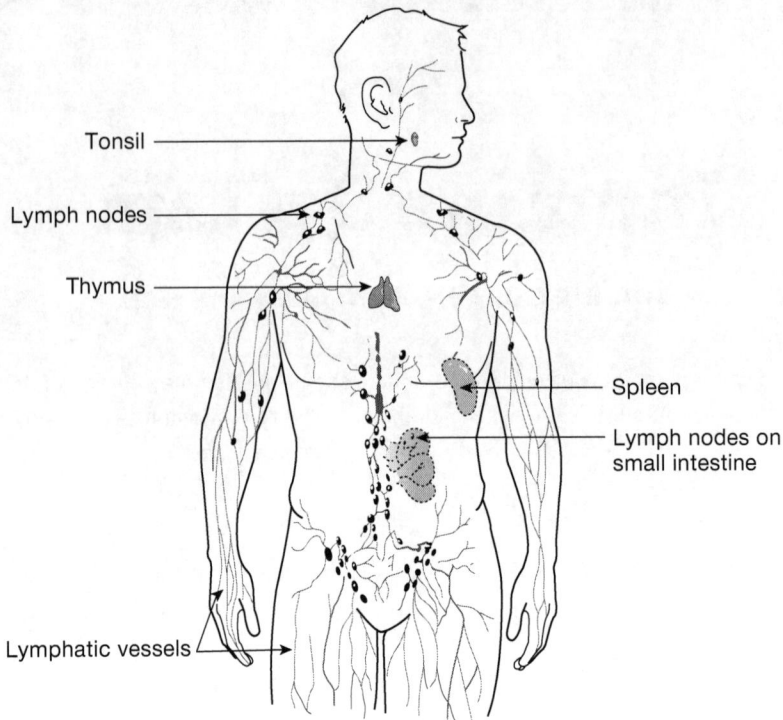

FIGURE 17-1. The lymphatic system (©*Alex's Lemonade Stand Foundation, 2025*)

Damage to the spleen and immune system

Much is still not known about immune status and risk of infections in childhood cancer survivors. By far, the best-documented threats to the body's immune system are removal of the spleen or high-dose (4000 centigray [cGy] or more) radiation to the abdomen. In the past, both of these treatments have been used to treat thousands of children and adolescents with Hodgkin lymphoma. It is not standard treatment today to remove the spleen, although some survivors may have experienced this due to other medical reasons. Patients with solid tumors are also sometimes treated with high-dose radiation to the spleen. In this book, the term *asplenia* refers to either the absence of the spleen or a spleen that no longer functions after high-dose radiation.

Susceptibility to infection is also a problem for survivors treated for chronic graft-versus-host disease (GVHD) after a stem cell transplant (e.g., bone marrow, cord blood, or peripheral blood). The doses of total body radiation used to prepare children for transplantation do not destroy the spleen, although they do destroy bone marrow function. This is discussed later in the *Bone Marrow* section of the chapter.

Signs and symptoms of deficient immune system

Susceptibility to viral and bacterial infections is the hallmark of survivors with lowered immunity due to asplenia. These infections can progress rapidly and, in some cases, are life-threatening. Signs and symptoms of infection may vary among survivors, but the most common are as follows:

- Fever
- Sore throat
- Cough
- Shortness of breath
- Enlarged lymph glands
- Fatigue
- Chills
- Red vesicles that break open, then crust over (i.e., chicken pox)
- Red vesicles that travel in lines along the paths of nerves (i.e., shingles)

Screening and detection

Survivors without spleens or with nonfunctional, irradiated spleens need an annual exam that includes a detailed history of infections and illnesses. Methods to screen for and detect infections that require antibiotics and/or hospitalization should be part of a plan that you and your healthcare provider work out.

Medical management

Survivors with asplenia are at increased risk for bacterial infections that overwhelm the immune system very quickly. Infections with certain types of bacteria can become life-threatening in a matter of hours. For this reason, children with asplenia are given daily preventive penicillin (or erythromycin if they are allergic to penicillin) and their parents are told to call the doctor immediately if the child develops a fever of 101°F (38.3°C) or higher. The Children's Oncology Group's (COG's) guidelines recommend that survivors with a temperature above 101°F (38.3°C) be given a long-acting, broad-spectrum antibiotic (e.g., ceftriaxone) and be closely monitored while awaiting the results of blood cultures.

If you are an adult survivor with asplenia, your follow-up program will likely instruct you to call your healthcare provider immediately if you develop a fever higher than 101°F (38.3°C). Because bacterial infections are very dangerous for survivors who have asplenia, you will be prescribed long-acting, broad-spectrum antibiotics even before tests show what type of organism your body is fighting.

You should have a thorough discussion with your primary care provider when you are well about her approach to dealing with patients with asplenia. You should have a plan to follow in case of illness and fever.

For additional information about testing and intervention for asplenia, you and your healthcare provider can refer to the COG's survivorship guidelines at www.survivorshipguidelines.org. On homepage, under Health Links, see *Immune System:Splenic Precautions*.

Because fevers can develop any time, such as when you are on vacation or traveling for business, make a plan for dealing with illness when away from home. One way to do this is to carry a wallet card with pertinent information about your history and risk and/or wear a medical alert emblem (see **Figure 17-2**, Wallet card for patients without a functioning spleen).

The following are additional suggestions for survivors with asplenia:
- Get the pneumococcal vaccine (prevents some types of pneumonia)
- Get the Hib vaccine (to prevent Hemophilus influenza B)
- Get the meningococcal vaccine (to prevent meningitis)
- Get the annual flu vaccine
- Make sure your healthcare providers know you don't have a functioning spleen before you have dental work or an invasive procedure such as a colonoscopy

Physician Phone: _____

Physician Name: _____

Patient Name: _____

Asplenic Patient

MEDICAL ALERT

MEDICAL ALERT: Asplenic Patient

This patient is asplenic and at risk for potentially fatal, overwhelming infection. Immediate medical attention is required for fever of ≥101°F (38.3°C) or other signs of serious illness. Suggested management includes:

1. Physical exam, CBC and blood culture.

2. Administration of a long-acting broad-spectrum parenteral antibiotic (e.g., ceftriaxone) accompanied by close clinical monitoring while awaiting blood culture result.

3. Hospitalization and broadening of antimicrobial coverage (e.g., addition of vancomycin) may be necessary under certain circumstances, such as the presence of marked leukocytosis, neutropenia, or significant change from baseline CBC; toxic clinical appearance; ≥104°F; meningitis, pneumonia, or other serious focus of infection, signs of septic shock, or previous history of serious infection.

FIGURE 17-2. Wallet medical alert card for patients without a functioning spleen. *Source:* Long-Term Follow-Up Guidelines for Survivors of Childhood, Adolescent, and Young Adult Cancers, Version 6.0 (October 2023). http://www.survivorshipguidelines.org/ Healthlinks, Immune System: Splenic Precautions.

LYMPH NODES

The lymphatic system is composed of vessels, nodes, and organs. Lymph vessels are delicate tubes that branch, like blood vessels, into all parts of the body. They carry lymph—a thin, colorless fluid that contains white blood cells called lymphocytes. Throughout the network of vessels are groups of small, densely packed areas of tissue called *lymph nodes*. Clusters of lymph nodes are found in the neck, underarms, and abdomen. White blood cells are stored in lymph nodes, and from there they are sent out to attack substances or organisms they identify as foreign to the body. To maintain blood volume, the fluid that routinely leaks from capillaries is collected by the lymphatic system, cleaned, and returned to the circulatory system. Two ducts under the collarbone connect the lymphatic system with large veins in the circulatory system (see **Figure 17-1**). Muscular contractions move lymph through the vessels, and one-way valves direct the flow.

Damage to lymphatic system

Some children and teens with cancer have lymph nodes removed for biopsy. In some cases, this can result in permanent late effects, such as:

- **Hydrocele.** Occurs when fluid collects in the scrotum (most often in males who had abdominal surgery).
- **Lymphedema.** Occurs when lymph backs up into an extremity, causing swelling, pain, and loss of function (very rare with modern therapy).
- **Impotence.** Occurs in males when lymph node removal or radiation interferes with the nerves that control erections (very rare with modern therapy).
- **Ejaculation problems.** Occurs in males who had a radical pelvic lymph node dissection (very rare with modern therapy).

Lymphedema in survivors is generally caused by obstruction due to infection or scar tissue. The most common locations are in the pelvis and legs, or under the arms. Extensive information about lymphedema is available online at the National Cancer Institute's website at www.cancer.gov (In drop down, select, *side effects*, then select, *lymphedema*) and the National Lymphedema Network's site at www.lymphnet.org.

Impotence, hydrocele, and problems with ejaculation are covered in *Chapter 15, Kidneys, Bladder, and Genitals*.

Signs and symptoms

Signs and symptoms of lymphedema are as follows:

- Limb feels full or heavy
- Skin feels tight
- Affected area feels painful and hot
- Limb has decreased flexibility
- Limb has swelling
- Indentations remain in skin when it is pressed (early in the process)

If untreated, the area can become very swollen and the tissues may harden.

Screening and detection

If you have lymphedema, your healthcare provider should take a history and do a careful evaluation of the involved areas. The history should include information about surgeries, radiation, infection, and when the lymphedema started. The circumference of the limb should be measured and circulation checked. Bring a list of your medications to show your healthcare provider, as other medical conditions such as diabetes, kidney problems, high blood pressure, congestive heart failure, or liver disease may contribute to the problem.

Medical management

Medical management of lymphedema includes treatments such as the following:

- Keeping the affected limb raised
- Wearing custom-fitted clothes that apply a uniform pressure
- Using manual lymphatic drainage

Healthcare providers should educate you about additional ways to prevent or control lymphedema, such as the following:

- Proper skin care
- Diet
- Exercise

- Ways to avoid injury or infection (for example, no blood drawing from the affected limb)

BONE MARROW

Bone marrow, the spongy material that fills the long bones in the body, is a blood-forming tissue. It produces white blood cells (which fight infection and disease), red cells (which carry oxygen and nutrients to body tissues), and platelets (which help form clots to stop bleeding). Decreases in cell production can cause lowered immune function, anemia, or bleeding problems.

Damage to bone marrow

Radiation to the bone marrow can affect blood cell production long after treatment ends. The amount of damage depends on the radiation dose and the amount of bone marrow in the radiation field.

Chemotherapy can also cause long-term effects in bone marrow function. Although the blood counts of most survivors return to normal within weeks after therapy ends, a few survivors treated with chemotherapy have problems with low blood counts for years after treatment.

Children who have undergone a stem cell transplant have lowered immune system function for months after treatment. The bone marrow of these children has been destroyed by chemotherapy and/or radiation to allow the healthy marrow or stem cells to grow. Re-establishing the immune function takes time. All stem cell transplant recipients have profound impairment of the immune system for up to a year. Transplant teams give families specific instructions about ways to prevent infections during that time.

Graft-versus-host disease

Graft-versus-host disease (GVHD) occurs when the bone marrow or stem cells provided by the donor (graft) attack the tissues and organs of the child receiving the transplant (host). It is a frequent complication of stem cell transplants when stem cells come from a donor (*allogeneic*). It does not occur in transplants when stem cells come from the patient's own body (*autologous*) or when stem cells come from the patient's identical twin (*syngeneic*). There are two types: **acute GVHD** and **chronic GVHD**.

Acute GVHD occurs within the first 100 days and chronic GVHD occurs or persists after day 100. Patients can develop one type, both types, or neither one. Approximately 30-50% of survivors who have a related human leukocyte antigens (HLA)-matched transplant develop some degree of GVHD. The incidence and severity of GVHD are increased for children or teens who receive unrelated or mismatched marrow, but are decreased if cells that cause GVHD are reduced prior to infusion. The majority of GVHD cases are mild, although some can be life-threatening.

> **Chicken pox and/or shingles can pose a threat to life if they are contracted when a child or teen is immunosuppressed.**

Chronic GVHD delays the return of normal immune function. Even when survivors with chronic GVHD have normal numbers of T and B cells, they may still be at risk for infection. Up to one-third of survivors with chronic GVHD develop serious, life-threatening infections.

Signs and symptoms of graft-versus-host disease

GVHD primarily affects the following parts of the body:

- Skin (itchy rash, discoloration or tightening of the skin, hair loss)
- Eyes (dryness, light sensitivity)
- Mouth and esophagus (dryness, tooth decay, difficulty swallowing)
- Intestines (diarrhea, cramping, weight loss)
- Liver (jaundice)
- Lungs (shortness of breath, wheezing, coughing)
- Joints (decreased mobility)
- Delayed immune response

Signs and symptoms of infection in those with delayed immune response

Children or teens who underwent autologous stem cell transplants (stem cells from their own body) do not develop GVHD, but they can have a *delayed immune response*. The signs and symptoms of infection are fevers, sore throat, and shortness of breath, often accompanied by fatigue. However, fatigue by itself is not a symptom of infection.

Chicken pox and/or shingles can pose a threat to life if they are contracted when a child or teen is immunosuppressed.

Screening and detection

Survivors of stem cell transplantations receive a multitude of tests that evaluate immune system function. Your institution will have its own list of tests and schedules, but it should include tests for both immune function and GVHD.

Medical management (after transplant)

Stem cell transplant survivors with GVHD may be treated with *corticosteroids* (known as steroids and which are used to treat inflammation) and other medications. All stem cell transplant survivors get *prophylactic antibiotics* (antibiotics given to prevent future possible infection) for at least 6 to 12 months, and those with chronic GVHD continue to take antibiotics until all GVHD therapy has ended. If the survivor has low levels of *immunoglobulin G (IgG)* (a type of antibody that helps prevent infection), she may get monthly IV IgG until her serum levels are normal for 2 months.

Prior immunizations are no longer effective after stem cell transplantation. Each treating institution has its own schedule for re-immunizing children and teens. Generally, survivors with no GVHD are given inactivated polio, influenza, and DPT (diphtheria-pertussis-tetanus) immunization after the first year. The MMR (measles-mumps-rubella) vaccine is usually given after the second year (survivors with GVHD do not receive the MMR). Find out when you (or your child) should get each immunization and talk with a healthcare provider about ways to avoid exposure to diseases until you are fully immunized. You also need to know how the treating institution manages chicken pox and shingles after a transplant.

Medical management (after treatment for any cancer)
Vaccines and Immunization:
Children who were treated when very young often miss immunizations and need to get them after treatment ends and their immune systems return to normal. Different institutions have different recommended schedules for re-immunizations. For example, your survivor's clinic may ask about immunization status and, if any are missing, advise that your child's pediatrician update them based on the Centers for Disease Control and Prevention (CDC) immunization schedules (www.cdc.gov/vaccines/hcp/imz-schedules/child-adolescent-age.html). The U.S. guidelines recommend re-immunization no sooner than 3 months after standard chemotherapy and no sooner than 12 months after a stem cell transplant. Both girls and boys are advised to receive the human papillomavirus (HPV) vaccine based on current recommendations. Parents should check with their child's treating institution to find out the preferred immunization schedule for their child.

> **Chemotherapy and radiation used to treat any childhood cancer can render prior immunizations ineffective.**

Chemotherapy and radiation used to treat any childhood cancer can render prior immunizations ineffective. More research is needed to better understand whether patients should be screened for antibodies against vaccine antigens (meaning whether immunizations given prior to treatment are still effective).

REFERENCES

Bisharat N, Omari H, Lavi I, Raz R. (2001). Risk of infection and death among post-splenectomy patients. *J Infect*. 2001 Oct;43(3):182-6. doi: 10.1053/jinf.2001.0904. PMID: 11798256.

Children's Oncology Group. (2023). *Long-Term Follow-Up Guidelines for Survivors of Childhood, Adolescent, and Young Adult Cancers*, v. 6 (www.survivorshipguidelines.org).

Chisholm JC. (2007). Reimmunization after therapy for childhood cancer. *Clin Infect Dis*. 2007 Mar 1;44(5):643-5. doi: 10.1086/511650. Epub 2007 Jan 24. PMID: 17278053.

Guilcher GMT, Rivard L, Huang JT, et al. (2021) Immune function in childhood cancer survivors: a Children's Oncology Group review. *Lancet Child Adolesc Health*. 2021 Apr;5(4):284-294. doi: 10.1016/S2352-4642(20)30312-6. Epub 2021 Feb 16. PMID: 33600774; PMCID: PMC8725381

Horwitz ME, Sullivan KM. (2006). Chronic graft-versus-host disease. *Blood Rev*. 2006 Jan;20(1):15-27. doi: 10.1016/j.blre.2005.01.007. Epub 2005 Apr 7. PMID: 16426941.

U.S. Centers for Disease Control and Prevention, *Human Papillomavirus* (www.cdc.gov/hpv/).

Van Tilburg CM, Sanders EA, Rovers MM, et al. (2006). Loss of antibodies and response to (re-) vaccination in children after treatment for acute lymphocytic leukemia: a systematic review. *Leukemia*. 2006 Oct;20(10):1717-22. doi: 10.1038/sj.leu.2404326. Epub 2006 Aug 3. PMID: 16888619.

RESOURCES

Website: ccgresources.org
All resources and references mentioned in this book are available on the website and will be routinely reviewed and updated.

Children's Oncology Group. (V6, 2023). *Long-Term Follow-Up Guidelines for Survivors of Childhood, Adolescent, and Young Adult Cancers*
Website: www.survivorshipguidelines.org
Under **Healthlinks**: *immune system, splenic precautions*

National Cancer Institute
Website at www.cancer.gov
Click, *About cancer, side effects, lymphedema*

National Lymphedema Network
Website: www.lymphnet.org

Passport for Care, Survivor Care Plans by Children's Oncology Group (V6, Nov 2023)
Website: https://cancersurvivor.passportforcare.org
Survivors and family can find online updated tailored long-term care plans which should be reviewed with their oncologist or health care provider.

U.S. Centers for Disease Control and Prevention
Website: www.cdc.gov
Search, *Immunization schedules for children and adolescents* or *vaccines and immunizations*

GLOSSARY

allogeneic stem cell transplant, when stem cells used for a transplant come from a donor

asplenia, the absence of the spleen or a spleen that no longer functions after high-dose radiation and results in deficient immune system

autologous stem cell transplant, when stem cells used for a transplant come from the patient's (host) own body

corticosteroids, medication used to enhance the body's ability to fight inflammation/infection; also known as steroids

ejaculation, sudden release of semen from the penis from sexual stimulation

graft-versus-host-disease (GVHD), a frequent complication of allogeneic stem cell transplants, when the bone marrow or stem cells provided by the donor (*graft*) attack the tissues and organ of the child receiving the transplant (*host*). GVHD may be acute or chronic. Acute GVHD occurs within the first 100 days after the transplant, while chronic GVHD occurs or persists after day 100.

hematopoietic stem cell transplant (HPSCT) also known as *stem cell transplant,* formerly known as bone marrow transplant, this procedure involves administering healthy stem cells (e.g., bone marrow, cord blood, or peripheral blood) to patients after the bone marrow has been destroyed by disease, chemotherapy (chemo), or radiation.

hydrocele, occurs when fluid collects in the scrotum (most often in males who had abdominal surgery).

immunoglobulin G (IgG), a type of antibody that helps prevent infection

immunosuppression, decreased immune function

impotence, often called erectile dysfunction is the inability for a male to achieve or maintain an erection long enough to engage in sexual intercourse

lymph nodes, small dense areas of tissue in the body's lymph system that store white blood cells (lymphocytes) which are sent throughout the body to fight infection or other substances/organisms identified as foreign to the body *lymphatic system,* a body-wide network of vessels, tissues and organs that play a critical role to help regulate fluid balance and protect the body from infection by filtering out pathogens

lymphedema, occurs when lymph backs up into an extremity, causing swelling, pain, and loss of function (very rare with modern therapy)

myelosuppression, decreased production of blood cells

prophylactic, intervention/medication given to help prevent an infection or other adverse reaction

prophylactic antibiotics, antibiotics given to prevent future possible infection

spleen, an organ in the upper abdomen that removes old red blood cells and platelets from the blood and also stores red blood cells and performs other important functions of the immune system.

stem cell transplant also known as *hematopoietic stem cell transplant (HPSCT)*, a procedure that involves administering healthy hematopoietic stem cells (e.g., bone marrow, cord blood, or peripheral blood) to patients after the bone marrow has been destroyed by disease, chemotherapy (chemo), or radiation.

syngeneic stem cell transplant, when stem cells used for a transplant come from the patient's (host) identical twin (donor)

thymus, a small organ beneath the breastbone that plays a role in helping white blood cells mature

tonsils, this tissue located in the back of the throat are part of the lymphatic system and function to help filter and destroy bacteria.

18
Muscles and Bones

LISA BASHORE, PhD, APRN, CPNP-PC, CPON

There are only two ways to live your life. One is as though nothing is a miracle. The other is as though everything is a miracle.
— *Albert Einstein*

CANCER SURVIVORS MAY experience a number of complications to their muscles and bones. Radiation and surgery can alter both the appearance and function of any part of the body. This chapter discusses the major late effects to the muscles and bones from amputation, limb-salvage procedures, radiation, and chemotherapy. It covers *osteonecrosis, osteoporosis, osteoarthritis*, and changes in body shape and size. Signs and symptoms, screening and detection, and medical management of these late effects also are presented.

MUSCLES

The muscles, together with other connective tissues (tendons and cartilage), form the support system for the skeleton. The muscular system enables body movement through a process of contraction and relaxation.

Damage to the muscles

Hypoplasia, or underdevelopment of soft tissue, is the most common late effect of radiation on muscles and soft tissue. Muscles that have been radiated do not grow as large or as strong as muscles that have not been radiated. For some survivors, hypoplasia is a problem more of appearance than function. For survivors who had high-dose radiation many years ago, the weakening of bone and muscle increases with age and can severely impact quality of life.

If you had radiation to one side of the body while you were growing, you may have less muscle and fat tissue in the areas that were irradiated. This can result in the side of your body that was irradiated appearing less developed compared to the side that was not treated. The difference in appearance between the two sides of your body is called *asymmetry*. The more weight you gain, the more noticeable the difference may become.

Some survivors who had radiation to muscle groups have persistent problems with muscle tone. Occasionally, lack of exercise during years of treatment can also cause loss of muscle tone.

Signs and symptoms of muscle damage

Signs and symptoms of hypoplasia (underdevelopment):

- Decreased muscle mass
- Asymmetry of muscle mass of treated and untreated areas
- Decreased range of motion
- Decreased strength of affected muscles
- Stiffness and pain

Follow-up screening and detection of muscle damage

An evaluation of late effects to the muscles includes a visual inspection of all muscle groups, looking for asymmetry, swelling, *atrophy* (wasting or thinning of muscle mass), *fibrosis* (scarring and thickening of muscle tissue), and strength.

Follow-up monitoring by your provider should include:

- careful measurements and comparisons of irradiated and untreated areas
- evaluation of tone, size, and strength for all muscle groups
- range of motion evaluated for affected muscle groups in arms or legs

You should discuss your ability to participate in daily activities such as going to work or school and taking care of your home. Talk about any limitations such as problems walking up stairs. Tell your healthcare provider about what types of exercise you do and how often. If you have late effects to the muscles that alter your appearance, discuss whether this affects your life in any way. Comprehensive care includes helping you adapt to changes in your body's appearance.

> I had physical and occupational therapy during the two years I received treatment. Because I slept most of the time, I lost strength in my legs and the rest of my body and had to use a walker, cane, and wheelchair. From two years of chemotherapy and steroids, I have developed avascular necrosis. This happens when the blood supply to your bones is cut off. As a result, my bone cartilage is deteriorating, leaving my joints to rub and bang together which is very painful. I have to get three joint replacement surgeries, one for each hip and one for my right shoulder.

Medical management of muscle damage

Reversal of late effects to the muscles isn't possible, but trying to prevent worsening is. The primary way to do this is through a reasonable exercise program that works for you and improves your range of motion and muscle strength. A physical therapist can help you design an individualized program to suit your needs.

BODY SIZE AND WEIGHT

Heights of survivors can be affected by radiation to the spine or alterations in hormone production (*Chapter 10, Hormone-Producing Glands*). Changes in body weight also can occur in small numbers of survivors. Long-term weight loss can be caused by malabsorption and other gastrointestinal problems (*Chapter 16, Liver, Stomach, and Intestines*). At the other extreme, some studies show that a percentage of survivors become obese.

Some studies show that survivors who were treated with doses of 1800 centigray (cGy) or more of cranial radiation have an increased likelihood of being obese. Risk factors include higher cranial radiation dose, surgical location, pre-cancer history of growth hormone deficiency, hypothyroidism, hypogonadism, not able to exercise (Children's Oncology Group, *Long-Term Follow-Up Guidelines for Survivors of Child, Adolescent, and Young Adult Cancers*, Version 6 (October 2023) Section 52, Overweight; Obesity (www.survivorshipguidelines.org)

Follow-up screening and detection for monitoring growth

Monitoring growth includes plotting your height and weight on a chart at regular intervals. Measurements should be taken every 2 to 3 months during therapy and for the first year after therapy, and then once or twice a year until growth is complete. Abnormalities in weight or height require a consultation with an *endocrinologist* or *gastroenterologist* experienced in treating survivors of childhood cancer. An endocrinologist is a doctor who specializes in the glands in the body that produce hormones and can diagnose and manage problems in their function. A gastroenterologist is a doctor who specializes in identifying and treating problems with the body's gastrointestinal system (the esophagus, stomach, small intestine, colon and rectum, pancreas, gallbladder, bile ducts, and liver).

For more information about growth, see *Chapter 10, Hormone-Producing Glands.*

Medical management of body size and weight issues

If you are underweight or overweight, you need a consultation with a medical specialist, such as a gastroenterologist or endocrinologist, as mentioned above. Growth hormone deficiency results in lack of full growth potential and also should be addressed. A discussion with a dietitian can also be very helpful in planning a healthy diet. A plan for weight loss usually includes an increase in exercise and changes in diet. Family participation in physical activities also helps survivors maintain a normal body weight.

> I now have been diagnosed with autoimmune disease which affects my muscles/joints and nerves. I take steroids to help that. I have myasthenia gravis which causes communication breakdown between the nerves and muscles, and my muscles feel weak and get tired easily. My eye-sight is blurry and my eyes droop. I do see a neurologist to help treat/manage it.

BONES

The human skeleton contains 206 bones, all held in place by connective tissues such as ligaments and tendons. The skeleton gives structure to the body and protects the internal organs. Bones determine our size and shape. The skeleton also works as a factory, making various blood cells in the marrow of the bones. Bones also store minerals such as calcium and phosphorus for use by the body.

The structure of bones changes as children grow. The skeleton of the fetus in the womb is made up mostly of cartilage. As pregnancy continues, bone develops, but even when the child is born, there are still areas that are a combination of bone and cartilage. At the end of long bones, such as those in the arms and legs, there are growth plates. *Growth plates* are where new bone growth occurs and have a high level of activity until the child stops growing, usually around 13 to 15 years for girls and 15 to 17 years for boys.

Damage to the bones

Survivors of childhood cancer can develop a number of complications that involve the skeleton. These can be caused by surgery, radiation, and/or chemotherapy.

Amputation

If a malignant tumor extends to vital structures such as major nerves and blood vessels, then *amputation* (surgical removal of a limb) may be necessary. The missing limb will be replaced by an artificial body part, known as a *prosthesis*. Survivors who had only the lower parts of leg extremities (below the knee) amputated usually function well after rehabilitation, though functional and physical activities could be impaired by poorly fitted prostheses or pain. Upper or lower limb amputees may experience psychological problems and impaired quality of life that require professional support. Generally, amputees can ski, run, hike, and perform other physical skills very well.

One major decision I made with my parents was to choose a below-the-knee amputation instead of a second bone-salvage surgery. When first diagnosed, my treatment plan laid out by my oncologist and surgeon consisted of eight rounds of chemo, a bone-salvage surgery to remove my tibia (where the tumor was) and replace it with a donor bone, and then 10 more rounds

(Continued)

(*Continued*)

of chemo following the surgery. A year after completing that treatment, the donor bone broke. My surgeon insisted that I undergo another bone-salvage surgery. This would have led to another 24-hour surgery, taking muscles and bone from other parts of my body to try and recover some semblance of function in my left leg, and this would still result in severe physical impairment for the rest of my life.

As an 11-year-old girl, I started doing independent research into other options. I discovered that amputation, while traumatic, would result in far better quality of life and allow me to go back to doing the things I loved, like dance and being active like a normal kid. My family and I decided to choose amputation below the knee, instead of the second bone-salvage surgery, and convinced my care team, even though it was not the original plan they hoped for.

Making these decisions and advocating for myself was never easy, but in the end resulted in the best quality of life for me. Fortunately, my support system and especially my parents allowed me to be a part of those decisions and gave me the confidence to continue to vocalize my needs and opinions when it comes to my continued long-term care.

These survivors may experience pain in the missing limb even though the limb is no longer present (known as *phantom pain*) and develop problems with calluses or pain in the stump. Those who had entire limbs removed or other portions of the skeleton removed (such as the pelvis) sometimes have ongoing problems with function and pain. Survivors requiring a *hemipelvectomy* (removal of all or part of the hemipelvis and the entire lower extremity) may have more functional problems.

The Amputee Coalition of America (ACA) provides extensive information about organizations and resources for amputees. https://www.amputee-coalition.org

Limb-salvage procedures

Growing numbers of survivors have *limb-salvage procedures* as an alternative to amputation. These procedures help save the limb by removing the part of the bone that is involved with the tumor. The bone is replaced with either a bone graft or a metal prosthesis. Another limb salvage procedure, known as *rotationplasty*, spares part of the lower leg so that the ankle can be rotated and used as a knee; below it, a prosthetic lower leg is surgically attached. In many cases, these surgeries are very successful, and the survivor's limb works very well. Other survivors require multiple surgeries and cope with pain, infection, and functional and physical activity limitations.

Limb radiation

Radiation to a limb will impact growth if a child has not completed puberty. If the growth plate is included in the field of radiation, the untreated limb will continue to grow, creating a length discrepancy in the child's limbs. This can be particularly problematic if the affected limb is a leg. The growth plate of the untreated leg may need to be surgically altered to stop growth to help keep the legs similar lengths.

In some cases, *limb-lengthening procedures* can reduce or correct the discrepancy in length between arms or legs while stretching the surrounding muscles and other soft tissues. This is a more involved process for the child and their family and can take six to nine months. The bone to be lengthened is cut and a lengthening device is surgically inserted between the cuts ends of the bone. In the next step, about a week later, the two ends of bone are slowly separated using the lengthening device. This is done by the family who have been trained by the surgeon how to use the device. This period, which usually takes a couple of months, is closely watched by the clinical team. After the limb has reached the desired length, the body takes over and new bone begins to grow and fill the gap.

Survivors who had radiation to a limb may be at risk for fractures without trauma, and fracture may occur after minor trauma that would otherwise not cause a fracture in an untreated bone. Fractures occur most often in children who received more than 4000 cGy to the bone. However, each survivor is different, so long-term follow-up is important.

Spine radiation

Some children with cancer get their entire spine irradiated. Others have a portion of the spine treated. *Scoliosis,* a sideways curvature of

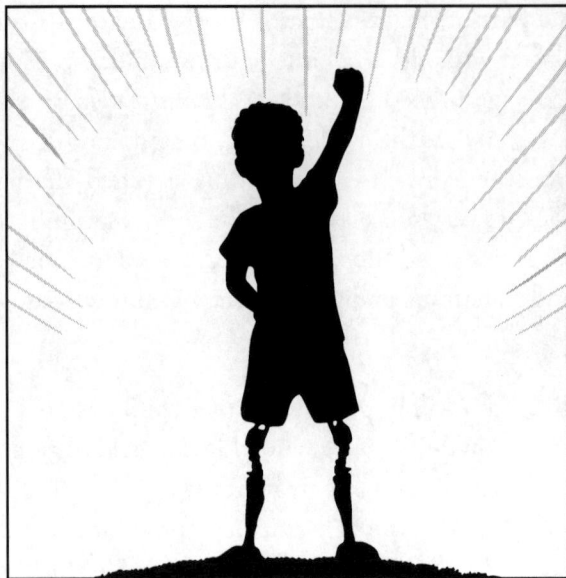

FIGURE 18-1. Survivors can continue to engage in physical activity and recreation, even run, hike, and ski. (©*Alex's Lemonade Stand Foundation, 2025*)

the spine (backbone), can be caused by receiving radiation to only one side of the spine that runs down the midline of the body. When the untreated side of the body continues to grow, the other side does not and the spine curves in the direction of the growing side (see **Figure 18-2**). Thankfully, children treated for cancer after 1990 will have a shorter trunk, but better spinal alignment. The damage is more pronounced for children treated when younger than age 6 years or during the growth spurt of puberty. A survivor whose whole spine was radiated also may develop scoliosis; this is thought to occur because damage to the muscles and soft tissue on the irradiated side of the body pull the spine out of alignment.

Other factors that may increase the risk of developing scoliosis are changes to the spine from tumor, osteoporosis, and the surgical fusion of two parts of the spine to one another to treat pain.

A rare side effect of radiation to portions of the spine is *kyphosis*, where the upper spine curves outward, giving a hunchback appearance. This can occur with scoliosis after radiation to portions of the spine. Severe kyphosis and/or scoliosis can affect the functioning of

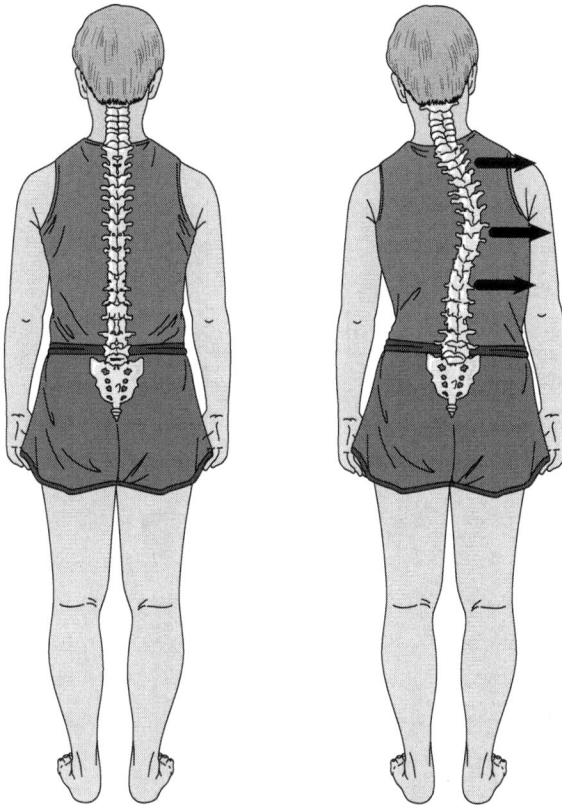

FIGURE 18-2. Scoliosis is curvature of the spine that occurs when one side of the body is irradiated and bones/muscles stop growing on one side of the body while the other side continues to grow causing the spine to shift and curve. (©*Alex's Lemonade Stand Foundation, 2025*)

other organs, such as the lungs, whose capacity can be reduced by the intrusion of the curved spine into the lung cavity.

If radiation to the whole spine is needed, current protocols attempt to spare adjacent tissues to decrease the risk of scoliosis and kyphosis. Better staging of solid tumors has also decreased the number of children and adolescents who require radiation. Radiation to the whole spine can stop or slow the growth of the spine. A short trunk (measured from the top of the head to the rump) occurs most often in brain tumor survivors whose entire spines were radiated with more than 3500 cGy. Total body radiation given prior to stem cell transplantation (i.e., bone marrow, stem cell, or cord blood) can also affect the growth of the spine, as well as growth of other bones exposed to radiation.

Osteochondromas are outgrowths of the bone that are sometimes seen in children who were treated with radiation. These bony projections often form where bones meet one another and can also form on the bones of your spine. The outgrowths are also known as *exostoses* (singular form: *exostosis*) and are commonly referred to as bone spurs. Young children who receive total body irradiation (TBI) can develop osteochondromas as they begin puberty. An x-ray is needed to confirm the diagnosis. These growths often do not require intervention. However, in a small number of cases, removal is necessary due to location and discomfort.

Slipped capital femoral epiphysis (SCFE) is a disorder sometimes seen in children whose hip was irradiated. *Epiphysis* refers to the area at the top or head (*capital*) of the long bone of the thigh (femur) where it attaches to the pelvis. It has a wide and rounded shape and fits inside an area of the hip where the pelvic bones form a cup-like space. The epiphysis is separated from the rest of the thigh bone below it by a growth plate. When the growth plate is damaged and weakened by radiation, the head of the femur stays in the cup of the hip joint, but the rest of the thigh bone can "slip" relative to the femoral head. SCFE is often seen at the beginning of the pubertal growth spurt. Survivors who received radiation and who have endocrine dysfunction are at higher risk (Hobbie et al., 2022).

Osteoporosis and osteopenia

Some childhood cancer survivors develop *osteoporosis*, a disease that occurs when the creation of new bone doesn't keep up with the loss of the old bone. When this happens, it causes the bone to lose density and to thin which make it weak, brittle, and more likely to break. This late effect (osteoporosis) is not well understood. It is known that survivors who took high doses of steroids (e.g., prednisone, dexamethasone), received high-dose methotrexate, had cranial radiation, had high-dose radiation to bones, or have low growth hormone seem to be most at risk. Young women who have an early menopause and men with low testosterone production also have a higher risk of developing osteoporosis.

Osteopenia is similar to osteoporosis but not as serious. Like survivors with osteoporosis, those with osteopenia have a lower-than-normal

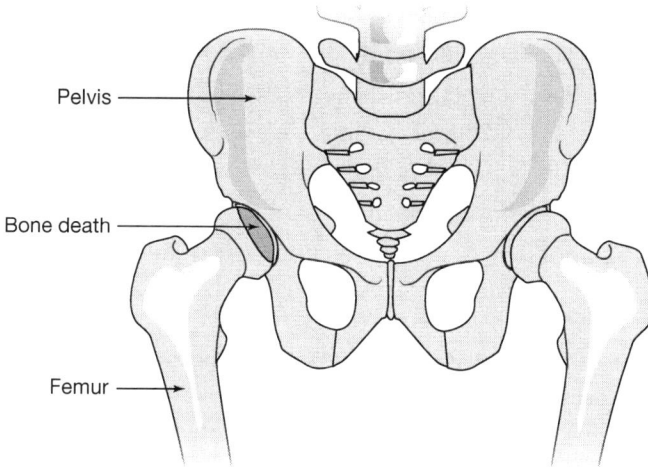

FIGURE 18-3. Osteonecrosis, or bone death, in the hip. (©*Alex's Lemonade Stand Foundation, 2025*)

bone density and experience a thinning and weakening of their bones. While the bones are not as strong as they should be, the loss of bone is not as great as it is in osteoporosis. Osteopenia can develop into osteoporosis.

Osteonecrosis

Osteonecrosis is the death of bone tissue due to a lack of blood supply which can lead to tiny breaks in the bone and cause the bone to collapse (see **Figure 18.3**). Other names for this condition are avascular necrosis (AVN) and ischemic necrosis. It is usually caused by radiation to bones and/or use of high-dose steroids (e.g., prednisone or dexamethasone).

Osteonecrosis is generally seen early rather than late—often within the first year after therapy. Adolescent girls are especially susceptible. Magnetic resonance imaging (MRI) is the best tool for diagnosis. As bone deterioration progresses, the bone may become weak and may eventually collapse. The course of the disease is variable. Some survivors have osteonecrosis for years with only minor problems with pain or movement, while others require surgery soon after diagnosis. Osteonecrosis can be very painful and sometimes leads to osteoarthritis (see below). The website for the Avascular Necrosis Support Group is located at www.facebook.com/groups/AVNInfo/.

Osteoarthritis

Osteoarthritis is a degenerative disease of the joints and occurs when the cartilage that protects and cushions the ends of bones wears down over time. It is characterized by pain with activity that subsides when resting. Survivors who had radiation to joints are at risk. People who have late effects that increase stress on the joints, such as osteonecrosis, may also develop osteoarthritis. Helpful information about arthritis can be found at the Arthritis Foundation's website—www.arthritis.org

Signs and symptoms of damage to the bones

Leg length discrepancy:

- Difference in length and muscle mass between two limbs
- Limping
- Lower back pain
- Hip pain
- Scoliosis

Fractures:

- Pain
- Deformity
- Swelling
- Bruising
- Loss of function

Scoliosis and kyphosis:

- Curved spine
- Uneven shoulder height
- Back or hip pain
- Limping
- Spinal shortening

Osteonecrosis, osteoarthritis, and SCFE:

- Pain in affected joint
- Limping
- Impaired function

Osteochondromas:

- Hard lump on any boney surface
- Possible pain (depending on location)

Osteoporosis and osteopenia usually have no signs or symptoms, and bone density changes might not show up on regular x-rays unless the affected bone gets broken or infected. Advanced osteoporosis can cause the bones in your spine to compress, causing shorter height. It can also cause kyphosis (a hump on the upper part of the back), discussed earlier.

Follow-up screening and detection of bone damage
Amputation or limb salvage
Survivors with amputations need an annual examination of the stump that includes a discussion about whether a prosthesis could be useful. Range of motion and function are evaluated. Survivors who had a limb salvage procedure should have both treated and untreated limbs measured every year (without clothes on to get accurate measurements), usually by an *orthopedic surgeon*. An orthopedic surgeon is a doctor who specializes in diagnosing and treating disorders involving the bones, joints, ligaments, tendons, and muscles, particularly performing surgery. A baseline and then annual x-rays are needed until growth is complete to assess the growth plate. Survivors should also have a discussion with their healthcare provider if they have any back pain, limb pain, limping, or changes in muscle mass.

As a below-the-knee amputee, a critical part to my physical mobility is my prosthesis. Unfortunately, high quality and customized prosthetics are poorly covered by insurance policies in the United States. There really is not a good option that provides amputees with quality prosthetics without paying enormous costs out of pocket for them. I have been very fortunate to have help from my family with covering those out-of-pocket costs to date, but there will come a time where I will be paying 5 figure costs for my prosthesis unless policies change dramatically. This is a huge ongoing issue, and a key focus of many advocates for amputees nationwide.

Scoliosis and kyphosis

A scoliosis check needs to be done every year if you are at risk. Your back will be examined while you bend over with your fingers touching your toes and your knees straight. Kyphosis is often seen on observation, but should be confirmed using X-rays.

If your child had radiation to the spine, several tests should be done to check for spinal abnormalities. Your child should have height checked while both standing and sitting, and the results should be plotted on a chart. Your child's healthcare provider should examine your child's spine every 3 months during puberty until growth is complete, and every year thereafter. A spine x-ray should be obtained for a baseline before puberty, then as needed.

Osteopenia, osteoporosis, and fractures

If you had more than 4000 cGy radiation to any bones, they are at risk for developing osteopenia and osteoporosis which can lead to fractures. Go to your healthcare provider if you have pain, swelling, or bruising in the areas that were irradiated. You may also be at risk if:

- You went into an early menopause (your periods stopped early).
- You are a stem cell transplant survivor who took high doses of steroids.
- You have any ovarian or testicular dysfunction.
- You have growth hormone deficiency.
- You have a family history of osteoporosis.

Discuss your risk with your healthcare provider to see whether you need bone density studies. X-rays or computed tomography (CT) scans may be done to assess the amount of damage.

A painful joint should be evaluated by your healthcare provider. You may need an x-ray or CT scan to check for osteoarthritis and osteonecrosis.

Medical management of bone damage
Amputation or limb salvage

Medical management of amputations includes a visual inspection and checks for range of motion and muscle contractures. You should have your prosthesis checked (if you use one) and have a discussion with your healthcare provider about any advancements in technology.

If you had limb salvage surgery or radiation and one limb is now longer than the other, discuss the treatment plan with your healthcare provider. Small differences in length of less than 2 centimeters (cm) usually don't require any treatment. Differences of 2-6 cm are treated with a shoe lift or surgery to stop the growth of the other limb. If the discrepancy is greater than 6 cm, other surgical steps may be necessary. These include shortening the untreated limb or lengthening the treated leg to restore a comfortable gait.

If you have an *endoprosthesis*, which is an artificial body part that is placed entirely inside your body (such as an artificial hip), you need to take antibiotics prior to dental work to prevent possible infection that could spread to the prosthesis.

Scoliosis and kyphosis

If you have any scoliosis or kyphosis, you should be referred to an orthopedic specialist with experience treating survivors of childhood cancer. If the curvature is noted during a period of rapid growth, such as puberty, do not delay seeing the specialist, because the curvature can increase rapidly during a growth spurt. Long-term survivors who have scoliosis or kyphosis often have back pain.

The following may help make the pain more manageable:
- Physical therapy
- Using a brace
- Moderate exercise
- Pain medication

If the curve in the back progresses (worsens) beyond 30 degrees (or curves 20 degrees with rapid progression), wearing a brace may be necessary. Curves greater than 40 degrees may require surgery. There are no standards for treatment of scoliosis after tumor surgery or radiation; the decision to use a brace or operate is performed based on the survivor's specific needs. Kyphosis treatment includes the use of any pain relievers as needed and exercises to strengthen the musculature around the spine. Possibly bracing may be used, but may not be an option for survivors. Surgical options are reserved for survivors with severe functional impairments.

Osteoporosis or osteopenia

If you have osteopenia or osteoporosis, your yearly examination should include education on the importance of:

- Weight-bearing exercise such as walking or running.
- A diet rich in calcium. This includes dairy products, shellfish, leafy green vegetables, and tofu. Your healthcare provider might also recommend taking supplemental calcium with added vitamin D.
- Adequate vitamin D. Some dairy products are fortified with vitamin D and the body makes some on its own when exposed to sunlight, but many survivors require supplementation. A nutritionist consultation may be helpful especially in the case of food allergies or to determine the best nutritional supplements.

Osteonecrosis

Treatment for osteonecrosis may include:

- Activity modifications
- Range of motion exercises
- Electrical stimulation
- Surgery to remove the inner layer of bone (*core decompression*) that involves drilling into the area of dead bone near the joint to reduce pressure and increase blood flow; sometimes a healthy piece of bone is inserted when the inner layer is removed. This procedure may slow or stop the osteonecrosis.
- Surgery to cut and realign a bone near a damaged joint (*osteotomy*) to reduce the weight bearing of the bone with osteonecrosis
- Pain and/or anti-inflammatory medication

Fractures

If you have a fracture in irradiated bone, most likely the fracture will occur where the bone was biopsied or at the site of tumor in the bone. These types of fractures may need surgery to insert a device to keep the bone aligned. Because the surrounding tissues were also irradiated, this surgery will be challenging. Make sure the surgery is done by an *orthopedic surgeon* with experience operating on irradiated bone and tissues.

Osteochondromas

Osteochondromas are generally noted first by the survivor or a family member. Once the diagnosis is confirmed by x-ray, management will be determined by the symptoms. If there is pain or if the osteochondroma is affecting other bone growth or joint function, a referral to an orthopedist is recommended.

REFERENCES

Children's Oncology Group. (2023). *Long-Term Follow-Up Guidelines for Survivors of Childhood, Adolescent, and Young Adult Cancers*, v. 6. (www.survivorshipguidelines.org)

Fernandez-Pineda I, Hudson, MM, Pappo AS, et al. (2017). Long-term functional outcomes and quality of life in adult survivors of childhood extremity sarcomas: A report from the St. Jude lifetime cohort study. *Journal of Cancer Survivorship, 11*(1), 1-12. https://doi.org/10.1007/s11764-016-0556-1

Hobbie WL, Li Y, Carlson C, Goldfarb S, et al. (2022). Late effects in survivors of high-risk neuroblastoma following stem cell transplant with and without total body irradiation. *Pediatric Blood & Cancer*, 69(3), e29537-n/a. https://doi.org/10.1002/pbc.29537

Paulino AC. (2004) Late effects of radiotherapy for pediatric extremity sarcomas. *Int J Radiat Oncol Biol Phys*. 2004 Sep 1;60(1):265-74. doi: 10.1016/j.ijrobp.2004.02.001. PMID: 15337565.

Together by St. Jude™, Spinal Problems in Childhood Cancer Survivors (https://together.stjude.org/en-us/treatment-tests-procedures/long-term-effects/spinal-problems.html)

RESOURCES

Website: ccgresources.org

All resources and references mentioned in this book are available on the website and will be routinely reviewed and updated.

Avascular Necrosis (AVN) Support Group
Website: www.facebook.com/groups/AVNInfo

Arthritis Foundation
Website: www.arthritis.org

Amputee Coalition
Website: www.amputee-coalition.org

Children's Oncology Group (V6, Oct 2023). *Long-Term Follow-Up Guidelines for Survivors of Childhood, Adolescent, and Young Adult Cancers.*

Website: www.survivorshipguidelines.org
Under Healthlinks: Under Musculoskeletal System,
Search topics: *amputation, bone health, limb-sparing proce-dures, osteonecrosis, scoliosis, kyphosis*

Passport for Care, Survivor Care Plans by Children's Oncology Group (V6, Nov 2023)
Website: https://cancersurvivor.passportforcare.org
Survivors and family can find online updated tailored long-term care plans which should be reviewed with their oncologist or health care provider.

GLOSSARY

amputation, removal of a limb from the body by surgery

asymmetry, when there is a noticeable difference in size between two parts of the body that are usually about the same size (e.g., hands, arms, legs).

atrophy, decrease in size and / or strength of tissue or an organ; also referred to as wasting or thinning

core decompression, a surgical procedure that involves drilling into the area of dead bone near the joint to reduce pressure and increase blood flow; sometimes a piece of healthy bone is inserted when the inner layer is removed

endoprosthesis, an artificial body part that is placed entirely inside your body (such as an artificial hip)

endocrinologist, a medical doctor (MD) who specializes in the glands in the body that produce hormones and who can diagnose and manage problems of gland/hormone function

exostosis (**plural:** *exostoses*), see osteochondroma

fibrosis, scarring and thickening of muscle tissue

gastroenterologist, a medical doctor (MD) who specializes in identifying and treating problems with the body's gastrointestinal system which includes the esophagus, stomach, small intestine, colon and rectum, pancreas, gallbladder, bile ducts, and liver

growth plates, growth plates are areas at the ends of bones in children where new bone growth occurs adding length and width to the bones. Growth plates eventually harden into solid bone and the bones stop growing, usually around age 13 to 15 years for girls and 15 to 17 years for boys.

hypoplasia, underdevelopment of soft tissues, such as muscle or an organ

kyphosis, when the top of the spine curves forward excessively and gives the appearance of a "hunched" back

limb-lengthening procedure, a procedure that can reduce or correct the discrepancy in length between arms or legs while stretching the surrounding muscles and other soft tissues. This process can take six to nine months. The bone to be lengthened is cut and a lengthening device is surgically inserted; the two ends of bone are slowly separated using the lengthening device. This is done by the family who have been trained by the surgeon how to use the device. After the limb has reached the desired length, the body takes over and new bone begins to grow and fill the gap.

limb-salvage procedure, a procedure that helps save the limb by removing the part of the bone that is involved with the tumor. The bone is replaced with either a bone graft or a metal prosthesis. Another limb-salvage procedure, known as *rotationplasty,* spares part of the lower leg so that the ankle can be rotated and used as a knee; below it, a prosthetic lower leg is surgically attached.

orthopedic surgeon, a doctor who specializes in diagnosing and treating disorders involving the bones, joints, ligaments, tendons, and muscles, and is specially trained to perform surgery

osteoarthritis, a degenerative disease of the joints that occurs when the cartilage that protects and cushions the end of bones wears down over time

osteochondroma (also known as an *exostosis* or a *bone spur*), a bony projection that may form where bones meet one another and can also grow on the bones of the spine. It usually does not require removal unless it causes pain or interferes with movement or bone growth.

osteonecrosis, the death of bone tissue due to a lack of blood supply which can lead to tiny breaks in the bone and cause the bone to collapse (also called *avascular necrosis (AVN)* and *ischemic necrosis*). (see **Figure 18-3**) *osteopenia,* a condition in which bone density is lower than normal and bones are beginning to thin and weaken. If not stopped, it can progress to *osteoporosis*

osteoporosis, a disease of the bones that occurs when the creation of new bone doesn't keep up with the loss of old bone. It causes the bone to lose density and to thin which make it weak, brittle, and more likely to break.

phantom pain, when a person feels sensations of pain in a missing or amputated limb even though the limb is no longer present

prosthesis, an artificial body part that replaces a body part that is missing or surgically removed

scoliosis, the sideways curvature of the spine caused by radiation to only one side of the spine. While the untreated side of the spine continues to grow, the treated side does not, instead curving in the direction of the growing side (see **Figure 18-2**).

slipped capital femoral epiphysis (SCFE), a hip disorder that occurs in some survivors whose hip was irradiated. This hip dysfunction is due to a damaged growth plate causing a *slip* between the thigh bone and the top of the femoral head.

19
Skin, Breasts, and Hair

JOANNE QUILLEN, MSN, APRN, PNP-BC

It's no use going back to yesterday, because I was a different person then.
— *Alice, Alice in Wonderland, by Lewis Carroll*

THE HUMAN BODY is wrapped in a waterproof covering called skin. Skin, hair, and nails are part of this covering, which is called the *integumentary system*. This system has several important functions. It protects the body by keeping fluids in and foreign organisms out. It insulates the body and helps regulate body temperature. Pigments in the skin help protect the body from sunlight's harmful ultraviolet rays. Nerve endings in the skin allow it to sense heat, cold, pain, and pressure.

Surgery, radiation, and chemotherapy can all cause short- and long-term changes in the skin, breasts, and hair. This chapter describes these changes, how they are diagnosed, and the most common methods used to manage them.

SKIN AND GLANDS

Skin is composed of two main layers: the epidermis and the dermis. The epidermis is a thin outer layer that is only 10 to 30 cells thick. The top layer of the epidermis is made up of dead cells full of keratin, a protein that keeps bacteria from entering the skin.

The thick, inner layer of the skin is called the *dermis*. Cells in the dermis produce *melanin*, a pigment that gives skin its color. Exposure to the sun increases the amount of melanin, causing a darkening of the skin. The dermis also contains nerve endings, blood vessels, and hair follicles. Sebaceous glands are usually attached to hair follicles in the dermis. These glands secrete oil that helps keep skin and hair from drying out.

Sweat glands produce a fluid containing water, salt, and waste products when the body is hot. When sweat evaporates, it cools the body. Blood vessels in the skin store blood to help regulate body temperature. During exercise, your skin appears flushed because the body pushes warm blood to the surface to cool off.

Damage to skin and nails

Skin can become discolored from some types of chemotherapy, higher doses of radiation, and *graft-versus-host disease (GVHD),* which occurs after some types of hematopoietic stem cell transplants.

Some children and adolescents treated with bleomycin or etoposide develop darkened areas of the skin (called *hyperpigmentation*). Pressure from trauma (such as removing a bandage from the skin) can result in darkened streaks in the traumatized areas. Bleomycin and etoposide can also cause darkening of the nail cuticles and creases on the palms. Dark bands on the nails may form as well. Doxorubicin (Adriamycin˚), daunorubicin, and idarubicin can also cause darkening in skin creases, nails, palms, soles of feet, and face. These changes usually disappear over time.

Moles

Children or teens who had radiation therapy sometimes develop large numbers of brown moles on their bodies, often in unusual places such as the scalp, hands, or toes. It is important to know the difference between a normal mole and a skin cancer, but your provider should evaluate any concerning skin lesion. Know the signs you should be looking for. (**See Figure 19-1 and Table 19-1**) Many survivors, like the general public, develop *dysplastic nevi* which is a

Table 19-1. ABCs of melanoma

	Melanoma characteristics	Moles, noncancerous
A = asymmetry	**A**symmetry – most melanomas are asymmetrical, if you draw a line down the center of the mole, each half looks very different from the other half.	Most are round and symmetrical. Look similar on both halves.
B = border	Melanoma borders are uneven and may have scalloped or notched edges.	Moles tend to have smoother, more even borders.
C = color	Multiple colors are a warning sign: different shades of brown, tan, or black colors. As it grows red, white or blue may appear	Benign moles usually one shade of brown.
D = diameter & dark	A warning sign if the lesion is ¼ inch (6 millimeters; about the size of a pencil eraser) or more in diameter or larger should be evaluated. Also regardless of size, a lesion that is darker than others.	
E = evolving	It is a warning if any spot on your skin changes size, shape, color or elevation (flat to raised) or if symptoms change such as itching, crusting, or bleeding. See your doctor right away.	

mole that does not look like a normal mole, has uneven edges and a combination of colors, ranging from pink to dark brown; may be larger than a normal mole, and is typically flat with a surface ranging from smooth to pebbly. Having at least 10 or more *dysplastic nevi* may increase your risk for developing skin cancer.

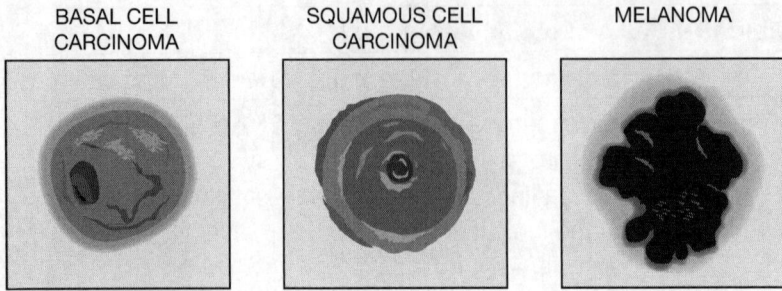

| BASAL CELL CARCINOMA | SQUAMOUS CELL CARCINOMA | MELANOMA |

FIGURE 19-1. Three types of skin cancer: A. basal cell carcinoma, B. squamous cell carcinoma, and C. melanoma. (©*Alex's Lemonade Stand Foundation, 2025*)

A. Basal cell carcinoma: Appearance: pearly, waxy bump with dark spot/red spot or flat brown lesion; Severity: least likely to spread; easy to treat.

B. Squamous cell carcinoma: Appearance: firm red pimple/nodule or scaly patch with darker crusted spot in center; Severity: easily treated if detected early; more likely to spread than basal cell carcinoma.

C. Melanoma. Appearance: black with very irregular borders with a lighter brown/red tone outline on the border, or a large brownish patch or smaller spot with black, red or white speckles. Other characteristics: an existing mole that bleeds, itches or changes shape/color. Severity: melanoma is the most serious form of skin cancer, needs diagnosis early, and can be difficult to treat and spreads easily/quickly.

Scarring and stretch marks

Most survivors have scars on their skin that serve as a daily reminder of their bout with cancer. Children or teens who had solid tumors may have extensive scarring from the tumor removal surgery. Those who had leukemia or lymphomas have scars from central line insertion and removal. Some children and teens who get severe cases of shingles have scarring along the nerve tracts. Mild and moderate cases usually heal without scarring.

Many survivors who had radiotherapy (except those who had cranial radiation only or total body irradiation) have permanent tattoos (small black dots) on their skin to outline the treatment areas. Some children and teens gain weight when they are on steroids (i.e., prednisone, dexamethasone) for extended periods of time. This can cause stretch marks. This is a variable side effect—some children gain weight but have no stretch marks, while others get them all over the body. Stretch marks sometimes fade with time.

> I always hated the way I looked and the scars I have. I came to realize that they meant I won a hard battle, but I didn't truly love them until I met my husband. He pointed out all the things he loved about me and my scars were one of them.

Radiation injuries to the skin

Survivors of childhood cancer who had high-dose radiation frequently have acute skin problems (e.g., redness, peeling) during treatment. Chronic radiation injury to the skin and underlying tissues can occur months or years after the radiation is given.

Signs and symptoms of radiation injury to the skin:

- Dry skin
- Dark and/or light areas on the skin
- Thinning of the skin
- A spidery pattern of capillaries visible in the skin (telangiectasia)
- Ulcers on the skin

The first late effect to the skin after radiation is usually a loss of elasticity. Areas of the skin can become tough (called *fibrosis*) and the tissues can contract. In some cases, *telangiectasia* appears, small red or purple clusters, often spidery in appearance on the skin.

Radiation can also cause the skin to age faster. Skin in the areas radiated may become drier and more wrinkled and may develop *age spots*. These late effects are much more likely in survivors who had high-dose radiation. Late effects to the skin depend on dose per *fraction* (the amount of radiation given at one time) and the total dose. Current technology uses megavoltage (skin-sparing) radiation to avoid severe damage to the skin.

Tissue damage under the skin can make the skin tighter and more vulnerable to breakdown. Factors that contribute to ulcers in the radiation field are trauma, pressure, ultraviolet light (from sunlight or tanning beds), and exposure to intense cold.

Damage to sweat glands, sebaceous glands and hair follicles

Radiation can also damage or destroy sweat glands, *sebaceous glands*, and hair follicles. Damage to these glands may be permanent. Itchy skin can persist for years after treatment with radiation. It is most common in those who had high-dose radiation or GVHD after an allogeneic bone marrow transplant.

Risk of skin cancer

A serious late effect to the skin after treatment for childhood cancer is skin cancer (although it can develop in people who never had childhood cancer). Radiation increases the risk and shortens the development time of skin cancers. Skin cancers can arise in irradiated or non-irradiated skin, and exposure to the sun may hasten their development. Having a family history of skin cancers and getting older also increase your risk of developing skin cancers. See *Chapter 20, Subsequent Malignancies*, for more information about skin cancers.

Medical management of damage to skin and glands

Careful evaluation of skin changes should be part of your yearly follow-up examination. In some cases, referral is made to a dermatologist for more frequent examinations. Any changes in color, scarring, dryness, fibrosis, or tightness should be identified and recorded in your medical chart. Reversal of late effects to the skin is not possible, but education about ways to slow the process can help.

Protect your skin from the sun. If you had radiation, you have a definite risk of cancers of the skin, especially in the irradiated areas. Try to limit your sun exposure, and use sunscreen of at least SPF (sun protection factor) 30 when you are out in the sun. If you had radiation to the chest or back, always wear a shirt when in the sun. If you had radiation to the arms or legs, keep them covered. Anyone who had cranial radiation or who has thin hair should wear a hat when outdoors.

Scars need extra protection from the sun. Normal skin sloughs off if sunburned, but scars cannot do that. They may remain darker. If you are going out in the sun for extended periods with your scars exposed, it's best to put zinc oxide on them.

Inspect moles regularly. If you have lots of moles on your skin, be sure to inspect them regularly. The moles probably won't become cancerous, but it is best to keep an eye on them. Always point them out to your healthcare provider at your follow-up visits, especially ones not normally noticed—for example, between your toes or on your scalp. Ask your healthcare provider to check areas you can't see such as on your back or back of the neck. If moles change shape, color, or size, make an appointment with a dermatologist. Some dermatologists take photographs of a survivor's moles so they can do a yearly comparison. Moles need continued surveillance, and you should always use sunscreen to protect your skin and moles from ultraviolet rays.

Dry skin and treatment for scars and/or stretch marks. If sebaceous gland damage makes your skin especially dry, using a moisturizing cream may make you more comfortable. Dermatologists sometimes treat scars, stretch marks, and other skin problems with medicated creams. If your scars and/or stretch marks bother you, check with your dermatologist to see if there are any medications available that might help to fade them. You could also consult a plastic surgeon to learn about any surgical options for removal of scars and/or stretch marks.

Precautions before surgery. Make sure to tell your surgeon about your cancer history if she needs to operate on previously irradiated skin. Special precautions must be taken as the tissue might be fragile and slow to heal.

BREASTS

Breasts arise from the epidermis during development in the womb. At birth, male and female breasts appear identical. During puberty, the female nipples, areolas, and breasts enlarge. The major part of female breasts is composed of mammary glands, which secrete milk after a child is born.

I am at a higher risk of developing breast cancer due to my radiation treatment. This has been a scary thought, especially because I am so young.

———

Because my ovaries were damaged during my radiation treatments, my hormones never fully triggered my breasts to develop. There aren't any medical issues with them, but it can be embarrassing to go through high school and college feeling like you look different than the other girls around you. Despite this, it's still important for me to get checked for breast cancer because I have a family history of it.

Damage to breasts

Radiation to a female's developing breast can affect its growth because the breast bud is very sensitive to radiation. However, each survivor is different, so long-term follow-up is important.

If you had radiation only on one side (e.g., flank radiation that included the breast tissue) before puberty, the irradiated breast may not grow as large as the non-irradiated breast.

Young women who had radiation to the center of the chest for Hodgkin lymphoma or non-Hodgkin lymphoma may notice underdevelopment of the breasts on the parts closest to the center of the chest. This can give the illusion of breasts that seem especially far apart.

When the developing breast is irradiated, it increases the risk of breast cancer. All survivors whose breasts were irradiated need lifelong surveillance for breast cancer (see *Chapter 20, Subsequent Malignancies,* for more information).

Also see breast cancer screening under **Hodgkin Disease Lymphoma** in *Chapter 7, Diseases.*

The scientific literature does not contain much information about breastfeeding after radiation for childhood cancer. (Ogg, 2020) More information will become known as more survivors grow up and have children. Survivors of breast cancer sometimes have problems breastfeeding from the irradiated breast. If only one breast was irradiated, women are usually able to breastfeed normally from the other breast.

Medical management of breasts

Your healthcare provider should carefully examine your breasts at each follow-up appointment if you had radiation to the chest area (mantle radiation for Hodgkin lymphoma, chest radiation for non-Hodgkin lymphoma, or total body irradiation prior to transplantation). You may need more frequent appointments during puberty.

Performing a monthly breast self-exam is one way to take care of yourself. This is especially important if your breasts were in the radiation field. Your healthcare provider should show you how to do a breast self-exam, as watching a video is usually not enough. You should do self-exams starting when you are a teenager and then every month for the rest of your life.

Survivors at increased risk for breast cancer need to have their first (baseline) mammogram done 8 years after treatment or by age 25, whichever comes last. So, if you had mantle radiation at age 15, your first mammogram should be done at age 25. If you had mantle radiation when you were 19, you should have your first mammogram at age 27. Follow-up mammograms are done on a schedule determined by your risk.

If you have breast hypoplasia or breasts that did not develop, you may choose to use prostheses like the ones worn by women who have had breast removal surgery. Some survivors choose to leave their breasts as they are, and others have their breasts surgically enlarged. This surgery should be done by surgeons who are experienced and familiar with operating on irradiated tissue.

HAIR AND NAILS

Hair and nails are made of dead cells from the epidermis (outer layer of skin). Individual hairs grow from living roots in hair follicles. Except for the root, the entire hair is made of dead cells. Nails grow from living roots underneath the cuticle (fold of skin at the base of nails).

My hair never seemed to fully come back after I lost it. It is very fine and thin, and that makes it difficult to style. I am hesitant to dye it or color treat it because I don't want to risk damaging the follicles even further and losing the hair completely.

My daughter had 30 rounds of proton radiation and 4 rounds of intense chemotherapy. She had radiation first which started the hair loss on her scalp and then chemotherapy which continued the hair loss all over her body including her eyelashes. Her hair started growing back about 4 weeks after chemo was finished. It is thinner than before treatment but most people don't notice it. She has a small bald patch behind her left ear where the focused radiation beam hit her. She also has a bald patch over the scar from her tumor resection on the back of her scalp about 4 inches long. It is not visible unless she has her hair in a higher ponytail.

Damage to hair and hair loss

Chemotherapy usually causes hair to fall out. When hair grows back after treatment, it can be a different color or texture than it was before diagnosis. Most survivors treated only with chemotherapy get a lush growth of hair after treatment ends.

Most children who have only chemotherapy prior to a stem cell transplant have full regrowth of hair. Very rarely, children who had busulfan and Cytoxan˙ to prepare them for a stem cell transplant have permanent baldness (called *alopecia*). Children and teens who take cyclosporine for extended periods of time can have excessive hair growth.

Radiation damages the hair follicles. The higher the dose, the more risk of permanent damage. Children or teens who had 1800 cGy or less radiation to the head usually have normal hair growth. Those who had more than 1800 cGy may have permanently thinned hair. Hair may not grow back in areas that had high-dose radiation (more than 3000 cGy). For instance, medulloblastoma survivors usually have bald areas on the back of the head where they got the most radiation. Survivors who had rhabdomyosarcoma of the parotid gland may have a hairless rim around the ears.

Medical management of hair damage or hair loss

Permanent loss of hair cannot be reversed; however, in the last decade, plastic surgeons have worked on new techniques to transplant hair. These hair transplants use micrografts from parts of the head that still have thick hair growth. If you are interested in exploring this option, ask your doctor for a referral to a plastic surgeon with extensive experience using these new methods.

Survivors share the following tips about managing hair:

- If your hair is thin or wispy, ask your hair stylist to recommend hairstyles and hair products that can help the hair appear fuller.
- Don't dye your hair, as this can dry out and damage the hair shafts.
- Don't use chemicals to straighten or curl your hair. If you do, ask your hairdresser to use the most gentle type to minimize breakage.
- If you have very thin hair, it looks fuller if you keep it cut relatively short.
- If you have scars or bald spots on your head, you can grow your hair to cover the area.

REFERENCES

Children's Oncology Group. (2023). *Long-Term Follow-Up Guidelines for Survivors of Childhood, Adolescent, and Young Adult Cancers*, v. 6. (www.survivorshipguidelines.org)

Fürst CJ, Lundell M, Ahlbäck SO, Holm LE. (1989). Breast hypoplasia following irradiation of the female breast in infancy and early childhood. *Acta Oncol* 1989;28(4):519-23. doi: 10.3109/02841868909092262. PMID: 2789829.

Henderson TO, Amsterdam A, Bhatia S, Hudson MM et al. (2010). Systematic review: surveillance for breast cancer in women treated with chest radiation for childhood, adolescent, or young adult cancer. *Ann Intern Med* 2010 Apr 6;152(7):444-55; W144-54. doi: 10.7326/0003-4819-152-7-201004060-00009. PMID: 20368650; PMCID: PMC2857928.

Ogg S, Klosky JL, Chemaitilly W, et al (2020). Breastfeeding practices among childhood cancer survivors. *J Cancer Surviv* 2020 Aug;14(4):586-599. doi: 10.1007/s11764-020-00882-y. Epub 2020 Apr 14. PMID: 32291564; PMCID: PMC7384306.

Rosenfield NS, Haller JO, Berdon WE. (1989). Failure of development of the growing breast after radiation therapy. *Pediatr Radiol* 1989;19(2):124-7. doi: 10.1007/BF02387902. PMID: 2922227.

Tosti A, Piraccini BM, Vincenzi C, Misciali C. (2005). Permanent alopecia after busulfan chemotherapy. *Br J Dermatol* 2005 May;152(5):1056-8. doi: 10.1111/j.1365-2133.2005.06469.x. PMID: 15888171.

Travis LB, Hill DA, Dores GM, et al. (2003). Breast cancer following radiotherapy and chemotherapy among young women with Hodgkin disease. *JAMA* 2003 Jul 23;290(4):465-75. doi: 10.1001/jama.290.4.465. Erratum in: JAMA. 2003 Sep 10;290(10):1318. PMID: 12876089.

RESOURCES

Website: ccgresources.org
All resources and references mentioned in this book are available on the website and will be routinely reviewed and updated.

Children's Oncology Group. (V6, 2023). *Long-Term Follow-Up Guidelines for Survivors of Childhood, Adolescent, and Young Adult Cancers*
Website: www.survivorshipguidelines.org
Under **Subsequent Neoplasms**, Search: *breast cancer, reducing subsequent cancers, and skin health*

Locks of Love
Website: https://locksoflove.org/
A nonprofit organization that provides hairpieces to financially disadvantaged children under the age of 21 suffering from long-term medical hair loss. (It does not provide hairpieces for temporary hair loss due to chemotherapy and radiation.)
234 Southern Blvd, West Palm Beach, FL 33405-2701
Phone: (888) 896-1588 or (561) 833-7962

Passport for Care, Survivor Care Plans by Children's Oncology Group (V6, Nov 2023)
Website: https://cancersurvivor.passportforcare.org
Survivors and family can find online updated tailored long-term care plans which should be reviewed with their oncologist or health care provider.

GLOSSARY

age spots, brown, tan or black spots on the skin a result of frequent sun exposure
alopecia, hair loss
asymmetry, one half of a cancerous spot or mole may not match the other if you were to split the mole in half
dermis, the thick inner layer of the skin

dysplastic nevus (plural: *dysplastic nevi*), a mole that does not look like a normal mole. It may have uneven edges and be a combination of colors, ranging from pink to dark brown. It may be larger than a normal mole and is typically flat with a surface ranging from smooth to pebbly.

epidermis, a thin outer layer of the skin that is only 10 to 30 cells thick

fibrosis, build-up of scar tissue and loss of elasticity in tissues

fraction, the amount of radiation given at one time

graft-versus-host-disease (GVHD), a frequent complication of allogeneic stem cell transplants, when the bone marrow or stem cells provided by the donor (*graft*) attack the tissues and organ of the child receiving the transplant (*host*). GVHD may be acute or chronic. Acute GVHD occurs within the first 100 days after the transplant, while chronic GVHD occurs or persists after day 100.

hematopoietic stem cell transplant (HPSCT), formerly known as bone marrow transplant, involves administering healthy stem cells (e.g., bone marrow, cord blood, or peripheral blood) to patients after the bone marrow has been destroyed by disease, chemotherapy (chemo), or radiation.

hyperpigmentation, patches of skin that are darker than the surrounding skin; can be a result of several conditions: "sun spots" or age spots from frequent sun exposure (brown, tan, or black spots); response to inflammation/injury to the skin; and melasma "the mask of pregnancy" (see *melasma* definition)

hypoplasia, when an organ or tissue does not develop completely

integumentary system, the body's largest organ of the body and includes the skin, hair and nails. It is the outer layer of the body and provides a protective covering and defense from the external environment.

melanin, a pigment that gives skin its color

melasma, a harmless skin condition that causes dark patches or spots usually on the face and affects mostly women with darker skin tones. It can occur on chest, upper arms and back and can be triggered by hormones (during pregnancy), sun-exposure, medications, and response to inflammation/injury to the skin.

sebaceous gland, gland in the skin connected to a hair follicle which releases *sebum*, an oily substance that helps prevent skin from drying out.

stem cell transplant, a procedure that involves administering healthy hematopoietic stem cells (e.g., bone marrow, cord blood, or peripheral blood) to patients after the bone marrow has been destroyed by disease, chemotherapy (chemo), or radiation.

telangiectasia, a skin condition which appears as small red or purple clusters, often spidery in appearance. This commonly appears on the face, nose, chin, and cheeks, but also on the legs, chest, back, and arms.

20
Subsequent Malignancies

LISA BASHORE, PhD, APRN, CPNP-PC, CPON

Nothing is to be more highly prized than the value of each day.
— *Goethe*

CHILDHOOD CANCER SURVIVORS may worry that treatment or *genetic predisposition* (risk of cancer due to our genes) or the combination of the two will result in a second cancer. *Second cancers* (or *subsequent malignancies*) are different than a recurrence of the first cancer. A second cancer occurs after treatment (e.g. radiation and/or chemotherapy) for a first (primary) cancer and is a new and different type of cancer which usually arises in a different organ or tissue from the first cancer (American Cancer Society, 2024). The chance of developing a second cancer depends on your original type of cancer, age of diagnosis, biological sex, types of therapy given, environmental exposures, genetic predisposition, and health behaviors. Overall, for most survivors, the chance of getting a second cancer is very small.

RISK OF GETTING A SECOND CANCER

You may wonder whether you are at increased risk of developing a second cancer. For most survivors, the answer is no. But the risk is not the same for everyone. Factors that determine risk include your genetic predisposition and whether or not you received radiation and/or certain chemotherapy drugs. Children with *cancer predisposition syndromes* are at higher risk of developing second cancers (Indelicato et al., 2021 and COG V 6.0 Section 7, Any Cancer Experience).

Your lifestyle and health behaviors can minimize or increase your risk, just as they can for people who never had cancer. For instance, if you had radiation to your chest, you have a small risk for developing throat and/or lung cancers. If you smoke, your chances of developing those cancers dramatically increase. If you don't smoke, don't drink alcohol, and eat a healthy diet, your risk decreases. See *Chapter 5, Staying Healthy*.

Much research is being done to maintain cure rates while lowering the toxicity of treatments to lessen the risk of second cancers. Pharmacogenetics (drug-genetic connection) is being used to identify the best cancer treatments while reducing the long-term effects including development of second cancers. Research is ongoing to identify those survivors most at risk so they can be followed appropriately. To find out your individual risk, talk to your healthcare provider during a follow-up visit. Before discussing your unique situation and risk, your provider will evaluate your original disease, the treatments you received, your age when treated, and your family history.

GENETIC PREDISPOSITION

Cancers with known genetic (hereditary) causes sometimes carry a greater risk of second cancers. For instance, survivors of the genetic form of *retinoblastoma* and those with Li Fraumeni Syndrome should be evaluated regularly for the rest of their lives, because they have a much higher chance of developing second tumors than do other survivors. See *Chapter 6, Genetic Testing and Childhood Cancer* for more information on the *cancer predisposition syndromes (CPS)* and why some children may be more at risk for cancers. One important thing to remember is that CPS place some children at higher risk for developing a primary (first new) cancer and not necessarily a second cancer. More information is being discovered about the genetics of cancer. However, there is more we need to learn about the relationship between chemotherapy, radiation and the development of second cancers in children with CPS.

Some types of cancer (colon, breast, and ovarian) run in families (hereditary), so it is important to discuss your family history with your healthcare provider. Speaking with a genetic counselor to discuss your personal or family history of cancer can help you to understand your risks of developing cancer. Genetic counselors can help with a risk assessment and walk you through genetic testing options. Knowing your risk factors can be helpful in determining your medical management moving forward. It is important to know that if you have a genetic mutation in a cancer predisposition gene, this does not mean you will develop cancer again. Survivors with many risk factors may live long and healthy lives and never get cancer again, while some people at low risk will get cancer. The facts your healthcare provider discusses with you are probabilities for large groups of people; no one can predict what will happen to you.

I have a family history of brain cancer, breast cancer, and thyroid issues. My doctors are aware of these and do checks when I go in for routine doctor's appointments. They also make me aware of any warning signs that I should be aware of so that I can schedule follow-up appointments if need be. I see my doctors regularly and am honest with them about my symptoms/how I feel. I am also very in tune with my body, and I just know when something feels off or wrong or unusual. When something concerns me, I go to the doctor, as I'd rather know that it's nothing to worry about than just worry about it on my own.

After chemotherapy, I had to do 14 rounds of proton radiation every day. I was extremely scared about this because of where my cancer was located. I had tumors in my chest and neck that needed radiation. My doctors warned me about the chance of developing breast cancer, heart disease and lung damage from the radiation. This has added to my anxiety. I have tried to be super proactive about following up with my doctors since ending radiation. I make sure I keep up with doctor appointments, scans, and annual exams to ensure the best chance possible of never getting any other sickness or disease. Although nothing can be promised, I feel better knowing I have surveillance of so many aspects of my health.

Advocating for myself has been one of the biggest things I have learned. It's so important to go to the doctors and get checked! You know your body best, and if something feels wrong or off,

(Continued)

just get it checked, because you never know. It's better to be safe than sorry. Advocating for yourself is one of the best things you can do for yourself.

My daughter was diagnosed with neuroblastoma at 2 ½ months. When she was 7 1/2, she was diagnosed with a secondary cancer, renal cell carcinoma. Doctors described it as a secondary cancer because it was caused by chemotherapy treatment from the first cancer. This was rare because renal cell carcinoma is not usually found in young children as a secondary cancer.

The risk of developing a secondary cancer sometimes scares me, but then I tell myself, let's go for round two -- I'm not scared; if I did it once, I'll do it again. I do everything I can to take care of my body and monitor myself thoroughly for any signs of secondary cancer.

I asked the doctor about potentially having a child with cancer before we started trying. They told me it was not a genetic illness, so that helped calm my fear. I worry about my son's health constantly. I am always wondering where a bruise came from or if he's eating enough. I think all moms are like that, though. I just am very extreme when it comes to worrying!

Risk of treatment

Survivors at highest risk for second cancers are those who:

- Were treated with radiation
- Received the following agents: classical alkylating agents (busulfan, carmustine, chlorambucil, cyclophosphamide (Cytoxan®), ifosfamide, lomustine, mechlorethamine, melphalan, procarbazine, thiotepa, heavymetals, carboplatin, cisplatin); Non-classical alkylators: (dacarbazine, temozolomide); anthracyclines (daunorubicin, doxorubicin, epirubicin, idarubicin, mitoxantrone) (COG V 6.0 section 16). Any of these medications can cause a secondary cancer, but higher doses of any or combinations of these drugs can increase the risk for second cancers.
- Have genetic diseases that carry an increased risk
- Are included in Section 7 of the COG Survivorship Guidelines (v6.0)

The screening allows for earlier detection and treatment should you develop another cancer, increasing your chance for early treatment and cure. It also gives you the opportunity to discuss ways of lowering your risks by making healthy lifestyle and behavior choices.

Radiation and some types of chemotherapy can increase the risk of second cancers. Combined radiotherapy and chemotherapy may play an additive role in the development of second cancers (Dracham CB, et al., 2018). Some types of second cancer are very easy to cure such as skin cancers and thyroid cancers.

Radiation

In general, higher doses of any radiation increase the risk of developing a second cancer. More recent protocols have used lower radiation doses (in some cases), more precise techniques, and radiation given in smaller fractions, allowing the healthy tissue to repair itself (COG V 6.0). It is hoped that the use of the new *proton-beam radiation therapy* will significantly decrease the risk of damage to healthy tissue. However, we do not yet know the long-term outcomes and whether the risk for secondary cancer will be significantly reduced in survivors who receive proton therapy (Indelicato DJ, et al. 2021).

Radiation kills cancer cells and may also cause changes in normal cells that are exposed to the radiation. In some cases, cancers can develop in the irradiated areas. For instance, female survivors of Hodgkin lymphoma (formerly called Hodgkin's disease) treated in the 1970s and 1980s who had more than 3600 centigrays (cGy) of *mantle (chest) radiation* have increased risk of developing breast cancer, often at an early age. *Scatter radiation* (radiation that escapes into areas around the tumor site) is less common now that radiation techniques have improved.

Thyroid tumors are common tumors that can develop following radiation delivered to the cranial/spinal region, head and neck, chest, or total body radiation given before a stem cell transplant. Younger children at time of treatment are at greater risk for thyroid tumors. Thyroid tumors can be either benign or malignant, and the malignant tumors are very treatable.

Radiation to the pelvis or abdomen (in higher doses) is associated with an increased risk of colon cancer. The current recommendation for follow up is to have a colonoscopy at age 35 or 10 years after the radiation, whichever occurs last.

Chemotherapy

Several chemotherapy drugs as listed above are associated with second cancers in some survivors. Examples include:

- **Alkylating agents:** procarbazine, nitrogen mustard, cyclophosphamide (Cytoxan®), ifosfamide, melphalan, and nitrosoureas. High doses of these drugs can cause *myelodysplastic syndromes* (bone marrow abnormalities that are similar to leukemia) as well as AML.

- **Epipodophyllotoxins:** VP-16 (etoposide), VM-26 (teniposide) (Smith MA, et al. 1999).

- **Platinum analogs:** cisplatin, carboplatin. Research has not clarified the risk of cancers after treatment with platinum analogs such as cisplatin or carboplatin. Most AML or myelodysplastic syndromes occur when these drugs are given in conjunction with alkylating agents or epipodophyllotoxins.

- **Anthracycline:** daunorubicin, doxorubicin, epirubicin, idarubicin, and mitoxantrone may be associated with the development of second acute myeloid leukemia.

- **Targeted therapies:** With the addition of *precision medicine* and testing for targeted genetic variants to help in the management of children with cancer, new agents (drugs) are being used and developed to treat the child's cancer. We do not have long-term outcomes on the Tyrosine Kinese Inhibitors (TKIS), CAR-T therapy, and other targeted medications and the long-term effects on childhood cancer survivors. Please discuss any long-term effects of these newer drugs/treatment with your provider. Each survivor is different, and long-term follow-up is important.

Children and adolescents who were treated with an immunosuppressant (e.g., cyclosporine or FK 506) have a small chance of developing disorders of the lymph system, including lymphoma. These disorders sometimes resolve without treatment when the immune system is no longer suppressed.

The bladder issue proved to be another blessing-in-disguise and led the doctors to discover her secondary cancer when she was seven and a half. The bladder defect caused her to have constant urinary tract infections (UTIs). It was while treating her for the UTIs that they discovered the solid mass which turned out to be Stage I renal cell carcinoma in her left kidney.

I tell everyone that our daughter is a survivor and she is here for a purpose. Her treatments for both cancers were quick and successful, so I just try to give everyone hope. Thankfully, she was fortunate enough to not have any late side-effects. So, I can truthfully tell others that she had a positive outcome from her treatments.

Follow-up exams, early detection and cancer prevention

Once you know what your risk might be, what do you do then? Practical ways to deal with this potentially upsetting information are to take precautions to prevent a second cancer and know the warning signs and attend follow-up survivor clinic visits every year. Notify your healthcare provider immediately if you have any changes in your health status or concerns.

Although you cannot change a genetic predisposition or undo the damage from radiation or chemotherapy, you can decrease your risk factors by making healthy lifestyle choices to reduce your risk. There are numerous ways to prevent cancer outlined in *Chapter 5, Staying Healthy*.

There are actions you can take to help control the risk factors for developing second cancer, for example, making sure you have periodic healthcare check-ups and making healthy lifestyle choices. Your healthcare provider should perform a thorough assessment each year and discuss any risks you have. The factors that determine which specific tests you need each year depend on the specific treatments you received for childhood cancer, past or current behaviors that affect your risk, and your personal or family history of disease.

Your follow-up examinations should include updating your family medical history with special attention to cancers that have developed in first-degree relatives (your mother, father, brothers, sisters, and children). This valuable information can be missed if family medical history is not updated at regular intervals.

All areas that were irradiated should be visually inspected. Areas where *scatter radiation* (radiation that escapes into areas around the tumor site) may have occurred also need to be examined. The necks of survivors who receive any head and neck radiation should be palpated (felt by hand) yearly. The results of a thorough physical evaluation and preliminary screening determine the need for additional tests. It's very important that female survivors who received chest, axilla, and or total body radiation get frequent follow-up care that includes annual mammograms starting at age 25, or 8 years after radiation, whichever comes later (Mulder et al., 2020). They also need to be taught breast self-examination because they can develop breast cancer at an early age.

You can help control some risk factors for developing second cancer, for example, yearly healthcare check-ups and follow-up screenings. Make healthy lifestyle choices and take preventive measures such as performing body self-checks, using sunscreen, eating healthy, and getting exercise.

Know your own body, and if you have any changes/concerns, check with your healthcare provider. Routine yearly examinations *will not* detect all subsequent cancers. Healthcare providers rely on you to bring concerns or abnormalities immediately to their attention. Try to feel confident in your ability to notice if something in your body does not feel right. If you have an ache or a pain that does not go away, it should probably be checked out. If you notice a lump in the area of your body that was irradiated, go immediately to have it evaluated. It probably will not be cancer, but having it evaluated will provide either reassurance or an early detection of a problem—both good outcomes.

Steps *you* can take for prevention and early detection/ treatment

- **Making healthy lifestyle choices** (See *Chapter 5, Staying Healthy*)
- **Yearly check-ups** at your survivors' clinic or long-term follow-up clinic
- **Periodically perform body self-checks** for skin cancers or lumps and have these checked by your healthcare provider. If you had *retinoblastoma* and radiation treatment to the orbit, regularly examine the socket yourself for any changes. By examining the orbit regularly, you are taking good care of yourself and making an investment in your future.
- **Routinely use sunscreen of at least 30 SPF** when you are going to be exposed to sun for long periods of time and try to avoid prolonged direct sun exposure during hours of 10 to 4 pm
- **Check-in with your healthcare provider if you have any concerns**

Take care of your emotional/mental health

Another way to think of this issue is to try to find a place in your life to remember your cancer history without letting it control your life or future plans. Don't trivialize or dismiss what's happened to you and your family—it was a significant part of your life and shaped your interests and character. And yet, your cancer history is only one part of who you are, and shouldn't determine your future life, possibilities, and happiness. (For detailed discussion, See *Chapters 2 Emotions* and *Chapter 3, Relationships*)

REFERENCES

American Cancer Society (2024). Website: www.cancer.org Search, *childhood cancer,* then *late effects of childhood cancer treatment, second cancers*

Bhatia S, et al. (2007). Therapy-related myelodysplasia and acute myeloid leukemia after Ewing sarcoma and primitive neuroectodermal tumor of bone: A report from the Children's Oncology Group. *Blood,* 109(1): 46–51.

Children's Oncology Group (V6, Oct 2023). *Long-Term Follow-Up Guidelines for Survivors of Childhood, Adolescent, and Young Adult* Cancers. Website: www .survivorshipguidelines.org

Dracham CB, Shankar A, Madan R. (2018) Radiation induced secondary malignancies: a review article. *Radiat Oncol J.* 2018 Jun;36(2):85-94. doi: 10.3857/roj.2018.00290. Epub 2018 Jun 29. PMID: 29983028; PMCID: PMC6074073.

Goshen Y. (2007). High incidence of meningioma in cranial irradiated survivors of childhood acute lymphoblastic leukemia. *Pediatr Blood Cancer*, 49(3): 294–297.

Indelicato DJ, Bates JE, Mailhot Vega RB, et al. (2021). Second tumor risk in children treated with proton therapy. *Pediatric Blood & Cancer*, 68(7), e28941-n/a. https://doi.org/10.1002/pbc.28941

Mulder RL, Hudson MM, Bhatia S, et al. (2020). Updated breast cancer surveillance recommendations for female survivors of childhood, adolescent, and young adult cancer from the international guideline harmonization group. *Journal of Clinical Oncology*, 38(35), 4194-4207. https://doi.org/10.1200/JCO.20.00562

National Cancer Institute, website: https://dceg.cancer.gov, Search *research, what-we-study, second-cancers*

Smith MA, et al. (1999). Secondary leukemia or myelodysplastic syndrome after treatment with epipodophyllotoxins. *J Clin Oncol*, 17(2): 569–577.

RESOURCES

Website: ccgresources.org

All resources and references mentioned in this book are available on the website and will be routinely reviewed and updated.

Alex's Lemonade Stand Foundation
Website: www.alexslemonade.org
Search, *childhood cancer families*
Alex's Lemonade Stand Foundation (ALSF) is changing the lives of children with cancer by funding impactful research, raising awareness, supporting families, and empowering everyone to help cure childhood cancer. ALSF offers many programs and tools to help families navigate the challenges of childhood cancer.

American Cancer Society (2024)
Website: www.cancer.org
Search, *childhood cancer*, then, *late effects of childhood cancer treatment, second cancers*

Children's Oncology Group (V6, Oct 2023). *Long-Term Follow-Up Guidelines for Survivors of Childhood, Adolescent, and Young Adult Cancers.*
Website: www.survivorshipguidelines.org
Click below to download Individual Health Links:
Subsequent neoplasms: *breast cancer, colorectal cancer, reducing subsequent cancers, skin health*

National Cancer Institute, Division of Cancer, Epidemiology and Genetics
Website: https://dceg.cancer.gov
Search, *childhood cancers, second cancers*

Passport for Care, Survivor Care Plans by Children's Oncology Group (V6, Nov 2023)
Website: https://cancersurvivor.passportforcare.org
Survivors and family can find online updated tailored long-term care plans which should be reviewed with their oncologist or health care provider.

GLOSSARY

cancer predisposition syndromes (CPS), a group of inherited genetic disorders that increase an individual's risk of developing certain types of cancer. These syndromes are caused by mutations in specific genes, which can be passed down through generations, leading to a higher likelihood of cancer occurrence in affected families.

genetic predisposition, the increased chance of developing a disease based on one's genetic makeup

healthy lifestyle choices, choices all survivors can make to lead a healthy, safe lifestyle to promote their health and do everything they can to prevent future cancer or health problems (see *Chapter 5, Staying Healthy* for detailed information)

hereditary health traits, diseases/disorders that tend to run in families; inherited genetic traits which an individual cannot control, such as genetic traits for cancer, diabetes, heart disease and other

mantle radiation, a radiation technique used in 1970s to the 1990s which treated a large area of the neck, chest, armpits and mediastinum (area between the lungs) in order to cover all areas with cancer involvement. This technique is **rarely used** today in current treatment.

myelodysplastic syndromes, bone marrow abnormalities that are similar to leukemia; a group of disorders caused by blood cells that are poorly formed or don't work properly

precision medicine, tailoring cancer therapy according to the genetic and molecular characteristics of the specific cancer using genetics testing and molecular biomarkers

proton-beam radiation therapy (also called charged-particle radiation therapy or *proton therapy*), a relatively new form of radiation therapy that uses high-powered energy from positively charged particles (protons) to treat cancer and some noncancerous tumors. Studies suggest that proton therapy may cause fewer side effects than traditional radiation, since doctors can better control where the proton beams deliver their energy.

retinoblastoma, a malignant tumor of the retina in the eye that occurs in four stages from 0-IV, with Stage 0 having a good outcome with treatment, and Stage IV retinoblastoma with metastases a poor prognosis.

risk factors for second cancer, factors that can influence likelihood of developing a second cancer; includes genetic factors (diseases/disorders that have a tendency to run in families) and more importantly health factors that the individual *can* control, such as living a healthy lifestyle (not smoking or alcohol consumption, healthy diet, physical activity, and taking precautions and medications)

scatter radiation, radiation that spreads out in different directions from where a radiation beam interacts with tumor site. Scattered radiation has lower energy than the original radiation beam but can still accumulate in the body over time, leading to severe and chronic health conditions.

second cancer, cancer that occurs after treatment (e.g. radiation and/or chemotherapy) for a first (primary) cancer and is a new and different type of cancer, which usually arises in a different organ or tissue from the first (primary) cancer (American Cancer Society, 2024)

subsequent malignancy (also referred to as, *second cancer*), cancer that occurs after treatment (e.g. radiation and/or chemotherapy) for a first (primary) cancer and is a new and different type of cancer, which usually arises in a different organ or tissue from the first (primary) cancer (American Cancer Society, 2024)

thyroglobulin level (blood test), a blood test used to detect the recurrence of cancer. The thyroglobulin test can be used as a tumor marker when already diagnosed in conjunction with a biopsy of the tumor to make the diagnosis

About the Editors

Lisa Bashore

My passion for pediatric oncology and survivorship began when I was a young girl and my friend's brother was diagnosed with acute lymphoblastic leukemia. Unfortunately, he experienced a recurrence of his leukemia and had to undergo a bone marrow transplantation that included radiation. As a result, he experienced many late effects of his disease and treatment.

The journey that brought me to focus on childhood cancer survivorship started with my professional encounters with the many children and adolescents for whom I cared early in my career. Their long-term struggles with medical late-effects drove my desire to focus on childhood cancer survivorship. My first encounter was with a childhood cancer survivor (actually an adolescent) who died suddenly due to a cardiac event. This tragic encounter just after I began my career in survivorship fueled my ongoing passion for survivorship and research to try to make a difference. As a pediatric oncology nurse practitioner, I had the privilege to design a childhood cancer survivorship program in the South that continues to flourish today. After 24 years in practice and now with a special focus on how genetics impacts cancer care and survivorship, I have never looked back on my career decision.

Throughout my career, I met the most amazing professionals and people (more than that of a Hollywood celebrity) many who changed the trajectory of childhood cancer diagnosis, treatment, and survivorship ---physicians, scientists, and nurses in particular. One of those is Wendy Hobbie, a pioneer in nursing care and study of childhood cancer survivors and an original author of this book. I spent several days with her at the *survivorship program* at the Children's Hospital of Philadelphia and took home with me a fraction of her vast knowledge of childhood cancer survivorship. The original authors of the first editions did a fabulous job writing and revising over the years. Now ALSF will continue to share this book with new, updated information to guide survivors and families on their survivorship journeys moving forward.

Joanne Quillen

As an oncology nurse practitioner, I often share this book with my patients, but I received my first copy by a strange happenstance about 22 years ago, and it changed my life and career goals.

I have seven siblings and two of my sisters developed Hodgkins disease, one at age 12 and the other at age 14. My older sister was later diagnosed with late-effects breast cancer and heart failure in the 1990's. During that difficult time, while I was on a flight to a Childrens Oncology Nursing Conference to present a poster, I began chatting with another nurse (Sue) sitting across the aisle. She told me about a Survivorship Clinic at Children's Hospital of Philadelphia (CHOP) where she worked, and spoke about this book and Wendy Hobbie, coauthor of the first editions. I was uncomfortable about attending this conference and leaving my older sister who was so ill at that time. When I returned home from the conference, a copy of *Childhood Cancer Survivors: A practical guide to your future*, was waiting for me. Sue had thoughtfully mailed me a copy along with Wendy's contact information. In a few days, I called Wendy and she began to explain about late effects of cancer treatments and the importance of long-term comprehensive follow-up care for survivors. When I started reading the book, I could not put it down –such a helpful resource and guide. I used it like the Bible and found answers to so many questions for my sisters and me.

My experience on this cancer journey with both of my sisters, reading this book, and seeing the impact of that Survivorship Clinic at CHOP changed me in a profound way. Soon after this encounter with Wendy and reading the book, I enrolled in the Pediatric Oncology Nurse Practitioner Program at University of Pennsylvania. I have been a Pediatric Neuro-oncology/Survivorship Nurse Practitioner for 19 years. In 2008, I started the first Survivorship Program in Wilmington, Delaware at the Nemours Children's Hospital. I continue to share this book with my patients and see how it continues to offer valuable support, guidance, and knowledge to both survivors and their families throughout their cancer journey.

Index

guilt
  because of survival, 43
  of siblings, 64
GVHD. *See* graft-versus-host disease
gynecology, gynecologist, 22, 29,
  380, 382

H

hair, 439–441
hand/eye coordination problems, 261
health insurance, 20, 88, 107–115
  resources for, 127–131
  glossary terms for, 132–136
Health Insurance Marketplace Exchange,
  107
health care team, 22-25
Health Insurance Portability and
  Accountability Act of 1996, 114
healthy lifestyle choices, 451–453
healthy lifestyle, 345
hearing loss, 198, 208, 214, 313–318
heart attack, 347
heart valves, 348–349
heart, 335–350,
heavy metals, 448
hemangiopericytoma, 221
hematopoietic stem cell transplant
  (see also stem cell transplant), 216,
  232, 277, 287, 359, 365, 388, 432
hemorrhagic cystitis, 372
hepatitis, 386–387
    hepatitis A, 386
    hepatitis B, 387
    hepatitis C virus (HCV), 387
hepatoblastoma, 219
hepatocellular carcinoma, 219
histiocytosis, 218
Hodgkin lymphoma, 200–205
Holter monitor, 193, 200
hormone-producing glands, 275–305
human genome, 163
Hydrea. See hydroxyurea (Hydrea)
hydrocortisone, 188, 192, 261, 300
hydroxyurea (Hydrea), 216
hyperprolactinemia, 279, 284, 295
hyperthyroidism, 286–287
hypothalamic-pituitary axis (HPA), 275–276
hypothyroidism, 286–287

I

idarubicin, 82, 190, 193, 200, 207, 210,
  213, 219, 228, 231, 432, 450
IEP. *See* Individualized Education Plan
ifosfamide, 79–80, 200, 206, 213–214,
  219, 226, 291, 369, 448, 450
    and bladder damage, 372–373
    and Ewing sarcoma family of tumors,
      198
    and hepatocellular carcinoma,
      219
    and infertility, 78, 79
    and Hodgkin luymphoma, 200
    and kidney damage, 366
    and neuroblastoma, 165
    and osteosarcoma, 211
    and rhabdomyosarcoma, 225
    and second cancers, 449
    and sperm production, 291
ifosfamide (Ifex)
illegal drugs, 343
imatinib mesylate (Gleevec), 215
immune system. *See* bone marrow; lymph
  nodes; spleen
immunosuppression, 397
immunotherapy, 188, 202, 240
impotence, 296, 402
Individualized Education Plan (IEP), 93,
  94–97
Individualized Transition Plan (ITP),
  97–99
Individuals with Disabilities Education
  Act, 91
induction, 187, 192, 218
infections
    in bladder, 374
    in ears, 307, 313–318
    heart, 349
    hepatitis, 386–387
    in kidneys, 371
    in sinuses, 325, 330
    in survivors without spleens, 399
    pneumonia, 359, 362
    sexually transmitted illnesses, 29,
      138, 151–159
    shingles, 399, 405, 406, 407, 434
    warts, 151
    See also lymph nodes; spleen